New Perspectives on Post-2020 Healthcare Reform:

Opportunities and Challenges

Raj Selladurai
https://orcid.org/0009-0008-4049-3942
Indiana University Northwest, USA

Charles Hobson
https://orcid.org/0009-0001-5520-5002
Indiana University Northwest, USA

Roshini Selladurai
https://orcid.org/0009-0001-7340-508X
Mayo Clinic, USA & Mayo College of Medicine, USA

Tony Spaulding
https://orcid.org/0009-0006-4071-9206
Mayo Clinic, USA

IGI Global
Scientific Publishing
Publishing Tomorrow's Research Today

Vice President of Editorial	Melissa Wagner
Director of Acquisitions	Mikaela Felty
Director of Book Development	Jocelynn Hessler
Production Manager	Mike Brehm
Cover Design	Jose Rosado

Published in the United States of America by
IGI Global Scientific Publishing
701 East Chocolate Avenue
Hershey, PA, 17033, USA
Tel: 717-533-8845 | Fax: 717-533-7115
Website: https://www.igi-global.com E-mail: cust@igi-global.com

Library of Congress Cataloging-in-Publication Data

Names: Selladurai, Raj, 1954- editor | Hobson, Charles J. editor | Selladurai, Roshini Isabell, 1991- editor | Spaulding, Tony editor
Title: New perspectives on post-2020 healthcare reform : opportunities and challenges / edited by: Raj Selladurai, Charles Hobson, Roshini Selladurai, and Tony Spaulding.
Description: Hershey, PA : IGI Global Scientific Publishing, [2026] | Includes bibliographical references. | Summary: "The book explores post-2020 healthcare reform by presenting emerging challenges and opportunities, proposing sustainable and optimal healthcare system models, and highlighting the insights of diverse stakeholders across medical, academic, private, public, and business sectors"-- Provided by publisher.
Identifiers: LCCN 2025054383 (print) | LCCN 2025054384 (ebook) | ISBN 9798337325774 hardcover | ISBN 9798337325781 paperback | ISBN 9798337325798 ebook
Subjects: LCSH: Health care reform--United States | Artificial intelligence--Medical applications
Classification: LCC RA395.A3 N46 2026 (print) | LCC RA395.A3 (ebook)
LC record available at https://lccn.loc.gov/2025054383
LC ebook record available at https://lccn.loc.gov/2025054384

British Cataloguing in Publication Data
A Cataloguing in Publication record for this book is available from the British Library.

Quotes and Testimonials

ENDORSEMENT

This work is intended to identify a number of rapidly changing attributes and properties of an increasingly volatile industry: healthcare. The collection of chapters helps identify some of the critical changes that are taking place within the medical industry, what the probable effects of these changes may be, and offers potential solutions to those problems they bring to all parties in the healthcare partnership. Some of these issues include: (1) a shrinking supply of medical professionals, (2) "burn-out" of overworked staff and physicians, (3) rising costs in all areas with shrinking budgets (demands for more efficiency), (4) the rapid increases in use of various AI and telemedical techniques, and (5) the well-intentioned, but not always helpful intrusions from all levels of government.

The authors of these outstanding and insightful essays are working doctors, healthcare administrators, and experts in a variety of organizational and professional processes and systems. They address many issues facing modern healthcare in rural, suburban, and urban areas and how to adapt to the needs of the local client base, the patients. The use of "wheel" models for more rural hospital systems is examined for example, as well as emerging treatment protocols such as Medically-Supervised Fasting (MSF), and improved training in highly urban systems that can make use of heavily team-based treatment systems with high demands for effective interprofessional communication.

I highly recommend this significant collection of research and analyses for anyone working in the highly charged healthcare arena of today.

Cuthbert L Scott

Indiana University Northwest, USA

Editorial Advisory Board

Table of Contents

Detailed Table of Contents

This chapter explores recent developments in US healthcare and those anticipated for 2026 and beyond. It will examine recent healthcare initiatives, including those focused on cost reduction, greater consumer choice, and further deregulation. The One Big Beautiful Bill Act (OBBBA) was signed into law by President Trump on July 4, 2025. It introduced sweeping changes across different areas, including healthcare reform to Medicaid, Medicare, and the Affordable Care Act (ACA). These healthcare reforms aim to lower premium costs and federal spending. Interviews were conducted with US stakeholders from multiple organizations and industry segments to gauge their views on healthcare reform. Several significant outcomes are addressed, including reducing healthcare costs for these stakeholders, enhancing access to healthcare, improving efficiency, enhancing the quality and delivery of healthcare services, increasing patient satisfaction, and advancing overall sustainability.

This chapter explores, analyzes, and discusses the challenges and potential recommendations for the unprecedented physician shortage affecting US healthcare systems. As a result, patients are waiting long periods to get an appointment, and in many cases, even longer to see a physician. Especially older patients who may need immediate attention and medical care end up waiting several weeks. Healthcare seems to be facing a crisis that is getting worse by the day. How did we get here, why, and what do we do about it are some of the questions addressed in this chapter.

Section 2
Newer, Innovative Perspectives in Healthcare

This chapter will explore how telemedicine can increase access to care, address the physician shortage, reduce healthcare costs, support patients in managing chronic diseases, and improve the patient experience. Today, with so much growth and reliance on technology, healthcare reform requires understanding how to incorporate technology to optimize the patient experience and outcomes. This chapter will focus on how best to harness the benefits of technology to provide optimal healthcare in a post-2020 world, from a clinician's perspective.

This chapter provides a high-level overview of clinical informatics (CI) and artificial intelligence (AI) in healthcare. It covers foundational concepts such as electronic health records (EHRs) and data standards, current applications including Clinical Decision Support Systems (CDSS) and ambient scribing/documentation, and near-term directions for both clinicians and patients. The chapter also introduces how foundational CI systems and healthcare data are leveraged to develop AI solutions, ranging from traditional machine learning to large language models, while addressing key issues such as bias, generalizability, and regulatory considerations. Finally, the chapter examines a potential future in which decentralized AI models augment clinicians in their daily work, generate deeper clinical insights, and transform patient care through advanced predictive models and digital twins.

The author reviews the development of artificial intelligence (AI) and how it has impacted patient care, including pediatric patient care. While there have been positive developments, such as better diagnostic options, unknown risks remain, such as data

This chapter reviews mental healthcare reform in the US, highlighting transinstitutionalization due to inadequate community support post-deinstitutionalization. It details legislative efforts, persistent access barriers (financial, attitudinal, structural, stigma), and the societal costs of delayed treatment. Proposed reforms include prioritizing affordability, combating stigma, strengthening primary care, and investing in early intervention. The text also explores nutritional psychiatry, the gut-brain axis, and the transformative potential of precision psychiatry via biomarkers and AI. Despite implementation hurdles, it advocates for collaborative efforts to achieve personalized mental healthcare and treat mental illnesses as brain diseases, not personal failings.

Section 3
Practices and Applications

Several reports show a shortage of primary care physicians in the US, and it seems likely to worsen as the population continues to grow and age. Therefore, it is critical to train the next generation of physicians and healthcare providers to effectively meet the needs of the US population. Alongside this structural challenge, the medical profession is also confronting a cultural one—an erosion of professionalism characterized by declining responsibility, integrity, and communication (Foster, 2019). In teaching and training resident physicians and medical students, some of these skills can be taught, but these skills are usually better "caught" than taught. This chapter presents two physicians' personal experiences in medical education. It discusses the significance of role modeling and best practices for effectively transmitting professionalism, competence, and communication to the next generation of resident physicians, medical students, and healthcare providers.

Foreword

The post-2020 era marks, I feel, a structural inflection point in U.S. healthcare. Pandemic disruption, workforce destabilization, technological acceleration, and declining public trust have exposed foundational weaknesses that demand substantial adjustments. New Perspectives on Post-2020 Healthcare Reform: Opportunities and Challenges engages this moment with uncommon coherence, advocating for substantial, systems-level, multidisciplinary, and values-driven changes. For decades, healthcare reform in the United States has long been characterized by cyclical urgency, fragmented interventions, and an uneasy tension between market forces, professional identity, and moral purpose. Now, pandemic disruption, demographic transition, workforce destabilization, rapid digitization, and renewed ideological contestation have converged to expose structural weaknesses that can no longer be addressed solely through policy adjustments.

We appropriately begin with the workforce crisis, offering a rigorous analysis of physician shortages and tracing their origins to training constraints, maldistribution, burnout, and policy misalignment. Chapter 2 situates reform within the contemporary policy landscape, critically examining post-2025 legislative changes and their consequences for patients, providers, and systems.

Technology offers both promise and risk. Chapter 3 examines telemedicine from the clinician's perspective, emphasizing pragmatic integration that enhances access without compromising professional judgment. Chapter 4 provides a sophisticated overview of clinical informatics and artificial intelligence. Chapter 5 extends this analysis to pediatrics.

Chapter 6 reimagines rural healthcare ecosystems through AI, reframing rural care as a connected network. Chapter 7 advances a bold economic argument for medically supervised fasting, directly engaging anticipated institutional and cultural resistance. Chapter 8 addresses mental healthcare reform, integrating historical policy failures with emerging opportunities, biomarkers, and AI.

Section III grounds reform in organizational practice. Chapter 9 on effective teamwork and communication, and advancing the Quadruple Aim. Chapter 10 elevates supply chain management to a strategic asset. Chapter 11 focuses on the transmission of clinical wisdom, professionalism, and communication skills.

We conclude with strategic reflection and a call to recover our foundational purpose, restore trust, and improve outcomes. In an era when healthcare reform is often reduced to slogans or short-term fixes, New Perspectives on Post-2020 Healthcare Reform offers something rarer: a thoughtful, integrative, and forward-looking contribution that will remain relevant well beyond its immediate policy context. I am very pleased to offer it to you with my very highest recommendation!

Edward E. Rylander
American Board of Family Medicine, USA & American Board of Hospice and Palliative Medicine, USA & In His Image Family Medicine Residency, Ascension Riverside Family Medicine Clinic, USA & Transitions LifeCare Hospice, USA

Preface

Hope is a psychological need that universally impacts every human heart. Perhaps it is the most dominant of all psychological, spiritual, and medical needs. Dr. McNair Wilson stated in his autobiography, Doctor's Progress, "Those who require heart surgery need hope. Hope is the medicine I use more than any other – hope can cure nearly anything" (Wilson, 1938). Also, a more recent Harvard Medical School report says that "medicine promises people hope. Hope rooted in the discoveries of the past and felt in the therapies of the present. Hope that is inspiring the future" (Beltran, 2017). Dr. Wilson's and Dr. Beltran's inspirational comments on *hope* are still so appropriate today for all our physicians and medical professionals in healthcare to remember and emulate as they continue to serve their patients with dedication, passion, and patience around the world!

The purpose of our book, "New Perspectives on Post-2020 Healthcare Reform: Opportunities and Challenges," focuses on our continual hope that it would add value to our nation's healthcare system reform, complex as it may be, toward developing a more optimal, sustainable healthcare system to benefit all the stakeholders in the US. Although it is not the perfect system, it is considered one of the best in the world today, given all the various dynamic factors that impact our healthcare system, including the large number of stakeholders, complexity of healthcare, size of the country, various costs and quality-related issues, and partisan groups' conflicting priorities.

The unique aspect of this book is that several authors have written chapters based on their personal experiences and perspectives with the US healthcare system. It includes contributions from authors, reviewers, editors, and editorial board members from academic, medical, healthcare, business, nonprofit, and professional disciplines and specialties at several institutions, including the world-renowned Mayo Clinic and Mayo College of Medicine in Rochester, MN, and the Duke University School of Medicine.

The publication will focus on the opportunities and challenges of healthcare reform - post-2020. This book will be a follow-up to our first healthcare reform publication,

"Evaluating Opportunities and Challenges of Healthcare Reform," published in Feb. 2020. In addition, some newer topics have been included, especially those related to the current administration's healthcare reform plans, with a focus on strategies to lower costs and increase efficiency in healthcare. Our publication would impact the research and academic community by providing ongoing, more comprehensive, and up-to-date coverage of healthcare reform. The audience would include academicians and practitioners interested in healthcare, as well as the general US audience, since everyone will be affected by the increase in healthcare costs and related costs for medicine, drugs, and other services.

The objectives of our healthcare reform book include:

- To present new perspectives on Post 2020 healthcare reform in terms of various challenges and opportunities.
- To develop new models of healthcare system/s toward sustainable, optimal healthcare.
- To present the views and perspectives of key stakeholders, including scholars, academicians, physicians, dentists, physician assistants, nurses, healthcare leaders, and practitioners from a variety of fields – medical, healthcare-related, private, public, academic, business, and other areas.

TARGET AUDIENCE

Our publication would impact the research and academic community by providing ongoing, more comprehensive, and up-to-date coverage of healthcare reform. The audience would include academicians and practitioners interested in healthcare, as well as the general US audience, since everyone will be affected by the increase in healthcare costs and related costs for medicine, drugs, and other services. The target audience would include all key stakeholders in the U.S interested in medicine and healthcare. These would include scholars and practitioners from the academic community across a variety of fields – academic, business, industry, medical, healthcare-related, private, public, and others - as well as physicians, healthcare leaders, administrators, and professionals. Our book would be useful to the general public, too, who will be most affected by current and future healthcare plans for themselves and their family members. It would also be beneficial to government leaders and policymakers, such as the U.S. Congress, state legislatures, and other government agencies. Physicians and other healthcare personnel would use the book to understand better the "big picture" of why many changes are necessary and being implemented, especially to improve quality and reduce costs. The book would help all interested key stakeholders and policymakers make better-informed decisions related to healthcare reform and policy development for the United States, and help all individuals and families make optimal healthcare plan choices.

Our book is divided into four sections. Section 1 explores two chapters on Current Topics in 2026 and Beyond. In Chapter 1, "Exploring Recent Developments in US Healthcare – 2025 and Beyond," author Raj Selladurai explores the recent developments in US healthcare and those anticipated for 2026 and beyond. The chapter examines recent healthcare initiatives, including those focused on cost reduction, greater consumer choice, and further deregulation. The One Big Beautiful Bill Act (OBBBA) was signed into law by President Trump on July 4, 2025. It introduced sweeping changes across different areas, including healthcare reform to Medicaid, Medicare, and the Affordable Care Act (ACA). These healthcare reforms aim to lower premium costs and federal spending. Interviews were conducted with US stakeholders from multiple organizations and industry segments to gauge their views on healthcare reform. Several significant outcomes are addressed, including reducing healthcare costs for these stakeholders, enhancing access to healthcare, improving efficiency, enhancing the quality and delivery of healthcare services, increasing patient satisfaction, and advancing overall sustainability.

In Chapter 2, "Physician Shortage in US Healthcare," authors Raj Selladurai and Tony Spaulding discuss the physician shortage crisis facing the nation. This chapter explores, analyzes, and discusses the challenges and potential recommendations for the unprecedented physician shortage affecting US healthcare systems. As a result, patients are waiting long periods to get an appointment, and in many cases, even longer to see a physician. Especially older patients who may need immediate attention and medical care end up waiting several weeks. Healthcare seems to be facing a crisis that is getting worse by the day. How did we get here, why, and what do we do about it are some of the questions addressed in this chapter.

In Section 2, Newer, Innovative Perspectives in Healthcare are analyzed and presented. Chapter 3, "Telehealth: Today' House Call," by author Roshini Selladurai explores how telemedicine can increase access to care, address the physician shortage, reduce healthcare costs, support patients in managing chronic diseases, and improve the patient experience. Today, with so much growth and reliance on technology, healthcare reform requires understanding how to incorporate technology to optimize the patient experience and outcomes. This chapter focuses on how best to harness the benefits of technology to deliver optimal healthcare in a post-2020 world from a clinician's perspective.

Chapter 4, titled "Clinical Informatics and Artificial Intelligence in Healthcare," by authors Jason Greenwood and Ray Qian, provides a high-level overview of clinical informatics (CI) and artificial intelligence (AI) in healthcare. It covers foundational concepts such as electronic health records (EHRs) and data standards, current applications including Clinical Decision Support Systems (CDSS) and ambient scribing/

documentation, and near-term directions for both clinicians and patients. The chapter also introduces how foundational CI systems and healthcare data are leveraged to develop AI solutions, ranging from traditional machine learning to large language models, while addressing key issues such as bias, generalizability, and regulatory considerations. Finally, the chapter examines a potential future in which decentralized AI models augment clinicians in their daily work, generate deeper clinical insights, and transform patient care through advanced predictive models and digital twins.

Author Susan Zinner, in Chapter 5, "Challenges and Opportunities Posed by Artificial Intelligence for Pediatrics," reviews the development of artificial intelligence (AI) and its impact on patient care, including pediatric care. While there have been positive developments, such as better diagnostics and treatments, unknown risks remain, including data breaches, privacy and confidentiality concerns, and poor modeling. AI will likely impact informed consent, and the author considers both the positive and negative ramifications of allowing AI to play a larger role in this process. She concludes with recommendations for integrating AI into pediatric healthcare to protect vulnerable children.

In Chapter 6, "Reimagining rural healthcare ecosystems in the age of AI and other enabling technologies," author Abburi Anil Kumar discusses reimagining rural healthcare as an integral part of a connected network of regional and national healthcare systems. An analogy for such a system is the telecommunications ecosystem, which, in addition to being a network of networks, also incorporates evolution, protocols, and regulations, while keeping the customer at the center. In the United States, over 60 million Americans rely on local healthcare facilities. There are several challenges facing rural healthcare systems, including disruptions in continuity of care, increased costs, and an additional toll on physical and emotional well-being. Emphasis is placed on the modern technologies, especially AI (Artificial Intelligence) and IoMT (Internet of Medical Things). Several medical innovations are discussed along with an international perspective. Specific issues with broadband connectivity, AI implementations, and the associated security risks are also discussed, along with suggestions for mitigating those risks. The chapter closes with a potential approach towards establishing a viable healthcare ecosystem.

Authors Charles Hobson and Crystal Shannon, in Chapter 7, "Medically Supervised Fasting (MSF) as a Way to Curb U.S. Healthcare Expenditures--A Call to Action," have introduced and discussed Medically supervised fasting (MSF) as an evidenced-based frontline treatment for a broad range of human diseases that is efficacious, safe, and very cost effective, compared to traditional medical practices. A specific call to action is presented involving the federal government, healthcare providers, health insurance companies, businesses, and a public service information campaign. Finally, anticipated obstacles are identified and discussed, including the pharmaceutical industry, OTC manufacturers, the hospital industry, the medical profession, and the public's lack of knowledge/misperceptions.

In Chapter 8, "Opportunities in Mental Healthcare Reform," authors Mahendra Ramachandran and Sarah Prabhu review mental healthcare reform in the US, highlighting transinstitutionalization resulting from inadequate community support after deinstitutionalization. It details legislative efforts, persistent access barriers (financial, attitudinal, structural, stigma), and the societal costs of delayed treatment. Proposed reforms include prioritizing affordability, combating stigma, strengthening primary care, and investing in early intervention. The text also explores nutritional psychiatry, the gut-brain axis, and the transformative potential of precision psychiatry via biomarkers and AI. Despite implementation hurdles, it advocates for collaborative efforts to achieve personalized mental healthcare and treat mental illnesses as brain diseases, not personal failings.

In Section 3, the book moves to Practices and Applications in healthcare. Chapter 9 focuses on "Role Modeling in Medical Education Training." Authors Lawrence Lee and Roshini Selladurai state that several reports indicate a shortage of primary care physicians in the US, and this shortage is likely to worsen as the population continues to grow and age. Therefore, it is critical to train the next generation of physicians and healthcare providers to effectively meet the needs of the US population. Alongside this structural challenge, the medical profession is also confronting a cultural one—an erosion of professionalism characterized by declining responsibility, integrity, and communication. In teaching and training resident physicians and medical students, some of these skills can be taught, but these skills are usually better "caught" than taught. This chapter presents two physicians' personal experiences in medical education. It discusses the significance of role modeling and best practices for effectively transmitting professionalism, competence, and communication to the next generation of resident physicians, medical students, and healthcare providers.

Chapter 10 addresses the teamwork model and applications in healthcare settings. Authors Raj Selladurai, Tony Spaulding, and Charles Hobson discuss "Impacting Factors, Effective Teamwork, and Healthcare Outcomes: Mayo Clinic Applications." This chapter focuses on key factors that impact effective teamwork in healthcare organizations, including a case study on the applications of a teamwork model at Mayo Clinic in Rochester, MN. Studies have found that patients are more satisfied when they engage with providers who understand and express their 'soft-skill' competencies. Effective teamwork and communication have been found to positively impact the quadruple aim, which encompasses patient experience, high-quality and safe delivery of patient care, lower costs, and provider satisfaction.

Authors Joe Dudas and James Francis, in Chapter 11, Supply Chain Leading Practices: "The Mayo Clinic Journey," provide an overview of Mayo Clinic's history, achievements, and supply chain management (SCM) strategies. As a prominent academic medical center in the United States, Mayo Clinic operates major campuses in Minnesota, Florida, and Arizona. The organization manages an annual supply expenditure of $6.8 billion and employs approximately 1,300 SCM staff. Mayo Clinic SCM leading practices encompass a vision, mission, and strategic plan; active engagement of senior leadership; clinical practice–supply chain integration; talent recruitment, development, and retention; partnerships (strategic) and supplier relationship management; commitment to service excellence and continuous improvement; digital information technology (IT) platform and strategy; innovation and automation; benchmarking; and business continuity.

In section 4, we look at the Strategic Process: Foundations and Practices in Healthcare. The authors, Barry Doublestein, Walter Lee, and Richard Pfohl, discuss two chapters on the strategic process along with three interesting case studies. In Chapter 12, "Healthcare at its Foundations - Recovering Purpose and Meaning," the authors argue that meaningful healthcare reform requires returning to foundational questions about purpose and structure rather than incremental system adjustments. Three critical fractures impede reform: eroding public trust (declining from 51% to 32% between 2020 and 2025), failure to progress beyond goods-and-services delivery to patient transformation, and consolidation-driven system design that undermines patient-centered care while fueling physician burnout. Before proposing solutions, the authors insist that healthcare leaders must address five worldview questions: What is healthcare for? What is a patient? What good are we pursuing? What does it mean to be a healer? What system best serves human dignity? Only then can leaders effectively apply the six-component Strategy Development Process: Strategic Foresight, Strategic Thinking, Strategic Innovation, Strategic Planning, Strategic Implementation, and Strategic Analysis and Assessment. This framework enables continuous adaptation in an era of exponential change while maintaining moral clarity and operational excellence.

Finally, in Chapter 13, the authors continue their discussion of the strategic process with "Foundations in Practice: Practical Applications of Strategy Development." This chapter examines how foundational worldview questions and a structured strategy development process translate into practical healthcare transformation. Through three detailed case studies, the chapter demonstrates how identity, purpose, moral vision, vocational understanding, and structural design shape effective strategic outcomes. The analysis highlights behavioral health integration, value-based care innovation, and community-centered transformation as examples of strategies grounded in philosophical coherence rather than in technical optimization alone. Across diverse organizational contexts, common themes emerge, including clarity of identity, workforce engagement, balanced measurement systems, and the integration of aspiration with pragmatic implementation. The chapter argues that healthcare strategy must unite analytical rigor with philosophical depth, showing how organizations that align mission, culture, and operational structures are better positioned to achieve sustainable transformation that supports patients, clinicians, and communities.

In conclusion, our book integrates comprehensive, up-to-date efforts to explore, analyze, discuss, and present the opportunities and challenges of healthcare reform in the post-2020 period, 2026, and beyond, which will impact millions of US stakeholders. It includes scholarly and practical perspectives from several stakeholders, including physicians, scholars, academicians, healthcare leaders and professionals, from various fields –medical, healthcare, private, public, academic, business, non-profit, and other areas. Our book also includes current, newer, innovative practices, perspectives, and reforms in healthcare, such as telehealth, AI-driven technology, the One Big Beautiful Bill Act (OBBBA), and related policies, provisions, and guidelines. Further, applications such as teamwork, role-playing in medical education and training, operations and supply chain management, and the foundations and implementation of strategic processes are appropriately supplemented with excellent case studies on Mayo Clinic (Rochester, MN), Providence St. Joseph Health, and Geisinger Healthcare System. We believe that this synergistically produced compilation of chapters on healthcare reform in our book project would make exceptional contributions to optimal and sustainable healthcare reform in the US. Currently, efforts and initiatives aim to lower overall healthcare costs and prescription drug prices, reduce healthcare premiums, increase price transparency, and improve the quality and delivery of patient care for all US stakeholders.

Our editorial team would like to invite our readers to join us in this significant process of discussions and deliberations on healthcare reform in the US. We welcome your input, opinions, thoughts, and suggestions as we work to enhance value to healthcare reform and support and assist our leaders and policymakers in developing an optimal, sustainable healthcare system that benefits all stakeholders in the US.

We look forward to hearing from you! Thank you.

Raj Selladurai
Indiana University Northwest, USA

Charles Hobson
Indiana University Northwest, USA

Roshini Selladurai
Mayo Clinic, USA

Tony Spaulding
Mayo Clinic College of Medicine and Science, USA

REFERENCES

Beltran, W. (2017). *The promise of hope.* Retrieved from The Promise of Hope | Harvard Medical School

Wilson, M. (1938). *Doctor's progress: Some reminiscences.* Retrieved from Doctor's progress; some reminiscences, by R. McNair Wilson | Catalogue | National Library of Australia

Acknowledgment

Raj Selladurai

School of Business and Economics, Indiana University Northwest

I am indeed grateful to my co-editors, Dr. Charlie Hobson, Dr. Roshini Selladurai, and Professor Tony Spaulding, for their advice, recommendations, assistance, and support with our healthcare reform book. It was indeed a rewarding academic and professional experience working with them on this healthcare book project. I wish to acknowledge my dean, Dr. Cindy Roberts, for her encouragement and support of my research interests and efforts in healthcare management and this healthcare project.

I would like to acknowledge every author who contributed a valuable chapter and helped with our book project. Also, I wish to thank all the Editorial Advisory Board members for their wisdom, advice, and guidance given toward this project. I like to thank all our reviewers for taking the time to review and evaluate the various chapters in our book.

I would like to thank my wife, Revathi Rebecca, my daughter, Roshini Isabell, and my son, Roshan Isaac, for their total, continually growing love, patience, support, and encouragement.

Above all, I would like to thank my Lord Jesus for everything, and I wish to dedicate this book to Him all for His glory -- Colossians 3:17, 23-24.

Charles J. Hobson

School of Business and Economics, Indiana University Northwest

I would like to acknowledge the inspirational leadership and vision of our Senior Editor, Dr. Raj Selladurai, in making this second edition a reality. Without his tireless dedication to the revision, the project would never have been completed. Thanks!

Roshini Selladurai

Mayo Clinic & Mayo College of Medicine, Rochester, MN

I'm grateful to my Heavenly Father for giving me such a brilliant and innovative earthly father who created the concept for this book and has carried it to completion. I've seen the long hours my dad (Dr. Raj Selladurai) has poured into this book, his encouragement to the various authors, his persistence in facilitating conversations on this topic, and his desire to do his part to make this world a better place--this time through writing a textbook on the healthcare reform. I'd like to acknowledge and celebrate all of his hard work, as well as the contributions of all involved in this project--including my co-editors, the various authors, advisory board members, and chapter reviewers.

Thank you also to my husband Bo for his support and to my wonderful mom and brother. And thank you to my son Theo Oliver who made a surprise early entrance into the world as we were completing this project—his appearance made finishing this book extra memorable!

Tony Spaulding

Mayo Clinic, Rochester, MN

I would like to extend my deepest gratitude to my co-editors, Dr. Raj Selladurai, Dr. Charles Hobson, and Dr. Roshini Selladurai, for their outstanding leadership and unwavering efforts. Their professionalism, commitment, and dedication have been instrumental in shaping this project, and their collaborative spirit has resulted in an excellent book. It has been an honor to work alongside such distinguished colleagues, and I am truly appreciative of their contributions to this achievement.

Section 1

Current Topics: 2025 and Beyond

Chapter 1
Exploring Recent Developments in US Healthcare:
2025 and Beyond

Raj Selladurai
http://orcid.org/0009-0008-4049-3942
Indiana University Northwest, USA

ABSTRACT

This chapter explores recent developments in US healthcare and those anticipated for 2026 and beyond. It will examine recent healthcare initiatives, including those focused on cost reduction, greater consumer choice, and further deregulation. The One Big Beautiful Bill Act (OBBBA) was signed into law by President Trump on July 4, 2025. It introduced sweeping changes across different areas, including healthcare reform to Medicaid, Medicare, and the Affordable Care Act (ACA). These healthcare reforms aim to lower premium costs and federal spending. Interviews were conducted with US stakeholders from multiple organizations and industry segments to gauge their views on healthcare reform. Several significant outcomes are addressed, including reducing healthcare costs for these stakeholders, enhancing access to healthcare, improving efficiency, enhancing the quality and delivery of healthcare services, increasing patient satisfaction, and advancing overall sustainability.

INTRODUCTION

Healthcare reform involves challenges and complexities due to the very nature of the subject – ensuring that all people have access to and receive useful, high-

DOI: 10.4018/979-8-3373-2577-4.ch001

quality healthcare, which is an essential part of human life. Further, as one gets older, healthcare becomes increasingly critical for a good quality of life. However, despite having the best healthcare system in the world, the US still faces ongoing problems, complexities, high costs, and challenges related to universal access and coverage. Before the passage of the Affordable Care Act (ACA), several estimates showed that approximately 50 million Americans were not insured; healthcare costs were increasing tremendously; and about 50% of the American adult population suffered from chronic problems such as diabetes, blood pressure, and heart-related conditions and diseases. Hence, the US healthcare system was not sustainably optimized, and some form of healthcare reform was necessary to address these problems. Following a series of heated debates in the US Congress over healthcare, the Affordable Care Act (ACA) was passed in 2010. It was supposed to be a more sustainable healthcare system, designed primarily to address the lack of healthcare insurance coverage for the millions of uninsured Americans. But several years later, despite providing expanded coverage for millions of Americans, the ACA faces significant challenges and shortcomings. Studies showed that many people still cannot access affordable healthcare insurance, that healthcare costs are skyrocketing in many states and regions of the country, and that several insurance companies are exiting unprofitable markets, leaving millions stranded to fend for themselves (Education Workforce, 2022).

In 2025, the US Congress and the current administration are still grappling with many challenges and working on several healthcare reform proposals, including initiatives aimed at significant healthcare outcomes. The One Big Beautiful Bill Act (OBBBA) of 2025 addresses lowering healthcare costs, offering more choices for consumers, introducing further deregulation, enhancing the quality and delivery of healthcare services, improving patient satisfaction, and promoting overall sustainability for various stakeholders.

BACKGROUND

Issues, Controversies, Problems

Healthcare reform has been a contentious issue for many years, sparking several controversial debates. After much planning, collaboration, and lengthy discussions in various settings, including the US Congress, the Affordable Care Act (ACA) healthcare bill was passed in 2010. It was considered the right first step in making healthcare more affordable and accessible for lower- and moderate-income segments of the US population (Jost & Pollack, 2016). Also, one of the critical factors/promises of the new ACA health care package proposal was that if American citizens "wished to keep their plans, keep their doctor," they could. This promise did not fully materialize as intended, and so further plans and discussions to repeal, modify, revise, and enhance the current healthcare system have emerged. One such concerted effort over several weeks resulted in a narrow, unsuccessful vote in the US Senate in 2018. However, this ACA healthcare law remains controversial, and the broader healthcare issue is expected to gain momentum again in every election year.

In 2025, the US faced a 43-day federal government shutdown from October 1 through November 12, with healthcare among the top contending issues (Kelly & Tangalakis-Lippert, 2025). Studies show that in the US, around 177 million Americans (more than half of the country) pay for and rely on private health insurance provided by their employers, a group or organization, or an insurance company (McCarthy, 2018). And recent Gallup polls have shown that most Americans (around 59%) rated the quality of their private healthcare plans positively, and 28% said they are satisfied with their healthcare costs (Cooper, 2025).

MAIN FOCUS OF THE CHAPTER

The chapter focuses on recent developments in the US healthcare system, including updates on initiatives related to the passage of the One Big Beautiful Bill Act (OBBBA) in July 2025 and its implications for US healthcare systems and multiple US stakeholders in 2026 and beyond.

ANALYSIS

As of December 2025 and into the next year, Republican-led initiatives under the Trump administration remain the major focus of healthcare reform. The initiatives are aimed at reducing healthcare costs, offering consumers more choices, and advancing greater deregulation. In 2025, the profit incentives in US healthcare, continuing high costs for the insured and the uninsured, and the wide disparities in healthcare access and affordability continue to pose challenges for the US (Betancourt, 2025). It appears that in the US, healthcare is prioritizing revenue and profits over patients, causing widespread anger and frustration among many people, including patients. The United Healthcare tragedy led to public outrage and expressions of frustration and anger over the business-as-usual practices of healthcare insurance companies that resulted in delayed or denied care with enormous financial and often life and death consequences. Also, the failure of Steward Healthcare, the nation's largest for-profit system, led to lower standards of quality, safety, and patient care, causing problems for patients in multiple states (Betancourt 2025). Further, increasing evidence suggests that consolidating large healthcare systems does not provide substantial improvements in quality, safety, or patient care. Yet, healthcare providers are organizing and unionizing in unprecedented numbers to prioritize the business of healthcare and profits over patients and patient care. It will need exceptional courage for healthcare stakeholders and organizations to change this spiraling trend.

Also, many people who do have insurance are unable to get the proper healthcare they need due to high costs or a shortage of providers in their communities (Zucker, 2025). Furthermore, nearly 25% of working adults had insurance coverage but were underinsured, with high out-of-pocket costs that made it difficult to afford patient care. Often, people skip necessary care, avoid specialist visits, fail to fill their prescriptions, and make compromises between critical treatments and necessities like food and rent (Betancourt, 2025). Such situations lead to poorer health outcomes that are certainly avoidable. Another alarming factor is that, although more money is spent on healthcare in the US, the benefits do not seem to justify the costs. The US seems to have more chronic disease and health disparities than other countries across the world, and also within the US in several states, in terms of health outcomes, access to patient care, quality, and equity. In addition to the physician shortage crisis facing the nation, another key factor is the investment in primary care. Other nations invest about 15 percent of their healthcare expenses in primary healthcare, but the US spends a measly four (4) percent (Betancourt, 2025). Such issues and concerns are major challenges that require stakeholders to have the courage to change their priorities, consider proven alternative models, and follow extensive evidence and emerging research.

Currently, major legislative and policy changes are being considered in the US, including the implementation of the OBBBA in 2026 and beyond toward sustainable healthcare reform (The White House, July 4, 2025).

Highlights of the OBBBA for healthcare reform

The OBBBA's major healthcare reform focus is on Medicaid, Medicare, the Affordable Care Act (ACA), Health Savings Accounts (HSAs), Prior Authorization and Insurance Reforms, and the Rural Health Transformation Program (RHTP). According to AdvisoryBoard (2025), the measure leads to more than 1 trillion dollars in cuts to federal healthcare programs, including major cuts to Medicare, Medicaid, and the ACA through reductions in reimbursements and enrollment, driven by administrative restrictions and beneficiary affordability reductions.

Table 1 below shows the major OBBBA healthcare policies and their potential impacts.

Table 1. OBBBA Healthcare policies and potential impacts

Major OBBBA healthcare policies	Potential Impacts [1]
Marketplace tax credit restrictions and Medicaid cost sharing Reduce affordability	**14.2 million** Projected increase in uninsured people (includes sunset subsidies)
Medicaid work requirements Increase admin burden Medicaid and Marketplace enrollment restrictions and eligibility verification barriers Increase admin burden	*Potential consequences:* Uncompensated care ( ) Exacerbated health conditions () Elective volumes () Health plan enrollment ()
State Medicaid financing restrictions Reduce federal funding to states	**$910 billion** Estimated direct reimbursement reduction (includes sequestration cuts)[2]
Medicare sequestration trigger Reduces federal spending	

1. Projected 10-year (2025-2034) impacts.

2. Summation of estimated Medicare sequestration impacts and major Medicaid state financing restrictions provisions (state-directed payments, MCO taxes, and provider taxes).

Source: H.R.1. 119th Congress. July 3, 2025; CBO. Estimated Budgetary Effects of Public Law 119-21, top Provide for Reconciliation Pursuant to 2. Title II of H. Con. Res. 14, Relative to CBO's January 2025 Baseline. July 21, 2025; CBO. Estimated Effects on the Number of Uninsured People in 2034 Resulting From Policies Incorporated Within CBO's Baseline Projections and H.R. 1, the One Big Beautiful Bill Act. June 4, 2025. CBO. E&C Reconciliation Recommendations. May 11, 2025; CBO. Dynamic Estimate: H.R.1, One Big Beautiful Bill Act. June 18, 2025.

From Table 1, the highlights of the OBBBA include:

Medicaid: Work requirements apply to adults ages 19 to 64 without disabilities or dependents, requiring beneficiaries to document at least 80 hours of work or other qualifying activities per month. It also requires adults covered under ACA Medicaid expansions to have their eligibility redetermined every six months. Furthermore, the new bill requires healthcare providers not to offer abortion services while receiving Medicaid payments in keeping with the current administration's pro-life, anti-abortion policies. To enhance program cost optimization, new state provider taxes are disallowed, and existing taxes are reduced from 6% of a provider's net patient revenue to 3.5% over several years. The states are required to conduct quarterly checks using the Death Master File to ensure that Medicaid enrollees are not deceased and to disenroll them if confirmed, again to lower overall costs (H.R.1, 119th Congress. July 3, 2025; McDermott+. Summary of Health-Related Provisions in the Final Reconciliation Package. July 7, 2025).

Also, the cuts to Medicaid will impact several other groups, including mental health care providers, patients, participants, and stakeholders. Although these new changes and policies may widen disparities and affect cost-effective mental health systems that are showing positive results, proactive planning and quick adaptation to new developments are critical for mental healthcare providers to ensure service continuity and address clients' needs effectively. Delaying action may lead to sudden staff reductions, overwhelmed services, and diminishing patient trust (MATERNAL MENTAL HEALTH LEADERSHIP ALLIANCE, 2025).

Medicare: The new bill also increases Medicare physician reimbursements by 2.5% in 2026, addressing physicians' concerns about lower Medicare reimbursements. Moreover, the bill allows $16 billion in cuts to Medicare disproportionate share hospital payments for three years (rather than deferring, as previously done), an administrative-related cost-cutting measure. Another efficient, cost-cutting measure is the new rule that blocks easy eligibility in Medicare Savings Programs for people enrolled in both Medicare and Medicaid. It also restricts most illegal immigrants, including those who have received asylum, from receiving Medicare benefits. It requires states to ensure that deceased individuals are not receiving Medicare benefits, another cost-cutting initiative. Further, the Inflation Reduction Act's Medicare Drug Price Negotiation Program is modified by broadening the orphan-drug exemption, ensuring that more drugs designated for rare diseases are excluded from price negotiation if they meet certain criteria (H.R.1, 119th Congress. July 3, 2025; McDermott+. Summary of Health-Related Provisions in the Final Reconciliation Package. July 7, 2025).

Affordable Care Act Marketplace: Under the new measure, stricter eligibility and income verification requirements apply to people who receive ACA exchange subsidies, as well as new checks for low-income enrollees with zero-premium plans. It also ends eligibility for premium tax credits during special enrollment periods and stops the ACA initiatives aimed at encouraging states to expand Medicaid. The measure prevents premium tax credits from being provided to most migrants or enrollees whose status is in doubt. Further, individuals who lose Medicaid coverage due to noncompliance with work requirements are still considered to have had minimum essential coverage for tax purposes, which could affect their eligibility for ACA subsidies. It ends the auto-reenrollment and provisional enrollment for ACA plans starting in 2028. The measure requires pre-verification of eligibility before receiving advance premium tax credits (APTCs). It treats Bronze and Catastrophic-level ACA plans as high-deductible health plans starting in 2026 (H.R.1, 119th Congress. July 3, 2025; McDermott+. Summary of Health-Related Provisions in the Final Reconciliation Package. July 7, 2025).

Also, the bill includes a rural health fund that will provide $50 billion to rural hospitals and community health centers over five years, addressing a much-needed, rural-community-wide healthcare need now. In addition, the measure establishes a new program within the Children's Health Insurance Program to support rural hospitals and providers with funds for care coordination, telehealth, workforce development, and alternative payment models (note: this program is distinct from the rural health fund). The measure expands eligibility for health savings accounts and allows funds to be used to pay for direct primary care arrangements. It also places a moratorium on a Biden-era regulation that set minimum staffing requirements for nursing homes. The measure permanently extends the safe harbor for high-deductible health plans to cover pre-deductible telehealth services (H.R.1, 119th Congress. July 3, 2025; McDermott+. Summary of Health-Related Provisions in the Final Reconciliation Package. July 7, 2025).

Impact: Overall, the OBBBA-related projected 10-year deficit impacts for 2025-2034 result in:

$4.5 trillion Net tax cuts (healthcare and other impacts).
$0.9 trillion Spending increases.
$3.4 trillion Total deficit change ($4.5 trillion deficit cuts – $0.9 trillion (spending increases) -- estimated attributable to economic effects and interest rate increases).
-$1.2 trillion Healthcare spending cuts.
-$2.1 trillion in other impacts.
-$3.3 trillion Total spending cuts (H.R.1, 119th Congress. July 3, 2025; McDermott+. Summary of Health-Related Provisions in the Final Reconciliation Package. July 7, 2025).

Some provisions of the OBBBA bill have taken effect immediately, though many of the healthcare cuts will be phased in over the coming years. Several major changes to eligibility, enrollment, and affordability will take effect over the next few years. The changes to Medicare and Medicaid by the states will be phased in over several coming years. As states begin to implement the changes in the coming years, the impact on healthcare margins will increase and compound as the changes interact with legislative and executive branch actions. Healthcare leaders have projected that the OBBBA, with $1.2 trillion healthcare spending cuts, will be the biggest single legislation to impact healthcare other than the BBA (Balanced Budget Act) of 1997, which then projected cuts of $390 billion (equivalent to $780 billion in today's 2025 dollars) to Medicare and Medicaid (Advisory Board, 2025). The bill makes major changes to the federal government's direct healthcare funding, its policy and regulatory activities, and its actions across the general business economy. Though some actions will still face legal challenges and Congressional pushback, the OBBBA healthcare reform will transform healthcare and shape operating conditions for many years to come.

Table 2. Operating Conditions and Healthcare Policy

Industry Funding	**Funding restrictions - research funding cuts, coverage erosion** **Federal budget – Medicare, Medicaid, ACA funding cuts**
Business Environment	Cost drivers – immigration and tariffs Market regulation – anti-trust, pricing, transparency, Medicare Advantage risk adjustments Economic indicators – inflation, employment, interest rates, and credit stability
Health Regulations	Department of Government Efficiency (DOGE); Make America Healthy Again (MAHA)– layoffs, data redaction, and program changes Health and Human Services (HHS) operations – restructuring, core program functions, and patient care guidelines

Source: Advisory Board, 2025

To better prepare for the new healthcare reform changes, healthcare systems should be proactive and more adaptable. Regarding capital and scenario planning, they should reevaluate their strategic planning and impact analyses. They must rationalize and optimize their services and infrastructure footprints. When feasible, they must acquire hospitals and free-standing infrastructure. They may wish to coordinate on rural and safety net support providers. To lower costs and increase efficiency, they must improve clinical operations; optimize supply management and contracting; and leverage existing and new technologies. Healthcare providers and systems must be proactive in their revenue-loss mitigation strategy by enhancing revenue cycle performance, attracting volume growth, and exploring and focusing on alternative line-of-business growth investments. They need to manage their workforce more efficiently in terms of capacity and retention, address any gaps in access and preventive patient care, and leverage partnerships with similar and common-cause organizations. Healthcare plans must be more efficiently managed by minimizing public insurance enrollment losses through partnerships with state agencies.

They must develop preventive coverage policies and negotiate commercial network rates to balance affordability and sustainability. Overall, they must reassess how healthcare policies affect their strategic planning, evaluate flexibilities in provider contracting to lower costs, and review and develop new sales and marketing strategies to improve efficient patient service delivery and patient satisfaction.

Many proponents believe that the unprecedented OBBBA healthcare reform would lower premiums and increase taxpayer savings. In contrast, critics argue it would undermine equity, potentially leading some states to implement cuts sooner than scheduled. Though healthcare enrollment projections at this time are mixed, periodically updated policies and implementation efforts in the coming years may provide optimal access to affordable healthcare for all Americans, which is the ultimate goal of sound healthcare reform (Advisory Board, 2025).

Health Savings Accounts (HSAs): The OBBBA would increase HSA eligibility to 7.3 million Americans in bronze and catastrophic ACA plans in 2025, potentially growing to 10 million people. So, millions of Americans who purchase low-premium plans in the individual market will be able to save tax-free for care and protect themselves against unexpected medical bills—an option previously accessible mostly to large employers. The HSA would provide them with tax-advantaged savings for medical expenses, which aligns with Republican support for consumer-driven healthcare (US House Committee on Ways & Means, 2025). Also, the expiring Tax Cuts and Jobs Act provisions would raise health-related tax expenses by 16% ($51 billion) in 2026 if not renewed, affecting employer-sponsored insurance and HSA incentives. Senator Rick Scott's bill, introduced in the Senate, proposes "Health Freedom Accounts," an HSA model to help fix Obamacare by empowering individuals to manage costs (Scott, 2025).

Prior Authorization and Insurance Reforms: In June 2025, major healthcare insurers pledged to implement six reforms under the leadership of HHS, led by R.F. Kennedy, Jr., and Dr. Oz, to reduce delays in approvals for imaging, surgery, and therapy. Such proactive decisions, which enhance transparency and accelerate approvals, would benefit 260 million insured Americans. The addressed concerns include:

> -Standardize electronic prior authorization submissions using Fast Healthcare Interoperability Resources (FHIR)-based application programming interfaces.
> -Reduce the volume of medical services subject to prior authorization by January 1, 2026.
> -Honor existing authorizations during insurance transitions to ensure continuity of care.
> -Enhance transparency and communication around authorization decisions and appeals.
> -Expand real-time responses to minimize delays in care with real-time approvals for most requests by 2027.
> -Ensure medical professionals review all clinical denials" (US Department of Health and Human Services, 2025, para 5).

Another bipartisan bill, H.R. 2433 (Reducing Medically Unnecessary Delays in Care Act), requires board-certified physicians for Medicare and Medicaid reviews to reduce delays in healthcare (Congress.gov, 2025). These developments reflect the move toward more market-driven solutions and fiscal pressures, but implementation will vary by state. For all stakeholders, the reforms emphasize the need for proactive advocacy to balance innovation with greater access.

The Rural Health Transformation Program (RHTP): The most significant recent reform is the RHTP program, launched under the OBBBA bill in July 2025. It is the largest federal government investment in rural healthcare in several decades, totaling

$50 billion over five years, with $10 billion allocated annually. All 50 states received awards for 2026, averaging $200 million based on rural population, state policies and guidelines, and proposed initiatives. State-led changes and transformation are focused on expanding access, improving the quality of patient care, strengthening the workforce, modernizing facilities and technology, and adopting innovative models such as preventive care, chronic disease management and control, behavioral and mental health, and maternal care. Implementation efforts for the program would include funding for telehealth expansion, workforce training and retention, new healthcare access points, and more effective coordination among providers. States must spend the 2026 funds by the end of 2027 to encourage rapid innovation. The program aims to emphasize "Make Rural America Healthy Again" priorities, such as personal health and fitness, nutrition, and root-cause interventions (CMS, 2025).

Overall, the OBBBA and the 2025 healthcare reforms have shifted the focus more toward market-based strategies and spending cuts, achieving unprecedented record coverage highs pre-expiration (300+ million insured). The Republican initiatives of lower healthcare costs, more choice, and more control for working families are emphasized in the bill. Accountability and fairness to the healthcare marketplace are being implemented through program integrity reforms that save taxpayers billions of dollars and drive down costs for everyone, such as:

- "Full income and eligibility verification before subsidies are issued, ensuring assistance goes only to those who qualify.
- Ending "anytime" enrollment abuse that fueled fraudulent sign-ups and drove premiums higher for everyone.
- Closing loopholes that allowed illegal immigrants and other ineligible groups to access taxpayer-funded health benefits" (para 4).

The Congressional Budget Office has found that these measures have already produced $185 billion in savings for taxpayers and reduced premiums by 0.6 percent, which is real savings for working families who will now have more control over their healthcare costs and spending (US House Committee on Ways & Means, November 13, 2025).

Furthermore, the CMS confirms that, in 2026, Obamacare enrollees will have more access to affordable health plans at lower costs.

- "Nine in ten enrollees will continue to receive subsidies for reduced-cost coverage in 2026.
- The average Obamacare premium after subsidies is $50 per month for the lowest cost plan – nearly 30 percent cheaper than in 2020.

- About 60 percent of eligible re-enrollees will have access to a plan at or below $50 per month.
- The average enrollee has between 6 and 7 issuers available, and 95 percent of enrollees have access to three or more issuers" (US House Committee on Ways & Means, November 13, 2025, para 5).

Also, the bill promotes Direct Primary Care (DPC) arrangements as qualified medical expenses, allowing American families to spend HSA funds on innovative, low-cost primary care that prioritizes access, prevention, and more time with their doctor. These DPC services deliver better outcomes, enabling patients to achieve 30 percent savings on medical costs and 54 percent fewer emergency room visits, thereby contributing to lower healthcare costs. Telehealth flexibility is being promoted and made permanent, ensuring that high-deductible health plans (HDHPs) can continue covering telehealth visits before deductibles are met. The employer-sponsored health plans are now more current, updated, and technology-based, allowing rural and working families better access to quality healthcare. As more than half of working families are enrolled in HDHPs, 85 million working families have easier access to telehealth services and benefits. And pre-dedictible telehealth allows the patients to see their doctor right away without incurring high out-of-pocket expenses (US House Committee on Ways & Means, November 13, 2025).

However, some may continue to raise concerns of perception about affordability and access disparities, especially for low-income, rural, and some immigrant populations. Stakeholders must continue to advocate for a balance between cost control, equity, and accessibility for all people living in the US, especially as healthcare is the most important human priority and the US is the world's leading source for high-quality physicians, healthcare professionals, medical services, and providers.

SOLUTIONS AND RECOMMENDATIONS

This section focuses on solutions and recommendations for recent developments in the US healthcare system, including updates on initiatives surrounding the passage of the One Big Beautiful Bill Act (OBBBA) in July 2025 (The White House, July 4, 2025). Also, the implications for US stakeholders and healthcare systems in 2026 and beyond are addressed, including healthcare outcomes such as cost containment, affordability, flexibility, accessibility, feasibility, lifestyle changes, government policies, limited healthcare plans, and implementation issues, from the stakeholders' perspectives.

What do Americans think of US healthcare?

The author conducted interviews on healthcare reform with several Americans representing different segments of the US population, stakeholders, and a variety of industries, including business, finance and banking, healthcare, transportation, oil and gas, nonprofit, government, railroad, IT, and education. Though the sample size is small, the consensus of opinions on the major challenges in healthcare reform enhances their reliability and validity, as they are very similar despite being expressed independently. However, these perspectives are not intended to be generalized to the entire US population without further replication of the interviews with a larger, more representative sample size.

The major concerns and perspectives toward healthcare that many Americans focus on, along with some potential solutions and recommendations to address them, include:

High cost of healthcare

In the US today, almost all Americans, if not most, agree that the US has the best healthcare services and medical treatments in the world. The top three hospital systems in the world for high-quality healthcare are in the US: Mayo Clinic-Rochester, Cleveland Clinic, and Johns Hopkins Hospital (Kayser, 2025). Yet, the major concerns, perceptions, and opinions of almost all surveyed participants clearly point to the high cost of US healthcare, decreased affordability, and lack of flexibility. For example, a CEO of a small-to-medium-sized transportation company headquartered in North Carolina says his company is grappling with the exorbitant, skyrocketing costs of its fully insured healthcare plan, especially for pharmaceuticals (C. Clark, personal communication, July 18, 2025). He explains that, for three employees alone, the company is paying upwards of $1 million annually in healthcare expenses for their medications. And in a domino effect, this also increases the medical insurance premiums for other employees. He describes a systemic problem/issue in the process in which the doctor prescribes a brand-name medication (even if a generic is available), along with a manufacturer's coupon that allows the employee to pay a nominal $5 to $10 to the pharmacy for the medication. However, the manufacturer company charges the employees' insurance company the full cost of the brand-name medication, which may amount to hundreds of thousands of dollars! Clark strongly recommends potential solutions for the high costs of healthcare pharmaceuticals, such as not allowing coupons to be given to the patients when lower priced generics are available, greater transparency into the actual prices charged (retail and costs), and having employers consider offering more incentives to employees to use medical services more efficiently, since someone is paying for the high healthcare costs. It may not be the employees, but their employer does! The healthcare system seems broken and needs reform so that people can ask and know how much a healthcare procedure or treatment costs at a facility before using healthcare services. Also, they can compare prices and service quality, as is done in most other service and consumer purchases, to pay the optimal price for the desired level of service quality (C. Clark, personal communication, July 18, 2025).

Another business leader in the oil and gas industrial services industry recommends an alternative, innovative solution to the high costs of healthcare (K. Hand, personal communication, June 26, 2025). He says consumers and employees (in most cases) can and should take greater personal responsibility and accountability for their health by taking better care of themselves by avoiding smoking, exercising more, eating more healthily, controlling their weight, etc. And so, by maintaining good health, their need for frequent doctor visits may be reduced, thereby lowering their overall healthcare costs, including the cost of their healthcare insurance and the group plans for the whole company and organization. Also, he suggests some relatively less expensive treatments and medicines that employees and patients could use, such as telehealth visits and obesity medicine (rather than more expensive hospital and clinic visits and tests unless absolutely needed), which would also lower their healthcare costs considerably without compromising their health. Further, other cost-cutting measures include changing government and healthcare regulations to allow patients to visit a PA (physician's assistant) or a nurse practitioner for routine healthcare visits at a lower cost than a physician, unless a routine or nonroutine healthcare condition requires a physician (K. Hand, personal communication, June 26, 2025).

High healthcare costs are on everyone's mind, as most people, if not all, would need proper healthcare at some time in their lives. A former Senior Vice President of a leading national banking institution, now retired, expresses his concerns about the high cost of healthcare (C. Pratt, personal communication, June 1, 2025). He says that his share of the healthcare premiums over the past 15-20 years has been skyrocketing more than 100 percent from about $300/month in the late 90s to early 2000s, to $1100/month in 2014, to $2000/month in 2025 for Medicare (C. Pratt, personal communication, June 1, 2025). So, the high costs of healthcare must be addressed, and solutions must be found to lower them and make healthcare more affordable. He commends the current administration for the public policy initiatives it is taking to address the high cost of healthcare through the One Big Beautiful Bill Act (OBBBA), including Medicare and Medicaid.

As of December 19, 2025, in an unprecedented move toward cutting prescription drug prices, 14 major pharmaceutical companies, including Pfizer, AstraZeneca, Eli Lily, and others, have made voluntary agreements to provide Most Favored Nation (MFN) drug pricing to American patients (White House Executive Order, May 12, 2025). This is another significant measure from the Trump administration to lower healthcare costs and make healthcare more affordable. More recently, in another measure to lower healthcare costs, the US House advanced a GOP healthcare bill to the Senate that would allow American consumers to buy lower-premium health insurance through a group plan (Congress.gov, December 15, 2025).

Furthermore, as of January 15, 2026, President Trump unveiled The Great Healthcare Plan to lower costs and deliver money directly to the American people (The White House, January 15, 2026). The plan aims to lower prescription drug prices, cut insurance premium costs, and increase transparency in the healthcare system by requiring all providers and insurers to post their prices. Hence, there are no surprises in billing, and building on existing requirements for hospitals and insurers to disclose negotiated rates. This plan is based on executive actions from his administration, and asks Congress to pass legislation to implement these changes to make healthcare more affordable again. These are mostly bipartisan healthcare reform issues that would benefit all Americans by lowering costs. However, some critics and experts contend that although the plan has lofty objectives, it lacks specifics on implementation, timelines, and funding, which may pose some challenges in Congress, especially for political reasons. Ultimately, however, Congress, leaders, administrators, and policy-makers at federal, state, and local levels must abide by the will of the people for the benefit of all people.

Access to healthcare

Several participants raised another concern about the lack of easy access and long wait times for much-needed healthcare, especially for older people who may have more critical and frequent needs. Setting up doctor visits is becoming a laborious process, and in many cases, appointments are scheduled several months in advance (C. Pratt, personal communication, June 1, 2025). He says that his surgeon's office scheduled the knee replacement surgery for him seven months later, and about two months prior to his scheduled date, they called and pushed it back even further, another three months more! Healthcare providers have long appeared insensitive to their patients' pain, discomfort, and suffering, providing relief and comfort only when they can. He says he thinks there is a shortage of physicians in the US and disagrees with the AMA's position to restrict the number of medical students enrolled in medical schools. However, several initiatives are currently being discussed in Congress and state legislatures to address the critical physician shortage. He also says that public policy must address the tort situation affecting the medical profession. With many doctors being sued for exorbitant sums, some are leaving the profession abruptly or retiring sooner than expected, adding to the physician shortage crisis.

Another stakeholder from the corporate and financial background and his spouse, a local city council leader, contend that the US healthcare system is unique in that it is believed that all legal citizens must have equal access to healthcare and to equal healthcare outcomes (D. Sauerman and L. Sauerman, personal communication, July 9, 2025). But in most countries, like the UK, Canada, Singapore, and other socialist nations outside the US, human life is valued differently based on age, social status, long-term outcomes and benefits, and other factors. Also, in other countries like Singapore, most people have both personal and employer-based group insurance, as well as government insurance for their health coverage, which is overall less expensive than here in the US. Also, there is greater transparency in pricing for various healthcare services in Singapore, according to a Singapore citizen (T. Das, September 16, 2025).

D. Sauerman also asks the question, "Are all lives equal in value? Should the tort value be the same for a 75-year-old patient as for a 30-year-old patient in terms of compensation from a lawsuit if an error was committed? The difficulty is determining the complex value of human life. But value is also correlated with the contribution the patient has made to the system and the costs the patient has incurred. According to experts, 95% of healthcare expenses are incurred in the last 30-60 days of one's life (D. Sauerman, July 9, 2025). Also, the Sauermans say the system lacks transparency regarding its cost structure across various aspects, including doctors' backgrounds and experience, and the costs and quality of services provided. There is a real disconnect between demand and supply for healthcare services, with a lack of transparency about costs before procedures and after procedures and treatments. They believe that the free market is the optimal solution to such complex transparency-related issues (D. Sauerman & L. Sauerman, personal communication, July 9, 2025).

A more recent example of a healthcare organization providing prompt access, instant attention, and high-quality patient care occurred at Mayo Clinic Hospital, Rochester, in January 2026, at the birth of the author's first grandson. The author (and his spouse) observed, for the first time in his and her life, the highest level of personalized patient care through the integrative teamwork of physicians, nurses, medical, professional, and administrative staff, front desk personnel, security staff, and all others serving at the Mayo facilities. It was an amazing experience that personified excellent patient care in every aspect and detail, as modeled by the #1 hospital system in the world (Kayser, 2025), which this author observed firsthand for about two weeks! The thought, "I hope every patient in the world is blessed every time to get this type of unique, utmost patient care and service in the hospital, wherever located," has been etched in this author's mind. Mayo Clinic has certainly set a model of high-quality teamwork-based patient care for healthcare organizations worldwide to emulate.

Lifestyle changes

Furthermore, a Mayo physician who is board-certified in obesity medicine says that patients can also take better care of themselves through exercise, healthy eating, fasting, and other lifestyle changes. They can also make use of several effective weight management treatments that are more recently available and being offered by physicians specializing in obesity medicine (R. Selladurai, M.D., personal communication, December 3, 2025). Such lifestyle changes in patients help improve overall healthcare accessibility, enabling patients with the most critical healthcare needs to access physicians and other healthcare providers more easily and quickly. Also, by using telehealth appointments for patients, healthcare service delivery is optimized, and costs are reduced by minimizing time and resource use.

Further, more healthcare education is needed at various levels – schools, colleges, medical schools, healthcare training schools, clinics, hospitals, and community healthcare organizations- to support preventive medicine. Today, preventive medicine also includes obesity medicine to help weight control, and other such preventive medicine education by helping patients minimize the causes of common diseases such as hypertension and diabetes thereby taking better care of their health through exercise, eating healthy, weight control, abstaining from tobacco, alcohol, substance abuse and other related negative effects on health according to a Midwest healthcare provider's coordinator (V. Miller, August 2, 2025).

Government policies oriented toward healthcare reform.

Many strong opinions across the US recommend, including views from a non-profit organization church leader, that the government take impactful measures toward sustainable and long-term healthcare reform in terms of balanced national budgets, reducing national debt, and cutting costs, generating more revenue, and other fiscally responsible actions (B. Lagos, personal communication, July 25, 2025). Interestingly, this is exactly what the current administration is trying to accomplish through the OBBBA initiative of fiscal responsibility and sustainability. Further, successful efforts by the Trump administration to get pharmaceutical companies to offer lower prices for medicines to American patients do lead to lower healthcare costs and sustainable healthcare (White House Executive Order, May 12, 2025). Lack of oversight and proper accountability allows pharmaceutical companies and medical providers to charge exorbitant prices and adopt different pricing structures for very similar services across medical services, hospitals, and other healthcare facilities. So, the government, as the appropriate regulatory agency for healthcare, needs to regulate prices and require all healthcare providers to provide clear transparency to all stakeholders to help a broken system start functioning effectively

(V. Miller, August 2, 2025). She also adds that healthcare has become more over-commercialized and profit-maximizing rather than patient-centered, which should be the primary focus of all healthcare. Furthermore, mental healthcare should be a top priority for all stakeholders, and the government should carefully evaluate it and provide appropriate solutions and recommendations. The government also needs to integrate the healthcare system, with several of its complex components fragmented and operating in silos, to provide patients with an overall, integrated, sustainable healthcare system.

Another strong recommendation is for the government to radically overhaul and restructure the US rural healthcare system, perhaps through its Rural Health Transformation Program. The rural healthcare system could be reimagined as a "connected network of networks," akin to the evolution of the global telecommunications ecosystem, with patients and patient care at its center. The proposed strategy relies on integrating Artificial Intelligence (AI) and the Internet of Medical Things (IoMT). AI offers a solution to 30%-35% of healthcare costs related to administrative overhead and can help with the initial patient triage structure (AnilKumar, 2026; Slater & Schur, 2023). Further, routine services like blood tests and X-rays from more expensive urban may be relocated to cost-effective local hubs, while improving access and lowering costs. However, while the technologies exist, implementation faces significant challenges, including cybersecurity threats, algorithmic biases, and legal ambiguities regarding ownership of data generated by these devices.

Limited options for healthcare plans

Often, employees are limited by their employer-sponsored group healthcare plans and are locked into them, which can restrict mobility and career growth, according to a railroad company's senior manager (J. Miller, August 2, 2025). Also, because companies generally pay most healthcare costs as part of employee benefits, healthcare insurance companies and providers often have no incentive to offer lower costs to patients. As a major regulatory agency responsible for optimizing healthcare costs for all stakeholders, the government must find ways to provide stronger incentives for all relevant healthcare parties to ensure they provide more affordable, accessible healthcare for the American public (J. Miller, August 2, 2025).

FUTURE DIRECTIONS

Future research could focus on monitoring and evaluating these newly proposed healthcare reform policies and changes once implemented to assess their effectiveness and benefits in the short and long term. Research must also evaluate the potential impact on various stakeholders (including patients, physicians, the insurance company, healthcare providers, hospitals, and other healthcare-related organizations) in terms of the new policies being more optimal, sustainable, and beneficial to them. Research studies would need to develop strategies to improve existing and proposed healthcare models so that all US stakeholders benefit from a comprehensive, sustainable healthcare system. Further, research must explore whether healthcare in the US should continue as a private employer-sponsored program, a federally managed program, a state-managed program, or a combination of these.

CONCLUSIONS

This chapter reviewed and evaluated recent developments in US healthcare reform. Major emphasis was placed on the new OBBBA, which was passed into law on July 4, 2025. The potential impacts of the healthcare policy on benefits and cost reductions were discussed. What do most Americans think about healthcare reform? Several stakeholders from diverse walks of life shared their perspectives on challenges and opportunities in healthcare reform. Recommendations made ranged from lowering healthcare costs and increasing access to quality healthcare to making lifestyle changes, pursuing specific government action and reform, and offering more options for consumers to choose their healthcare plans as they see fit.

REFERENCES

Advisory Board. (2025). *One Big Beautiful Bill Act: Understanding the healthcare impacts.* Retrieved from One Big Beautiful Bill Act: Understanding the healthcare impacts

AnilKumar. A. (2026). Reimagining rural healthcare ecosystems in the age of AI and other enabling technologies. In R. Selladurai, C.Hobson, R. Selladurai, & T. Spaulding. (Eds.). (2026). *New perspectives on post-2020 healthcare reform: Opportunities and challenges.* Hershey, PA: IGI Global, Inc.

Betancourt, J. (2025). *Looking to 2025: Changing healthcare, and the need for courage.* Retrieved from Looking to 2025: Changing Health Care, and the Need for Courage – Commonwealth Fund | healthcarereimagined

Centers for Medicare and Medicaid Services (CMS). (2025). *CMS announces $50 billion in awards to strengthen rural health in all 50 states.* CMS Announces $50 Billion in Awards to Strengthen Rural Health in All 50 States | CMS

Congress.gov. (2025). H.R.2433 - *Reducing Medically Unnecessary Delays in Care Act of 2025.* Retrieved from H.R.2433 - 119th Congress (2025-2026): Reducing Medically Unnecessary Delays in Care Act of 2025 | Congress.gov | Library of Congress

Congress.gov. (2025). *Text – H. R. 1 – 119th Congress (2025-2026): An act to provide for reconciliation pursuant to title II of H. Con. Res. 14.* Retrieved from Text - H.R.1 - 119th Congress (2025-2026): An act to provide for reconciliation pursuant to title II of H. Con. Res. 14. | Congress.gov | Library of Congress

Congress.gov. (2025). *H.R. 6703 Lower health care premiums for all Americans Act.* Retrieved from H.R.6703 - 119th Congress (2025-2026): Lower Health Care Premiums for All Americans Act | Congress.gov | Library of Congress

Congressional Budget Office (CBO). (2025). *H.R. 1, One Big Beautiful Bill Act (Dynamic Estimate).* Retrieved from H.R. 1, One Big Beautiful Bill Act (Dynamic Estimate) | Congressional Budget Office

Congressional Budget Office (CBO). (2025). *Estimated budgetary effects of public law 119-21, to provide for reconciliation pursuant to Title II of H. Con. Res. 14, Relative to CBO's January 2025 baseline.* Retrieved from Estimated Budgetary Effects of Public Law 119-21, to Provide for Reconciliation Pursuant to Title II of H. Con. Res. 14, Relative to CBO's January 2025 Baseline | Congressional Budget Office

Congressional Budget Office (CBO). (2025). *CBO's Review of the Reconciliation Recommendations of the House Committee on Energy and Commerce.* Retrieved from CBO's Review of the Reconciliation Recommendations of the House Committee on Energy and Commerce | Congressional Budget Office

Congressional Budget Office (CBO). (2025). *Estimated effects on the number of uninsured people in 2034 resulting from policies incorporated within CBO's baseline projections and H.R. 1, the One Big Beautiful Bill Act.* Retrieved from Estimated Effects on the Number of Uninsured People in 2034 Resulting From Policies Incorporated Within CBO's Baseline Projections and H.R. 1, the One Big Beautiful Bill Act | Congressional Budget Office

Cooper, A. (2025). *How Many Individuals Are Content With Health Insurance?* Retrieved from How Many People Satisfied With Health Insurance.

Education Workforce (2022). *Five reasons Obamacare is a failure.* Retrieved from Five Reasons Obamacare is a Failure | Committee on Education & the Workforce

Jost, T. J., & Pollock, H. (2016). Making Healthcare Truly Affordable after Healthcare Reform. *The Journal of Law, Medicine & Ethics*, *44*(4), 546–554. DOI: 10.1177/1073110516684785 PMID: 28661251

Kayser, A. (2025). *World's best hospitals 2025 – United States of America.* Retrieved from World's Best Hospitals 2025 - United States of America

Kelly, A., & Tangalakis-Lippert, K. (2025). *The longest government shutdown in US history is over after 43 days.* Retrieved from The Longest Government Shutdown in US History Is Over After 43 Days - Business Insider

Maternal Mental Health Leadership Alliance (MMHLA). (2025). *The One Big Beautiful Bill Act (OBBBA) and its Impact on Maternal Mental Health.* The One Big Beautiful Bill Act (OBBBA) and its Impact on Maternal Mental Health — Maternal Mental Health Leadership Alliance: MMHLA

McCarthy, J. (2018, December 7). Most Americans rate still rate their healthcare quality quite positively. *Well-Being.* Retrieved from https://news.gallup.com/poll/245195/americans-rate-healthcare-quite-positively.aspx

McDermottt+ Consulting (2025). *Health-related provisions in the One Big Beautiful Bill Act.* Retrieved from Health-related provisions in the One Big Beautiful Bill Act - McDermott+

Scott, R. (2025). *Sen. Rick Scott introduces bill to fix Obamacare and drive down health care costs.* Retrieved from Sen. Rick Scott Introduces Bill to Fix Obamacare and Drive Down Health Care Costs.

Slater, B., & Schur, M. (2023). *The future of healthcare as an integrated ecosystem of health and care.* Retrieved from https://www.gensler.com/blog/future-of-healthcare-as-integrated-ecosystem

The White House. (2025, July 4). *The One Big Beautiful Bill.* Retrieved from The One Big Beautiful Bill – The White House

The White House. (2026). *President Trump unveils the Great Healthcare Plan to Lower Costs and Deliver Money Directly to the People.* Retrieved from President Trump Unveils The Great Healthcare Plan to Lower Costs and Deliver Money Directly to the People – The White House.

The White House Executive Order. (2025, May 12). *Delivering most-favored-nation prescription drug pricing to American patients.* Retrieved from Delivering Most-Favored-Nation Prescription Drug Pricing to American Patients – The White House

US Department of Health and Human Services (2025). *HHS Secretary Kennedy and CMC Administrator Oz secure industry pledge to fix the broken prior authorization system.* Retrieved from HHS Secretary Kennedy, CMS Administrator Oz Secure Industry Pledge to Fix Broken Prior Authorization System | HHS.gov

US House Committee on Ways & Means. (2025, November 13). *Republicans Deliver Lower Health Costs, More Choice, and Greater Control for Working Families.* Retrieved from Republicans Deliver Lower Health Costs, More Choice, and Greater Control for Working Families - Ways and Means

US House Committee on Ways & Means. (2025, December 30). *Ways & Means Committee delivered historic tax relief for families in 2025.* Retrieved from Ways & Means Committee Delivered Historic Tax Relief for Working Families in 2025 - Ways and Means

Zucker, H. (2025). Where have all the physicians gone? AARP.org/Bulletin. Retrieved from America Is Facing a Shortage of Doctors

ADDITIONAL READING

AAMC (2024). *New AAMC Report Shows Continuing Projected Physician Shortage* New AAMC Report Shows Continuing Projected Physician Shortage | AAMC

Armour, S. (2017, October 17). *Conservatives make new push to repeal Affordable Care Act.* Retrieved from https://www.wsj.com/articles/conservatives-make-new-push-to-repeal-affordable-care-act-1529400721

Collins, S., & Blumenthal, D. (2016, February 24). *New federal survey shows gains in private health coverage and fewer cost-related problems getting care.* Retrieved from https://www.commonwealthfund.org/blog/2016/new-federal-survey-shows-gains-private-health-coverage-and-fewer-cost-related-problems

DeJulio, B., Firth, J., Kirzinger, A., & Brodie, M. (2016). *Kaiser health tracking poll.* Retrieved from https://www.kff.org/health-costs/poll-finding/kaiser-health-tracking-poll-january-2016/

Jones, C., & Dolsten, M. (2024). *Healthcare on the brink: navigating the challenges of an aging society in the United States.* Healthcare on the brink: navigating the challenges of an aging society in the United States - PMC

KEY TERMS AND DEFINITIONS

Buy own health insurance: One can buy one's own health insurance and not have to get coverage through his/her employer. Depending on where one works, one may have the option of getting employer-sponsored health insurance, called group coverage.

Cost reduction: strategies to cut healthcare costs, currently at exorbitant levels.

Employer-sponsored healthcare plans: Healthcare insurance plans sponsored/offered by employers, which are currently the most popular type of healthcare coverage used by the majority of the US population.

Free choice in healthcare insurance plans: The "Freedom of Choice in Health Care Act" allows an individual to freely enter into contractual agreements with health care providers for health care services and coverage, without any mandate or penalty from state legislatures.

Healthcare reform: changes made to improve healthcare for all stakeholders, especially in terms of lowering costs and enhancing access to quality healthcare.

OBBBA: One Big Beautiful Bill Act passed into law in July, 2025 offering lower costs, more choices, and greater control over their healthcare.

Private and public healthcare: Private healthcare can be provided through "for-profit" hospitals and self-employed practitioners, and "not-for-profit" non-government providers, including faith-based organizations. The government usually provides public health care through national healthcare systems.

Universal healthcare access: This usually means everyone in a given country has access to and can enjoy the protection of health insurance, whether the country has a single-payer system, socialized medicine, an insurance mandate, or relies on a set of subsidies and other incentives.

Universal healthcare coverage: All legal residents of the country are included and can receive and benefit from healthcare through available plans or insurance.

APPENDIX 1.

Table 1. OBBBA Healthcare policies and potential impacts

Major OBBBA healthcare policies	**Potential Impacts** [1.]
Marketplace tax credit restrictions and Medicaid cost sharing Reduce affordability	**14.2 million** Projected increase in uninsured people (includes sunset subsidies)
Medicaid work requirements Increase admin burden Medicaid and Marketplace enrollment restrictions and eligibility verification barriers Increase admin burden	*Potential consequences:* Uncompensated care (up) Exacerbated health conditions (up) Elective volumes (down) Health plan enrollment (down)
State Medicaid financing restrictions Reduce federal funding to states	**$910 billion** Estimated direct reimbursement reduction (includes sequestration cuts)[2.]
Medicare sequestration trigger Reduces federal spending	

1. Projected 10-year (2025-2034) impacts.

2. Summation of estimated Medicare sequestration impacts and major Medicaid state financing restrictions provisions (state-directed payments, MCO taxes, and provider taxes).

Source: H.R.1. 119th Congress. July 3, 2025; CBO. Estimated Budgetary Effects of Public Law 119-21, to Provide for Reconciliation Pursuant to 2. Title II of H. Con. Res. 14, Relative to CBO's January 2025 Baseline. July 21, 2025; CBO. Estimated Effects on the Number of Uninsured People in 2034 Resulting From Policies Incorporated Within CBO's Baseline Projections and H.R. 1, the One Big Beautiful Bill Act. June 4, 2025; CBO. E&C Reconciliation Recommendations. May 11, 2025; CBO. Dynamic Estimate: H.R.1, One Big Beautiful Bill Act. June 18, 2025.

APPENDIX 2

Table 2. Operating Conditions and Healthcare Policy

Industry Funding	**Funding restrictions - research funding cuts, coverage erosion** **Federal budget – Medicare, Medicaid, ACA funding cuts**
Business Environment	Cost drivers – immigration and tariffs Market regulation – anti-trust, pricing, transparency, Medicare Advantage risk adjustments Economic indicators – inflation, employment, interest rates, and credit stability
Health Regulations	Department of Government Efficiency (DOGE); Make America Healthy Again (MAHA)– layoffs, data redaction, and program changes Health and Human Services (HHS) operations – restructuring, core program functions, and patient care guidelines

Source: Advisory Board, 2025

Chapter 2
Physician Shortage in US Healthcare: Challenges and Potential Solutions Toward Healthcare Reform

Raj Selladurai
http://orcid.org/0009-0008-4049-3942
Indiana University Northwest, USA

Tony Spaulding
http://orcid.org/0009-0006-4071-9206
Mayo Clinic, USA

ABSTRACT

This chapter explores, analyzes, and discusses the challenges and potential recommendations for the unprecedented physician shortage affecting US healthcare systems. As a result, patients are waiting long periods to get an appointment, and in many cases, even longer to see a physician. Especially older patients who may need immediate attention and medical care end up waiting several weeks. Healthcare seems to be facing a crisis that is getting worse by the day. How did we get here, why, and what do we do about it are some of the questions addressed in this chapter.

INTRODUCTION

The current US healthcare system is one of the largest in the world; however, it faces many problems and complexities, which necessitate that the nation's leaders and lawmakers continue exploring healthcare reform. Recent efforts in 2018 to change, modify, enhance, and reform the Affordable Care Act (ACA) federal

DOI 10.4018/979-8-3373-2577-4.ch002

healthcare program came close to being passed in the United States Senate but fell short by a few key votes. In 2026, Congress and the current administration are still grappling with many challenges and working on various healthcare reform proposals, including addressing the physician shortage facing healthcare organizations across the US. Significant outcomes—lowering healthcare costs, enhancing the quality and delivery of healthcare services, improving patient satisfaction, and promoting overall sustainability—are addressed, along with their implications for various stakeholders.

BACKGROUND

Healthcare reform involves challenges and complexities due to the very nature of the subject – ensuring that all people have access to and receive useful, high-quality healthcare, which is an essential part of human life. Further, as one gets older, healthcare becomes increasingly critical for a good quality of life.

And why did/does the US need healthcare reform in the first place? The current US healthcare system is among the largest and best in the world, given the country's size, population, and multiple healthcare private and public plans. According to the 2025 Newsweek report, the US healthcare system loop has over 6,000 hospitals and a total gross output of around 1,075 billion US dollars (Kayser, 2025). Also, among the best hospitals/healthcare systems worldwide offering the highest-quality medical care, the top three are Mayo Clinic-Rochester, Cleveland Clinic, and Johns Hopkins Hospital (Kayser, 2025). The US healthcare system is considered a source of many amazing innovations, especially in the medical field, and provides the best, high-quality care to those who need it at the right time. The US has some of the world's best physicians, nurses, researchers, and healthcare provider systems. People from all over the world, including leaders and influential figures, come to the US when they need critical lifesaving treatments, services, and surgeries. "It is here, in America, where treatments are discovered, methods are improved, and diseases are cured" (America Next, 2014, p. 3).

However, despite having the best healthcare system in the world, the US healthcare system still faces ongoing problems, complexities, high costs, and challenges related to universal access and coverage. One such significant issue is the shortage of physicians (Zucker, 2025). The physician shortage is resulting in unnecessary delays and longer wait times for patients. The average wait time for new patients to see their physician is about 26 days, and this is for healthy patients. For sick patients, it tends to get worse. For many critically ill patients aged 65 or older, the wait is about 30 days or more to get an appointment with a medical specialist (Keenan, 2025). The situation is certainly leading to a crisis quickly and becoming worse day by day. A physician, Clarel Antoine, professor of obstetrics and gynecology at New York City's NYU Grossman School of Medicine, says, "The backbone of our healthcare system, private practice, is on the brink of collapse. As a result, the nearly 70 million Americans on Medicare, many with chronic conditions, can expect longer waiting times for medical care" (Zucker, 2025, para 3). In another personal health experience, a business leader from Tennessee seeking an appointment with a specialist for his critical breathing issues was told to wait for six months. He asked in frustration, "What if I don't last that long?" (R. Harter, personal communication, April 20, 2024). Due to an aging population living longer thanks to improved medical treatments, medicines, technology, and services, better healthy diets and exercise, and several misguided professional steps and policies over the years, the current unprecedented physician shortage seems here to stay. This significant issue must receive serious attention. Also, this crisis is putting everyone in the US (especially the older patients and more critically ill people) at increased risk now and in the future, demanding immediate, swift responses and actions to counter it.

MAIN FOCUS OF THE CHAPTER

The main focus of this chapter is the physician shortage in the US healthcare system—how it happened, why, and how to help resolve the crisis by addressing the challenges it poses and offering recommendations for potential solutions in healthcare reform.

ANALYSIS

How Did We Get Here?

Several factors have caused the physician shortage in the US healthcare system. One major factor is that demand for physicians and surgeons currently exceeds supply. Although about 839,000 physicians were practicing medicine in 2024 (US Bureau of Labor Statistics, 2024), there was a shortage due to demand exceeding supply. The demand for physicians is projected to grow faster than supply, leading to a shortage of between 13,500 and 86,000 physicians by 2036 (Association of American Medical Colleges (AAMC), 2024). Primary care seems to be the hardest-hit area of the physician shortage. Over 92 million Americans live in the designated primary care Health Professional Shortage Areas (HPSAs) as of 2026, up significantly from prior years, and about 100 million people do not have a regularly scheduled primary care provider (Bebinger, 2025).

Another factor contributing to the physician shortage is the lack of a demand-supply equilibrium. To meet the growing demand from patients (AAMC, 2024), there must be an adequate increase in supply. But this is not currently happening, as shown in Table 1. Also, due to the extreme strain on doctors caused by the current shortage, many are choosing to leave, switch professions, or retire early. Furthermore, the AAMC cannot keep up with the need to graduate more doctors faster due to various constraints, including maintaining high-quality, professional standards, securing additional funding to cover the high cost of medical education, and meeting other healthcare requirements.

Table 1 below shows the projections of physicians' supply and demand in the US healthcare workforce.

Table 1. Projections of physicians' supply and demand

	2027	**2032**	**2037**
Supply	936, 530	936,590	949,360
Demand	1,060,710	1,103,620	1,136,490
Surplus/Shortage	(124,180)	(167,030)	(187,130)
Percent Adequacy	88	85	84

(Source: HRSA Health Workforce, 2024)

Percent adequacy is calculated by taking the projected supply in 2037 divided by demand in 2037.

Implications of the Physician Shortage

Often, patients experience unnecessary delays in scheduling appointments with their physicians, which is a major effect of the physician shortage. And then, further delays in receiving the right treatment from physicians are an even more drastic effect of the shortage. One of the many frustrating, sad, and horrific experiences that patients and their loved ones face due to physician shortages may be illustrated by Michelle, a New Yorker (Zucker, 2025). Marvin, her dad, an engineer, called her and said that he was experiencing the classic symptoms of a stroke -- speech slurring and facial drooping. She immediately directed him to go to a hospital. The doctors told him that he needed an MRI. But he had to switch his pacemaker to an MRI-safe mode. And despite Michelle's calls to every hospital and doctor—neurologists, cardiologists, and primary care physicians—no one could help him get the MRI completed that time. In the next few months, Marvin went through two more similar episodes, and subsequent tests revealed he had suffered two more strokes. Ultimately, he had open-heart surgery. "But it left us so angry and frustrated that he had to nearly die to get the care he needed," said Michelle (Zucker, 2025, para 13).

Similarly, another patient's experience highlights the implications of the physician shortage. Alli Phillips of Denver developed some swelling in her hands in April 2023; when she called her doctor for an appointment, she was told the earliest she could see the doctor was in June, about two months later. When she saw her doctor later, she was told she needed to see a specialist. But the specialist did not have an appointment until November of that year. Meanwhile, Allie's knees started to swell, and she had difficulty walking down stairs and turning doorknobs. When her appointment with the rheumatologist finally came, he prescribed some medicine that slightly improved her symptoms. Then, Alli consulted with a concierge doctor paying a hefty $3500 per year fee (not covered by her insurance). The concierge doctor spent some time with her, diagnosing the problem, and then recommended multiple treatment options and long-term care to get the health conditions under control. Alli wonders how people with few resources get around the system to get the healthcare they so badly need (Zucker, 2025).

Furthermore, the healthcare system needs immediate reform, as even doctors and other healthcare professionals face difficulties accessing quality healthcare services. A doctor working for a major medical facility in the South moved to the Northeast. In the moving process, his wife was diagnosed with cancer. In the new city, the insurer would not cover her cancer treatment until she obtained a referral from a new primary care physician. Though he was a well-known physician, he could not find another doctor in the area who would take on his wife as a new patient. So, they returned to their prior facility in the South to receive treatment for the wife (Zucker, 2025). Although she is doing much better and well now, thanks to the immediate treatment and care she received, the need for the right healthcare reform to address the critical physician shortage is a top priority for our nation.

Why Did We Get Here?

In 1980, a US government report stated that American teaching hospitals were graduating too many medical students, leading to a surplus of 70,000 physicians by 1990. Hence, in response, American medical schools imposed a 25-year moratorium on increasing class sizes, as regulated by the AAMC and the American Medical Association (Zucker, 2025).

However, a major flaw of the report that went unnoticed then was the nation's growing population, which is about 110 million more than it was in the 80s. In early 2005, as the population continued to grow and the physician shortage became more pronounced, the AAMC and the AMA revised their policies to encourage more young people to train as physicians and surgeons. Over the past 20 years, more doctors have been practicing medicine. Today, more than 97,000 students are enrolled in US medical schools, and the AAMC projects a shortage of 86,000 physicians by 2036 (AAMC, 2024). By then, the US population is expected to have increased by 8.4 percent since 2021; the 65+ age group would increase by 34 percent, and the 75+ age group would increase by 55 percent (AAMC, 2024). Though medical school enrollment has risen, the need to train more medical school graduates in residency programs continues to grow, and more government support is needed, according to David Skorton, president of the AAMC (AAMC, 2024).

Another factor that impacts the physician shortage is the cost of medical education and related implications. With many medical students carrying about $250,000 in student loan debt and the average primary care physician (PCP) earning an annual salary of $275,000, most medical students wish to enter specialties that allow them to make more than double the PCP's salary. PCPs are undervalued by government and insurance providers, as evidenced by their lower compensation packages. But demand for PCPs continues to grow, as patients must see a PCP before being referred to a specialist. Further, about 50% of medical students and residents choose not to enter direct patient care but instead pursue teaching or research (Elsevier Health Report, 2023). Some of them, due to stress or overwork, cut back on working hours, see fewer patients, or quit the medical profession.

Moreover, a few changing perspectives among physicians and the medical profession have contributed to the physician shortage. In the past, many young people dreamed of becoming doctors and surgeons from an early age. It was quite common to see doctors practicing medicine beyond their retirement age. However, over the years, and currently, many doctors wish to leave medicine within two to three years, and among the 55+ age group of physicians, it is about 50% who wish to leave medicine. A major cause of this attrition is the management of healthcare facilities by private equity firms and companies such as Amazon and CVS Health, which are increasingly buying out hospitals and private practices. Reports indicate that almost 80% of all physicians were employed by hospitals and corporations, a figure that has increased by 200% over the past ten years (Physician Advocacy Institute, 2024). The consequences of corporate ownership have led to more profit-oriented management policies, and it is all about money, which most physicians and medical professionals are not used to, given their strong "serving their patients" mentality. They dislike the total control management companies exercise over the time physicians can spend with their patients — often about 15 minutes — which they believe is not healthy for patients or their doctors. In a recent study, 61% of doctors surveyed said they found private equity ownership detrimental to healthcare (Zhu, Zeveney, & Reed, 2024).

Also, doctors are inundated with paperwork for various reasons, especially to meet electronic health record (EHR) requirements. And the paperwork reduces the time they need to spend caring for their patients. Doctors often point out that, though the EHR was meant to be a tracking system for patients' records and to allow easy access to other doctors and medical professionals, it has become more of a documentation process for insurers and regulators. Many physicians often cut back on their working hours, leaving even less time to see patients. A Mayo Clinic 2023 study found that about 40 percent of physicians intended to cut back on their working hours over the next 12 months (Shandafelt et al., 2023). The study further noted that reductions in working hours and the fact that about 26 percent of doctors said they planned to quit in the next two years would reduce the workforce by about 20,234 physicians, which equals all the medical school graduating classes combined (Shandafelt et al., 2023). Also, the physician-patient relationship clearly takes time to develop trust, which happens when patients share their personal and health information with their physicians – and that certainly takes more than just 15 minutes per visit.

Where are all the Physicians Going?

Among the factors that have caused a physician shortage in the US healthcare system, burnout is the most dominant cumulative result. The new takeover-related changes in corporate ownership of healthcare practices and facilities have forced doctors to practice medicine in ways that do not serve their patients well. And those who try to hold on to their private practices are finding it extremely difficult to continue due to several financial pressures and spiralling costs they must manage. After 45 years of serving his patients with passion and love for the profession, Michael Hotchkiss, M.D., had to quit his obstetrics and gynecology practice. He says, "I am no longer able to continue practicing medicine in a manner that aligns with my convictions regarding the best interests of my patients" (Zucker, 2025, para 34). Also, the doctor was horrified to report that, to make matters worse, he was unable to refer his patients to another doctor quickly. The situation was precarious and critical for patients in need of healthcare, especially as most were 50 years or older and very few physicians were accepting new patients. And when he found doctors willing to take new patients, they were not in the immediate vicinity, and so the patients had to drive 45 minutes or more to see a doctor.

The disturbing healthcare situation has turned into a disastrous, unexpected trend and a serious crisis – about 300-400 doctors now die every year from committing suicide, a figure which is significantly higher than the general US population (Davis, 2024). Physicians who enter the medical profession with a strong passion and dedication to serving their patients soon find themselves unable to do so satisfactorily. But they come under the control of corporate healthcare organizations, which dictate how much time they should spend with their patients (usually 15 minutes or less), require extensive paperwork, and impose more compliance and regulatory requirements. Further, the pandemic has pushed physicians into retirement early, others became more frustrated with the corporate ownership and the healthcare system, some became critically sick and needed disability, and many sadly died. And those who survive are in constant battle with insurance companies for approvals and compliance requirements – an exhausting task outside of their patient-focused healthcare goals and purposes, which motivated them to enter medicine in the first place.

SOLUTIONS AND RECOMMENDATIONS

Several potential solutions and recommendations for addressing the physician shortage crisis in healthcare, in the context of healthcare reform, will be discussed.

Some Newer Alternatives

Concierge Medicine

The appeal of concierge medicine is flourishing today. It is a USD 7.35 billion market in 2024, with about 7,000 physicians currently practicing, and this number is expected to grow (Grandview Research, 2025). The growth is phenomenal due to patient awareness of the benefits of concierge medicine, the increasing use by physicians, and the shortage of PCPs. For example, MDVIP, a Florida-based company, was founded in 2000 and has grown into a network of more than 800 physicians (Lincoff, 2015). In this type of practice, concierge doctors focus on preventive care more than traditional physicians do. "If you keep the patient out of the hospital or the ER, it saves patients much money. The people that buy into this model are really trying to buy into a personalized engagement model focused on prevention," said Bret Jorgensen, CEO of MDVIP (Lincoff, 2015, p. 6). In the concierge medicine model, the patient pays a yearly subscription-type membership fee to the physician's practice, ranging from about $ 2,000 to $10,000 per year, to receive personalized healthcare services, longer visits, and shorter wait times (Kiss, 2023).

Physicians have also turned to shift work, a model in which they care for patients in a hospital during specific set hours, protecting and continuing their time off. These hospitalists transfer their patient care to the next doctor on call when their shift ends. In 2000, there were only a few hundred hospitalists, but today there are over 60,000. They provide adequate patient care in the hospital; however, this trend reduces the number of physicians available for routine wellness visits (Zucker, 2025).

Physician Shortage and Impact on Older Patients

Older patients in the US are increasingly growing in number due to higher mortality rates, thanks to better medical treatments and medicines, a healthier lifestyle, including food habits, more attention to exercise, mobility, and walking. However, there are not enough geriatricians to adequately provide personalized healthcare for older people with specific needs. Also, by 2037, experts anticipate a shortage of more than 2,000 geriatricians to care for older patients (HRSA, 2024). "There is a perfect storm coming, with increased patient complexity, decreased reimbursements, and increased demand for prior authorizations from the insurance company. The combination of these makes it increasingly difficult for physicians to accept new patients and, in some cases, even keep their doors open. We cannot afford to lose even one more doctor," said Bruce Scott, president of AMA (Scott, 2024). Given the limited near-term potential for new geriatricians in healthcare, one option is to train primary care and specialty physicians in the specific challenges they would face in caring for aging patients. Also, healthcare leaders, educators, and administrators must redesign medical school and residency program curricula to meet the specific needs of elderly patients. Further, all Medicare-supported training must be mandatory, with an emphasis on older adults. The entire patient-care system for older adults must be well-integrated to smoothly provide home-based care, telehealth visits, hospice, emergency facilities, office practices, clinics, nursing homes, strengthening the training and skills of elderly caretakers, developing new models of geriatric patient care, and increasing and retaining the elderly workforce, and other related services.

Novel Approaches Toward Addressing the Physician Shortage in the US.

Federal and state lawmakers, including in at least 15 states, have introduced legislative initiatives to address the physician shortage in the US healthcare system.

Making some modifications to the process, such as practice under supervision and then completing a successful match, the model moves medical students from unsuccessful matches to supervised practice, then to completing residency requirements, passing license exams, and finally to completing state licensure requirements and board certification. Increased workforce availability is the intended outcome.

Currently, IMGs entering bypass pathways to independent practice require Educational Commission for Foreign Medical Graduates (ECFMG) certification, which, in turn, requires passing the United States Medical Licensing Examination (USMLE)

Steps 1 and 2, among other criteria. These licensing exams and certification criteria need to be continued and strengthened as necessary to ensure that IMGs meet the high competencies of US medical school preparation, training, and residency program requirements. Increased workforce availability is the intended outcome.

Congressional Initiatives Toward Minimizing the Physician Shortage

Congress has to act quickly to help minimize the physician shortage in the US and increase easier access to healthcare for millions of people, according to the AMA (Mukkamala, 2025). One immediate solution for Congress is to remove several administrative paperwork requirements that seem excessive, causing burnout and leading to early retirements among physicians. Another significant action needed is the updating of the Medicare payment system, which has seen physician reimbursement decline by more than 33 percent since 2001. Also, the Medicare-funded GME residency slots need to be expanded, especially in areas and specialties with critical shortages, such as primary care and psychiatry. The AMA also strongly supports the recently introduced Resident Physician Shortage Act of 2025, which would add 14,000 additional Medicare GME positions over seven years and codify the Rural Resident Planning and Development program. This bipartisan measure will enable patients to access healthcare more easily by expanding physician training in hospitals, both rural and urban, with the greatest workforce needs.

Furthermore, the AMA also supports the Specialty Physicians Advancing Rural Act, another bipartisan initiative under consideration. This bill will create a loan-repayment program for specialty medicine physicians who agree to serve for six years in a rural area experiencing a physician shortage. Also, the AMA has expressed serious concern over the changes to the federal student loan program in the 2025 budget reconciliation bill, which would make medical school unaffordable for many medical students, including the most qualified applicants (Mukkaala, 2025).

Recognizing the significance of and need for Graduate Medical Education (GME) funding, the 118th Congress convened the full Senate Committee on Health, Education, Labor, and Pensions on February 16, 2023, for a hearing titled "*Examining Health Care Workforce Shortages: Where Do We Go from Here?* In response to the major concerns expressed at the hearing about the physician shortage crisis facing healthcare in the US, Congress enacted the Consolidated Appropriations Act, 2024. By doing so, Congress extended funding for the HRSA's "Teaching Health Center Graduate Medical Education (THCGME)" program through December 31, 2024. This program supports the education and training of medical students in primary care residency programs in community-based ambulatory patient care centers (Adashi, O'Mahony, & Cohen, 2024). A bill is pending before Congress, the "*Resident Physician Shortage Act*" *of 2023*. If enacted, it will create 2,000 additional positions each year from 2025 to 2031. The newly appointed physicians will be placed in hospitals in the rural areas and other health professional shortage areas. Other initiatives being considered include making it easier for international medical graduates to continue their training in the US through the necessary, appropriate visa changes (Adashi, O'Mahony, & Cohen, 2024).

Telemedicine Helps Address the Physician Shortage

Although telemedicine may not directly solve the physician shortage crisis, it can act as a powerful augmentation tool by making the current workforce more efficient and reachable. It can help alleviate problems, especially in rural areas where physicians may be in short supply. By using telemedicine, physicians can see more patients more quickly, thereby reducing wait times. They can also effectively generate an alternative revenue stream while incurring lower overhead costs, and help their patients save time and money on travel to the physician's facility/office, hospital, or clinic. One physician can see more patients via telemedicine consultations across a wider area and multiple sites. So, telemedicine provides improved access to healthcare, optimizes existing workforce and resource utilization, and addresses geographic and specialty gaps among patient groups. Therefore, often telemedicine consultations turn out to be a win-win for both physicians and patients. Also, telemedicine allows physicians to refer their patients to other specialists when needed. This is especially critical in some shortage areas, such as neurology, cardiology, psychiatry, and endocrinology, where patients in rural or underserved areas may have quicker access to experts via telemedicine, which they may not have locally in person Furthermore, patients can receive more timely healthcare for non-emergency issues and conditions, follow-ups, and chronic conditions such as diabetes and high blood pressure via remote consultations (Advanced Medical Reviews, 2022).

Artificial Intelligence (AI) Helps Mitigate the Physician Shortage

Artificial Intelligence (AI) is being used to help manage the physician shortage crisis in healthcare. In 2026, AI adoption and use among physicians in healthcare are increasing rapidly, with about 67 percent of all physicians using some form of AI tools and about 90 percent of healthcare workers using it too (Meyer, 2026). AI does not replace physicians, but it can augment their capacity by enabling them to manage more patients effectively. A major part of the physician's time (up to 60 percent) can be consumed by administrative tasks related to scheduling, workflow management, patient care management, patient communication and education, ensuring the patient is following instructions and taking medication on schedule, prior authorization, and record management. However, AI-driven automation can streamline these tasks and operations efficiently, reducing human effort, errors, and time. In doing so, AI enables physicians and healthcare staff to focus on providing personalized, direct patient care, thereby improving both productivity and satisfaction, and helps reduce stress and burnout (Meyer, 2026). Also, several advanced AI-powered systems emerging can perform tasks that enhance productivity and efficiency, streamline workflows, and support faster decision-making in healthcare. AI clinical assistants can perform many administrative tasks, relieving physicians so they can see more patients per day, increasing revenue flow, and optimizing time use. They also support diagnostics and decision-making related to access to patients' health data and maintenance records. AI also helps expand access via virtual telehealth models in programs such as Mass General Brigham's Care Connect for urgent primary care needs, allowing the physicians to handle about 40-50 patients daily with AI assistance (Bebinger, 2025). AI-driven telehealth models can also generate an alternative revenue stream for physicians while incurring lower overhead costs. Physicians can help their patients save time and money by consulting with them remotely rather than having them travel to the physician's facility/office, hospital, or clinic. By leveraging technology, AI-powered telemedicine programs enable a single physician to see more patients via telehealth consultations across a wider area and multiple sites (Advanced Medical Reviews, 2022).

Moreover, AI-powered programs can improve working conditions by drastically reducing repetitive work and alleviating stress in high-demand areas, such as ICUs and primary care settings. They can potentially retain more physicians in the workforce, serving their patients effectively, and make their profession more attractive to future physicians entering the job market.

From Physicians: The Biggest Threats to Physicians in 2026 and Beyond

A recent survey of physicians identified the major threats they anticipate in 2026 and beyond (Newitt, 2025). They strongly contended that the erosion of trust in scientific expertise and evidence-based medicine is the greatest threat physicians will face and must overcome. A strong trust in science and medicine is foundational to public trust, informed consent, and shared decision-making for the benefit of all stakeholders. Yet, the decline did not occur on its own. The COVID-19 pandemic had a major adverse impact on the nation and, in fact, the whole world. It caused tremendous uncertainty and profound emotional, social, and economic strain on almost the entire global population. Nearly every individual and family experienced some impact and loss from the pandemic – perhaps the loss of a loved one or family member, and the unexpected, excessive burden on clinicians and hospitals was unprecedented. The pandemic event left lasting imprints on healthcare systems; it exposed vulnerabilities, required rapid contingency planning and adaptations, and demanded optimal decision-making amid uncertainty. Many people have become disappointed, cynical, and have begun to doubt whether the medical profession can provide the level of protection and certainty that society hoped for. Controversies emerged over misinformation from some experts with access to data, who often advanced unsupported narratives. The results, sadly, were confusion rather than clarity, polarization and division rather than partnership and unity, and delayed or declined critical interventions that could have improved healthcare outcomes for millions of stakeholders (Newitt, 2025).

Rebuilding trust in the medical profession and healthcare is more than a mere communication challenge; it requires a cultural change. It required acknowledging the hardships many have suffered over the past several years, honoring the experiences of families and patients, and remaining firm in the commitment that science and evidence-based medicine are the most reliable paths to improved health. The future of patient care and the practice of medicine depend on regaining public confidence and trust in healthcare systems. Clinicians and medical leaders who provide evidence-based advice on diagnosis, treatments, and lifestyle recommendations need the patient's acceptance of the information and a benevolent, helpful service intent. And any form of distrust or doubt would undermine healthcare providers' ability to influence and improve patient care and outcomes.

Further, allowing the physician shortage to continue and, in some cases, worsen will be detrimental to all healthcare stakeholders. Some state-level policies have negatively impacted the situation by passing legislation allowing physicians to be replaced by nonphysician practitioners, leading to malpractice conditions. Also, at the federal level, Congress has been slow to act on this significant issue. However, several pro-physician measures such as the Resident Physician Shortage Reduction Act (to increase residency positions), the Physician and Patient Safety Act (to ensure professional due process rights for physicians), the Specialty Physicians Advancing Rural Care Act (offer loan repayments to specialty physicians serving in rural areas), and the Restoring Rights of Physicians to Own Hospitals Act (to repeal the ACA ban on physicians to own hospitals) need to be passed quickly by Congress so that the country has an adequate number of qualified, trained physicians to continue providing high-quality healthcare to patients. And to ensure that the best and brightest candidates will continue to be recruited to the medical profession (Newitt, 2025). Healthcare reform focused on these four measures and similar ones; implemented quickly, they would certainly help resolve the physician shortage crisis (Newitt, 2025).

Also, a major issue is that, in 2026, physicians need to recognize the new importance of meeting patients where they are, using AI and related technologies to provide high-quality healthcare. This means reviewing the ChapGPT research with their patients, patiently and/or explaining the evidence-based rationale for some recommendations, and addressing any distrust or misinformation the patient may have. Or give them time to think and answer all the patient's questions about the treatment options or related healthcare matters. All these require physicians to be humble and patient with their patients, and a sharp contrast from how they may have practiced in the past. Further, concerns over reimbursement and payment policies and practices in many specialties are affecting the financial viability and continuity of these physicians' practices. Physicians and group practices must deal with regulations from government agencies, large insurance companies, corporate and private equity ownership, and governing companies, among others. Practitioners and hospitals in both rural and urban areas are being affected.

Another threat to healthcare systems would be the financial instability of hospitals due to the non-renewal of ACA subsidies, leaving more patients underinsured or uninsured. As many hospitals already operate on thin margins, any revenue loss will further strain hospital systems, leading to hiring freezes, delayed backfills, reduced budgets, and service consolidations. Anesthesia, labor and delivery units, surgery and operating room-related areas, ICUs, trauma, and other specialties that use hospitals to deliver their healthcare services will be drastically affected. Although the major impact will be felt in rural and underserved areas, it will extend across geographical boundaries, especially for a large proportion of Medicaid and uninsured patients. Urban community centers, and even academic medical centers, though strong in resources, can become vulnerable due to high costs, uncompensated patient care, and budget cuts (Newitt, 2025). Healthcare organizational leaders, federal and state-level policymakers, and other stakeholders need to come together to develop more comprehensive and workable solutions to address these threats to the physician shortage and to continue providing high-quality healthcare in the US—one of the largest and best healthcare systems in the world.

Practical Ways of Ensuring the Timely Healthcare That Patients Critically Need

According to Gallup polls (Saad, 2023), only 33 percent of all Americans have a high level of confidence in the medical system, but about 66 percent trust the physicians. When people realize that the doctor is retiring or has little to no time to see them, it is imperative to ensure patients receive the care they need as soon as possible. Some ways to do so include:

- To develop friendships with the nursing and scheduling staff to keep track and monitor any cancellations, and by keeping you on the waiting list, etc.
- Scheduling the next appointment at the end of the current one – great opportunity to secure a spot on their calendar.

- Make sure to complete all necessary paperwork before the visit so the patient can make the most of their time with the physician.
- Ask about telehealth options. Several surveys indicate that about 87 percent of doctors offer telehealth appointments, and many patients request telehealth visits with their physicians (R. Selladurai, M.D., personal communication, December 1, 2025). Yet, only about 37 percent of patients used this service in the last year (Zucker, 2025).
- Ask your doctor to give you a referral and reach out on your behalf.
- Ask your insurance company for a list of physicians and healthcare providers.
- Use the urgent care facilities as necessary.
- Monitoring your health at home. Blood glucose monitors, blood pressure monitors, and ECG-related devices for tracking heart rhythms are available for patient use. Calling your physician about changes in vital signs may help the patient get quicker appointments or receive directives to go to an emergency care facility sooner.
- Do your own research online and in other sources to learn more about healthcare services, including physician board certifications, specialty training, insurance plans, and hospital affiliations (Zucker, 2025).

As healthcare affects all stakeholders, their loved ones, and their friends, everyone needs to understand that the healthcare system is in crisis due to a physician shortage and must support all initiatives and efforts to improve it for everyone.

FUTURE DIRECTIONS

Future research could test these newly proposed healthcare alternatives and models to manage the physician shortage, when implemented, to measure their effectiveness and benefits in the short and long term. Research must also evaluate the potential impact on various stakeholders (including patients, physicians, the insurance company, healthcare providers, hospitals, and other healthcare-related organizations) regarding the new solutions and recommendations being more optimal, sustainable, and beneficial to them. Research studies would need to develop strategies to improve existing and proposed healthcare models so that all US stakeholders benefit from a comprehensive, sustainable healthcare system. Further, research must explore whether healthcare in the US should continue as a private employer-sponsored program, a federally managed program, a state-managed program, or a combination of these, and which of these would most likely minimize the physician shortage and crisis in the US healthcare system.

CONCLUSIONS

This chapter explores, analyzes, and discusses the challenges and potential recommendations for the unprecedented physician shortage affecting US healthcare systems. It addressed the implications of the physician shortage, including long wait times for patients to get an appointment and then receive services from physicians. Also, a recent survey of physicians who discussed the major threats facing their profession in 2026 and beyond was analyzed. Further, the use of AI and telemedicine to help manage and mitigate the physician shortage crisis has been discussed. Some practical ways were recommended for older patients who may need immediate attention and proper medical care. As healthcare faces a crisis that is worsening by the day, the chapter focused on how we got here, why, and what we must do about it as soon as possible to achieve optimal healthcare reform that ensures adequate patient care for all stakeholders in the US.

REFERENCES

AAMC (2024). *The complexities of physician supply and demand: Projections from 2021 to 2036*. Retrieved from The Complexities of Physician Supply and Demand: Projections From 2021 to 2036.

Adashi, E., O'Mahony, D., & Cohen, G. (2024). The national physician statement: The imperative of Congressional action. The National Physician Shortage: The Imperative of Congressional Action. [The National Physician Shortage: The Imperative of Congressional Action - The American Journal of Medicine]. *The American Journal of Medicine, 137*(11), 1030–1031. DOI: 10.1016/j.amjmed.2024.05.032 PMID: 38876332

Advanced Medical Reviews (AMR). (2022). Telemedicine: A solution to the predicted physician shortage? Retrieved from Telemedicine: a Solution to the Predicted Physician Shortage?

Abdel-Razig, S., & Stoller, J. (2024). Addressing physician shortage in the United States with novel legislation to bypass traditional training pathways: The fine print. [Retrieved from Addressing Physician Shortages in the United States With Novel Legislation to Bypass Traditional Training Pathways: The Fine Print - PMC]. *Journal of Graduate Medical Education, 17*(1), 16–19.

America Next. (2014). *The freedom and empowerment plan: The prescription for conservative consumer-focused health reform*. America Next.

Bebinger, M. (2025). *Can artificial intelligence help with a primary care provider shortage?* Rerieved from Can artificial intelligence help with a primary care provider shortage?: NPR

Davis, M. (2024). How many doctors commit suicide every year? *Advance Study.org*. Retrieved from How Many Doctors Commit Suicide Every Year? - Advance Study

Grandview Research (2025). *U.S. concierge medicine market size*. Retrieved from U.S. Concierge Medicine Market Size | Industry Report, 2030

HRSA Health Workforce (2024). *Physician Workforce: Projections, 2022-2037*. Retrieved from Physician Workforce: Projections, 2022-2037

Kayser, A. (2025). *World's best hospitals 2025 – United State of America*. Retrieved from World's Best Hospitals 2025 - United States of America.

Keenan, T. (2025). *Rural adults wait longer and travel farther for medical appointments. AARP.org*. Retrieved from Medical Appointment Waiting and Travel Time.

Kiss, J. (2023). *6 types of concierge medicine fees.* Retrieved from *6 Types of Concierge Medicine Fees*

Lincoff, N. (2015). *The future of healthcare could be in concierge medicine*. Retrieved from https://www.healthline.com/health-news/the-future-of-healthcare-could-be-in-concierge-medicine-063015

Meyer, H. (2026). AI in 2026: Combatting the healthcare staffing shortage. [Combatting the Healthcare Staffing Shortage - Providertech]. *AI*, •••, 2026.

Mukkamala, B. (2025). *The physician shortage will worsen – unless Congress acts now.* Retrieved from The physician shortage will worsen—unless Congress acts now | American Medical Association

Newitt, P. (2025). *The biggest threat to physicians in 2026.* The biggest threat to physicians in 2026 - Becker's Physician Leadership

Physician Advisory Institute (2024). *Over 77% of physicians are employed. Here's how that's shaping healthcare.* Retrieved from Over 77% of physicians are employed. Here's how that's shaping healthcare.

Saad, L (2023). *Gallup: Historically low faith in U.S. institutions continues*. Retrieved from Historically Low Faith in U.S. Institutions Continues

Saad, L (2023). *Gallup: Historically low faith in U.S. institutions continues*. Retrieved from Historically Low Faith in U.S. Institutions Continues

Scott, B. (2024). *Inaugural address at the 2024 AMA annual meeting.* Retrieved from There is a perfect storm coming, with increased demand for prior authorizations from the insurance company by Bruce Scott, MD - Search Videos

Shandafelt, T., Dyrbe, L., West, C., Wang, H., Carlasare, L., & Sinsky, C. (2023). Career Plans of U.S. Physicians After the First 2 Years of the COVID-19 Pandemic. *Mayo Clinic Proceedings*, p. 1629-1640. Retrieved from Career Plans of U.S. Physicians After the First 2 Years of the COVID-19 Pandemic - Mayo Clinic Proceedings

U.S. Bureau of Labor Statistics. (2024). Physicians and Surgeons: Occupational Outlook Handbook. Retrieved from Physicians and Surgeons: Occupational Outlook Handbook: U.S. Bureau of Labor Statistics

Zhu, J., Zeveney, A., Read, S., & Crowley, R. (2024). Physician perspectives on private equity investment in healthcare. [Retrieved from Physician Perspectives on Private Equity Investment in Health Care | Health Care Economics, Insurance, Payment | JAMA Internal Medicine | JAMA Network]. *JAMA Internal Medicine*, *184*(5), 579–580. DOI: 10.1001/jamainternmed.2024.0062 PMID: 38466275

Zucker, H. (2025). Where have all the physicians gone? AARP.org/Bulletin. Retrieved from America Is Facing a Shortage of Doctors

ADDITIONAL READING

Jones, C. & Dalsten, M. (2024). *Healthcare on the brink: navigating the challenges of an aging society in the United States.* Healthcare on the brink: navigating the challenges of an aging society in the United States - PMC

Walensky, R., & McCann, N. (2025). Challenges to the future of a robust physician workforce in the United States. [Challenges to the Future of a Robust Physician Workforce in the United States | New England Journal of Medicine]. *The New England Journal of Medicine*, *392*(3), 286–295. DOI: 10.1056/NEJMsr2412784 PMID: 39813651

KEY TERMS AND DEFINITIONS

Challenges: Complex issues, problems, and situations in healthcare that are difficult to manage.

Crisis: The physician shortage has become so acute that it is a crisis day by day.

Physician shortage: Patient demand for physician services exceeds the supply of physicians.

Potential solutions: Possible alternatives, short and long term, to meet the healthcare challenges.

Universal healthcare access: This usually means everyone in a given country has access to and can benefit from health insurance, whether the country has a single-payer system, socialized medicine, an insurance mandate, or relies on subsidies and other incentives.

Universal healthcare coverage: All residents of the country are included and can receive and benefit from healthcare through available healthcare plans or insurance.

Section 2
Newer, Innovative Perspectives in Healthcare

Chapter 3
Telehealth:
Today's "House Call"

Roshini Selladurai
http://orcid.org/0009-0001-7340-508X
Mayo Clinic, USA & Mayo College of Medicine, USA

ABSTRACT

This chapter will explore how telemedicine can increase access to care, address the physician shortage, reduce healthcare costs, support patients in managing chronic diseases, and improve the patient experience. Today, with so much growth and reliance on technology, healthcare reform requires understanding how to incorporate technology to optimize the patient experience and outcomes. This chapter will focus on how best to harness the benefits of technology to provide optimal healthcare in a post-2020 world, from a clinician's perspective.

INTRODUCTION

Today, telehealth (often used interchangeably with telemedicine) encompasses a range of tools, including virtual consultations, remote patient monitoring (RPM), and the delivery of healthcare services via technology (live video conferencing, phone messaging, remote monitoring devices), among other digital health technologies. It has developed from a pandemic-era need into a significant cornerstone of current healthcare. Telehealth accounts for more than 80% of all physician-patient consultations in office-based settings in the US, with some specialties, such as family medicine and mental health, exceeding 50% of visits (Peters, Lendon, Caffrey, Myrick, Mahar, & DeFrances, 2024). Among several measures that impact healthcare, two key policies have boosted telehealth growth. The 2025 Medicare Physician Fee Schedule permanently allows audio-only telehealth for home-based services when

DOI: 10.4018/979-8-3373-2577-4.ch003

patients lack video access or consent. And the 2024 Telehealth Modernization Act has facilitated cross-state licensing through compacts adopted by over 30 states, enabling providers to serve rural and underserved areas more efficiently (Telehealth. hhs.gov, 2025). Healthcare policy reforms, technological advancements, and greater emphasis on patient-centered care have driven this integration of telehealth into medicine and healthcare.

BACKGROUND

The primary model of medical care in the United States during the late 19th and early 20th centuries was the physician's house call. Almost 40% of physician-patient encounters in the 1930s were house calls (Kao, Conant, Soriano, & McCormick, 2009). The phrase "house call" conjures an image of a physician carrying a medical bag into a patient's home to provide personalized care. Though this model fostered strong relationships, it was inherently inefficient, as travel time limited the number of patients a physician could see in a day, and the portability of equipment limited diagnostic options. Advances in diagnostic testing and medical equipment outgrew the medical bag and required a different setting (Stevens, 1998). By 1972, house calls only accounted for 5% of care provided by health practitioners. That percentage decreased to less than 1% by 1980 (Fortin, Baca-Motes, Steinhubl, & Topol, 2019). The norm became centralized care, with physicians and patients traveling to hospitals or offices for health care.

However, as technology advanced, another shift enabled modern house calls. A milestone was achieved in the 1960s that helped pioneer remote patient monitoring systems: the space race led NASA to develop telemonitoring systems to ensure the health of astronauts in orbit (Jagarapu & Savani, 2021). This key milestone demonstrated how technology could be harnessed to advance healthcare.

Telehealth rapidly grew during the COVID-19 pandemic, which illuminated both its potential and its limitations. This caused healthsystems to re-evaluate the long-term role of remote care. Currently, more than 76% of hospitals in the US connect doctors and patients remotely via telehealth, up about 35% from 10 years ago (Harvard Health Publishing 2025). As healthcare systems advance beyond the pandemic era, telehealth remains a key tool at the center of healthcare reform.

MAIN FOCUS OF THE CHAPTER

The chapter focuses on the growing use of telehealth in healthcare systems and on how best to harness technology's benefits to deliver optimal healthcare in a post-2020 world, from a clinician's perspective.

ANALYSIS

Telehealth (often used interchangeably with telemedicine) refers broadly to the use of communication technologies to deliver medical care from a distance. Telehealth consultations could be through live video visits, remote monitoring, mobile health interventions, or asynchronous consultations (via recording forwarding).

Telehealth is a key tool in healthcare reform, offering benefits such as improved access, optimized efficiency, reduced costs, and enhanced quality of care.

Benefits

Improving Access and Equity

With technology, patients in underserved areas can receive healthcare without traveling long distances. This improves patients' access to healthcare who may otherwise be limited due to a rural location, low income, or mobility impairment. Telehealth improves access for patients – more than 80% of the respondents expressed satisfaction with the easier access (AMA, 2021). It also promotes digital equity for patients by assessing their digital readiness and determining whether telehealth is a viable option. Further, physicians may offer modality of choice and preparation – patients with low digital literacy may benefit from options such as video, audio-only, or in-person. Designing inclusive workflows such as consent forms and instructions being offered in patients' preferred language; tracking and monitoring digital metrics in terms of age, language, device, and payor, all of which enhance the use of telehealth services (Ivanova, 2025). Clinicians may also support advocacy efforts through community organizations and federal, state, and local organizations focused on digital technology and other telehealth tools.

Optimizing Efficiency

Telehealth can help reduce unnecessary in-person visits and save the time associated with travel. When feeling ill enough to need a visit but not ill enough to require an in-person visit, a telehealth visit can be the perfect solution to provide care without requiring the patient to leave their home. Additionally, triage can be done via telehealth to determine if the patient needs to be seen in person and in what setting (outpatient, urgent care, emergency department, or inpatient). Also, several reports show that telehealth innovation using Artificial Intelligence (AI) will promote greater efficiency (Whereby, 2025). By automating several routine tasks and analyzing large amounts of data, workflows will be streamlined for scheduling appointments, managing patient records, and transcribing virtual telehealth consultations, minimizing the burden on healthcare providers and optimizing their time and effort for patient care. AI algorithms can assist physicians in diagnostics by rapidly analyzing patient records and providing decision-making support to clinicians. Further, cumulatively, all this will promote greater efficiency, enabling physicians to focus more on patient care while leading to greater patient satisfaction.

Decreasing Costs

Telehealth focuses on increasing home monitoring for patients, thereby helping prevent complications and lowering healthcare costs, especially for older patients who may be monitored to ensure they are eating, sleeping, and taking their medications on time and as per schedule (Harvard Health Publishing, 2025). Additionally, telehealth visits offer lower-cost care compared to hospital or clinic visits.

Also, the current healthcare reform policies in 2026, under the One Big Beautiful Bill Act (OBBBA), allow Direct Primary Care (DPC) arrangements as qualified medical expenses, allowing American families to spend HSA funds on innovative, low-cost primary care that prioritizes access, prevention, and more time with their doctor. These DPC services deliver better outcomes, enabling patients to achieve 30 percent savings on medical costs and 54 percent fewer emergency room visits, thereby contributing to lower healthcare costs. Telehealth flexibility is being promoted and made permanent, ensuring that high-deductible health plans (HDHPs) can continue covering telehealth visits before deductibles are met. The employer-sponsored health plans are now more current, updated, and technology-based, allowing rural and working families better access to quality healthcare. As more than half of working families are enrolled in HDHPs, 85 million working families have easier access to telehealth services and benefits. And pre-dedictible telehealth allows the patients to see their doctor right away without incurring high out-of-pocket expenses (US House Committee on Ways & Means, November 13, 2025).

Improved Quality

Although telehealth started as a pandemic workaround method of patient care, several studies show that it delivers comparable - if not superior, in many cases–

outcomes to in-person care across several quality aspects of effectiveness, patient-centered focus, patient satisfaction, timeliness, efficiency, and safety (HHS.gov, 2025). Telemedicine enables more frequent patient engagement, timely access to specialists, remote monitoring that could identify problems earlier, and continuity of care (Harvard Health Publishing, 2025).

Also, studies have shown improvements in the doctor-patient relationship, including better communication, higher consultation quality, and greater opportunities for patient education and engagement. When well integrated, the advantages of telehealth provide an attractive option for many patients, especially older patients, thereby contributing to improved overall quality of patient care. Further, studies show that physician and patient satisfaction with telemedicine is high and mutually beneficial, indicating improved quality of telehealth healthcare. Several studies have shown high patient satisfaction with telehealth across various medical specialties, as reported in a systematic review and meta-analysis (Fadaiadeh et al., 2024). Also, physicians from different specialties, geographic and practice locations, and healthcare situations are generally satisfied with providing telehealth patient care. Patients indicated that telehealth consultations were a viable resource during and after the pandemic. Further, patients expressed higher satisfaction with the video technology used in telehealth consultations, as did the physicians, who indicated high levels of acceptability, appropriateness, feasibility, and satisfaction with this mode of technology in their consultations with patients. Video consultations can minimize the risks of exposure, contamination, and infection transmission for both patient groups and physicians while maintaining satisfaction. In addition, both physicians and patients strongly prefer the continued use of telehealth consultations. Therefore, with increased satisfaction for both physicians and patients, telehealth must be considered a standard, sustainable method of providing healthcare not only during a crisis but also beyond it, and adequate infrastructure, policies, regulations, and related changes must be implemented in healthcare systems. It does not replace in-person visits but supplements the telehealth physician-patient consultation and interactions in appropriate situations and when mutually preferred, convenient, and beneficial to both patient and physician.

Telehealth and Family Medicine

Telehealth has been used across several specialties of medicine, most frequently in family medicine. Meta-analyses and comprehensive scoping of multiple studies on the impact of telehealth in family medicine show several advantages and benefits: increased patient access to physicians and healthcare was reported in 38% of studies, and provider convenience and patient safety were reported in 32% of studies. Also, patient preference fulfillment and patient convenience were found to be strong in 30% and 27% of the studies, respectively (Mahdavi et al., 2025).

Several studies have highlighted that the primary advantage of telehealth is the increased access to patient care. Patient access enhancement is seen in many ways – increased access for patients with limited mobility, for patients living in remote areas, and through improved physical and economic access. Telehealth also enhances the continuity of patient care, especially in bad weather and during health emergencies, and for some groups, such as the elderly, students, and individuals who may struggle to take time off from work (Mahdavi et al., 2025).

Telemedicine also enhances family-centered patient care by actively involving the family members and caregivers in the patient care process. They may be involved in patient consultations, provide information that the patient may not share, though pertinent to the patient's health, and engage with the patient and physician in decision-making when necessary or appropriate. Video consultations give healthcare providers more insight into the patient's home and lifestyle, allowing them to make comprehensive, constructive assessments. Further, telehealth, by delivering healthcare remotely, provides patients and other family members with safety by avoiding exposure to diseases and health hazards – a primary reason and outcome for using telemedicine during the COVID-19 pandemic (Mahdavi et al., 2025).

Service providers also benefit in many ways from telehealth. Physicians find it more convenient, as telehealth allows consultations from home and promotes flexible scheduling. They like the greater physician satisfaction that comes from a better work-life balance, which allows them more family time and a better overall quality of life (DePuccio et al, 2022). Further, minimizing crowding in healthcare facilities and patient workload reduces workplace stress, the potential for violence and injury, and long patient wait times. Also, telemedicine enhances practice efficiency and adds value. Time saved by using telehealth for patient admissions, room preparation, and other routine administrative tasks can be redirected to patient consultations, and no-show appointments may be minimized, controlled, or avoided altogether (Mahdavi et al., 2025).

Telemedicine to Help Address the Physician Shortage

Telemedicine may be used as one strategy to help minimize the impact of the physician shortage crisis in the US. It helps make the existing workforce more efficient and accessible, especially in rural and underserved areas facing acute physician shortages. By using telemedicine, physicians can see more patients more efficiently and optimally, thereby reducing the wait times. Also, virtual telehealth models in programs such as Mass General Brigham's Care Connect for urgent primary care needs allow physicians to handle about 40-50 patients daily with AI assistance (Bebinger, 2025). They can also generate an alternative revenue stream while incurring lower overhead costs, and help their patients save time and money by consulting with them remotely rather than traveling to the physician's facility/office, hospital, or clinic. By using technology, telemedicine allows one physician to see more patients via telehealth consultations across a wider area and multiple sites. So, telemedicine provides improved access to healthcare, optimizes existing workforce and resource utilization, and addresses geographic and specialty gaps among patient groups. Therefore, often telemedicine consultations turn out to be a win-win for both physicians and patients. Also, telemedicine allows physicians to refer their patients to other specialists when needed. This is especially critical in some shortage areas, such as neurology, cardiology, psychiatry, and endocrinology, where patients in rural or underserved areas may have quicker access to experts via telemedicine than they would locally in person. Furthermore, patients can receive more timely healthcare for non-emergency issues and conditions, follow-ups, and chronic conditions such as diabetes and high blood pressure via remote consultations. Telemedicine also helps physicians minimize the stress and risks associated with in-person facility consultations, including exposure to contamination and infections from sick patients and healthcare staff (Advanced Medical Reviews, 2022).

Several surveys indicate that about 87 percent of doctors offer telehealth appointments today, and many patients request them. Yet, only about 37 percent of patients used this service in 2024 (Zucker, 2025). Therefore, as physicians increasingly adopt telehealth consultations, the potential for more patients to use telehealth visits would help strengthen the existing clinician workforce and help mitigate the shortage crisis considerably.

Potential of Telemedicine in Global Health

Telehealth can expand access to experts worldwide through virtual consultations (Kim & Zuckerman, 2019). In an unprecedented move, North Korean private citizens teleconferenced online with their counterparts in medical education in several countries outside their country to revamp their country's medical education system. The telehealth initiative sets a precedent for other global health efforts that can use telemedicine to improve the health of millions of people across physical, social, geopolitical, and economic distances, even reaching the most remote communities (Kim & Zuckerman, 2019). Today, telemedicine is better positioned to deliver healthcare globally and remotely through significant advances in information and communication technology (ICT), decreased overall costs, and the growing popularity of technological resources, even in low- and middle-income settings. Also, the infrastructure for providing global healthcare in developing countries has been continuously improved. According to the World Health Organization, most developing countries today can provide at least one mobile health program to their populations, delivering healthcare services ranging from health call centers to disaster and emergency relief programs. These exciting developments are providing impetus for medical communities worldwide to focus on telemedicine's potential to address global health issues, as well as the challenges of deploying it worldwide.

Telemedicine can significantly improve healthcare services globally for patients with limited access to medical care and do so cost-effectively across many medical specialties, from family medicine to dermatology and radiology, benefiting millions of patients who lack adequate healthcare (Kim & Zuckerman, 2019). Furthermore, telemedicine connects more patients in rural areas, nationally and globally, with specialists to provide much-needed healthcare services. Also, beyond access to healthcare specialists, global healthcare trends indicate a need for greater patient education and engagement with chronic diseases across income groups. Mobile health applications can provide treatment support, disease management, patient self-care, and education to impact positive behavior and healthy lifestyle changes. Telehealth programs and applications can, in most cases, minimize the high cost of hospitalization and help patients achieve their personal health goals through remote patient monitoring and family member support in the healthcare treatment process. Also, telemedicine is a viable option and a response to the need for healthcare networks to interconnect data for sharing and funding purposes during crisis management nationally and globally. Telehealth programs and applications bring the world closer together and will continue to grow, meeting the needs of millions of people more effectively than ever before (Kim & Zuckerman, 2019).

Challenges

Though telehealth offers many benefits, there are still challenges to address. For example, many states require providers to be licensed in the state where the patient is located at the time of the visit, which can restrict interstate telemedicine efforts. Insurance companies may have restrictions on which patients can be reimbursed for telehealth visits—though many of those restrictions were temporarily waived during the COVID pandemic. Also, challenges related to the lack of regulatory standards, biases against technology-based medicine, the need for additional policy changes, and overcoming inertia must be addressed and managed more effectively. Research healthcare communities must find sustainable models for telehealth programs that can integrate with existing healthcare systems. Further, relevant policies, standards, and regulations need to be formulated and implemented to achieve a sustainable vision and continued growth of telemedicine at the national and global levels. This will lead to changing the current fragmented perspective of telemedicine into an established, sustainable healthcare structure and system.

To utilize telehealth, patients need access to the internet, devices such as smartphones or computers, and some level of digital literacy. As a result, a "digital divide" can be created, with certain populations with lower access to telehealth unable to benefit from it. Also, the lack of physical "touch" and personal examination, along with perceptual and communication barriers (cited in 30 percent of the studies) for some patients, was a concern and may be viewed as a disadvantage. Patient privacy concerns were expressed in 24 percent of the studies, and inadequate access to current communication technologies was cited in 20 percent of the systematic review study (Mahdavi et al., 2025). Another disadvantage of telemedicine, due to the lack of physical examination, is its difficulty in treating complex health conditions and emergencies. However, a viable alternative would be to use hybrid consultations, where telehealth services are supplemented with in-person visits when the physician deems them necessary for the patient.

In many cases, patient diagnoses and clinical decisions cannot be made without a physical exam. For example, self-reported symptoms of skin rash or dizziness spells, and abdominal pain may be difficult to diagnose in a phone call, as well as complex medical conditions such as chest pain, heart-related, respiratory, and neurological issues may be treated more effectively by supplementing telehealth visits with a visual consultation and/or physical examination, too. Physical exam limitations can lead to inadequate clinical assessments, diagnostic issues, or delays if a patient is scheduled for an inappropriate telehealth visit.

Sometimes, limited interaction between the healthcare provider and patient can lead to lower trust in the doctor-patient relationship. Reduced patient participation in the care process can also be a concern; sometimes, the patient's perception of the acceptability of the telehealth visit may undermine it. The patient may make redundant or unnecessary appointments if he or she perceives the telehealth visit was inadequate. However, while telehealth enhances access to healthcare for most patients, it may remain less accessible for some segments of the population, such as low-income and marginalized groups with limited access to technology, worsening inequities in access (Mahdavi et al., 2025).

Multiple telehealth platforms exist, but all must meet the necessary privacy and security standards (such as HIPAA in the US), integrate with electronic health records (EHRs) to document the encounter, and be relatively user-friendly for both patients and providers. Internet connectivity can also influence the quality of the visit. Additionally, the whole healthcare team must adapt to a new workflow when telehealth visits are introduced into the schedule.

Despite some drawbacks, the advantages of telehealth clearly outweigh the disadvantages. With its growing popularity as a viable option and its adoption and use by more physicians, telehealth will continue to grow rapidly nationally and globally.

Infrastructure Requirements

The infrastructure needed for a successful implementation of telehealth consulting in family medicine includes technical, legal, and cultural changes and adaptations. The technical and communication technologies included information technology, adequate and efficient technical support, efficient communication networks, and reliable internet technology, especially in rural and remote areas. Legal frameworks must focus on the appropriate instructions and guidelines needed to define the scope of telehealth services and identify the right types of consultations for telehealth. Several studies have emphasized the need for a standardized platform for physician-patient interactions and consultation visits. Further, an efficient triage system is needed to assess which patients are suitable for telehealth appointments and consultations. Also, it is very important to ensure that all relevant patient information and records are updated, documented, and available prior to the virtual visits, and to schedule follow-up appointments for each visit (Mahdavi et al., 2025).

Furthermore, for the successful implementation of telehealth, a patient registration system must be set up with easy access, adequate support for patients to use, and dedicated staff promptly available to help manage any issues. The shift to virtual healthcare requires new workflows and appropriate changes in processes, staff training, and continuing patient education. Both providers and patients must have the necessary communication devices, tools, and technologies for telehealth. Also, for virtual care, patients may often need access to devices beyond a phone, such as a blood glucose meter or sphygmomanometer, especially for patients with specific health conditions. Also, providing appropriate technical support for specific patient groups, such as the elderly and rural populations, and improving patients' digital and health literacy are crucial for effective telemedicine services (Mahdavi et al., 2025).

Key Applications of Artificial Intelligence (AI) in Telehealth

Since the pandemic, telemedicine has become a viable option in healthcare. When integrated with AI, it becomes even more effective through smarter diagnostics, personalized care, and the efficient use of technology and resources. Today, AI is deeply embedded in telemedicine, and physician adoption has increased from 38 percent in 2023 to 66 percent in 2024 (Pratt, 2025). It has been used in a variety of medical applications, including administrative and clinical support, medical imaging analysis, virtual triage, diagnostics, disease management, and patient monitoring.

AI investment in telemedicine is increasingly spiralling upward by about 25 percent annually and is projected to exceed $156 billion by 2033 (Pratt, 2025).

AI is used frequently in contact center assistance. Healthcare assistants using AI can enhance patient contact and engagement by handling scheduling, answering medical-related questions, and reminding patients, especially older ones or those with memory issues, to take their medications regularly and on time. All these routine tasks would reduce the administrative burden on providers and allow them to spend more quality time with their patients. Also, patient engagement may be improved by chatbots that provide information and answer questions, manage scheduling, and handle patient intake before clinical visits. AI-driven chatbots can enhance communication and information flow between patients and providers, ensuring better adherence to treatment guidelines and instructions. Virtual triage and virtual assistants can use AI to determine whether a candidate is appropriate for telemedicine by asking health-related questions about symptoms and analyzing the patient's responses. Using AI, virtual care assistants can answer patients' questions, provide guidance, and schedule appointments with providers. AI can also help break down language barriers by enabling the virtual agent to speak the patient's preferred language, thereby increasing patient interactions and engagement (Pratt, 2025).

Further, by using AI to analyze patients' medical data, clinicians can interpret medical imaging results and make more accurate diagnoses, allowing the physician to determine whether the patient will be best treated at home, in a clinic, or in a hospital setting. Also, with the help of AI, the provider may recommend more effective treatment plans for the patient. By using AI and voice recognition technology, clinicians can summarize notes in the patient's records or for referrals to other providers. AI can be used for administrative tasks such as billing and claims processing, maintaining patient data, handling duplicate records, correcting inaccurate or incomplete information, and other workflow processes. Other AI applications include remote patient monitoring and clinical patient monitoring. AI can retrieve, analyze, and report the patient's readings from blood pressure cuffs, heart monitors, and other devices so that providers – physicians, nurses, and clinical staff can make appropriate decisions. In clinical settings, AI can process patients' health information and present it to nurses as documentation, so they can focus more on direct patient care, which may be perceived as better care because a live human being is looking at them rather than a computer. Also, chronic disease management, assessment, and prediction may be more effectively achieved through AI in patient monitoring, information processing, and provider feedback, supporting relevant healthcare responses and actions (Pratt, 2025).

Artificial Intelligence (AI) – Making Telehealth More Effective

AI is frequently used to address some of telehealth's challenges and drawbacks and enhance its effectiveness. Through machine learning and deep learning, AI facilitates workflow automation, medical image interpretation, predictive analytics for disease progression, management, and control, real-time patient monitoring, and decision support systems. Telemedicine relies heavily on vast amounts of patient health data, and if incomplete, inaccurate, or delayed, it can jeopardize the provider's assessments and treatment of patients. However, with the use of AI, which can analyze vast amounts of data quickly and accurately, physicians' assessments and treatments are rendered more effective. Also, AI applications have been used in telemedicine across various medical specialties. For example, AI-driven computer vision algorithms have been successfully used in dermatology, ophthalmology, and other specialties, achieving high sensitivity and specificity for melanoma and diabetic retinopathy. According to some studies, the performance and results of such uses are comparable to, or in some cases superior to, those of human specialists. Also, AI-powered chatbots and digital assistants have been used to triage patients, provide mental health support, and streamline telehealth consultations, especially in family medicine. While many of these AI applications are still in pilot or early-stage development, some have been validated and are being used successfully. For example, AI-driven triage assistants have accurately and successfully directed patients to the appropriate levels of care (Rossi & Rehman, 2025). Several wearable devices, along with AI, can continuously monitor the patient's vital signs and detect conditions such as cardiovascular and respiratory diseases earlier (Khan et al., 2025). Further, several clinical studies show that devices such as the Apple Watch and Kardia Mobile can detect atrial fibrillation symptoms with high sensitivity and specificity, and that wearable blood pressure monitors can detect hypertension, enabling providers to take timely, relevant action (Rossi & Rehman, 2025).

TELEMEDICINE DURING THE COVID-19 PANDEMIC AND IMPLICATIONS FOR REFORM

The COVID-19 pandemic was a natural experiment in accelerating the adoption of telemedicine. During the early months of the pandemic in the United States, telehealth visits increased by over 4,000% (Koonin et al., 2020). Telehealth use among Medicare patients increased 63-fold in 2020 compared with 2019, from 0.84 million to 52.7 million visits (Saharkhiz & Rao, 2024). Many regulatory barriers were temporarily waived, including expanded Medicare coverage that made non-rural patients eligible, audio-only visits being reimbursed, and relaxed state licensing requirements (CMS, 2020). Additionally, a patient's home was eligible to be an "originating site" for a visit.

The rapid expansion and utilization of telehealth during the pandemic helped foster a better understanding of the clinical applications of telehealth for the general public, such as the following:

Primary Care: Virtual triage, preventive screenings, chronic disease monitoring, and follow-up care can often be delivered through telehealth. Telehealth primary care can be clinically comparable to in-office visits for chronic diseases such as diabetes and hypertension. Virtual patient monitoring can improve outcomes in heart disease, chronic obstructive pulmonary disease, and diabetes by allowing frequent surveillance and early intervention (Inglis et al., 2015). Also, for patients with heart failure-related issues, the use of telemedicine consultations and non-invasive telemonitoring did reduce the overall risk of mortality and hospitalization. Studies showed that these interventions improved patients' health-related quality of life and heart care knowledge, as well as self-care behaviors, such as lifestyle changes toward healthier eating, low sugar intake, better diet control, blood pressure control, and and regular exercise. Further, the studies showed that patients were satisfied with these interventions and that the interventions were associated with the measured outcomes (Inglis et al., 2015).

Mental health: Telepsychiatry can be as effective as in-office care for many conditions, with the added benefits of convenience and reduced stigma (Hubley et al., 2016). It is an innovative approach to delivering mental health services that increases access to evidence-based healthcare. Telepsychiatric services are current uses of mental healthcare for patients, especially those living in rural areas who have difficulty accessing in-person services, including many older patients. Through video-based conferencing and similar modern technologies, telepsychiatry services have experienced accelerated growth and reach for many patients. Its use and popularity have spiraled upward, with many large and small healthcare organizations offering mental health services from the convenience of patients' homes, for patients and for mental health providers alike (Hubley et al., 2016).

Specialized Care: Tele-ICU programs can reduce mortality and length of hospital stay. As of 2018, about 18 percent of ICU beds were covered by tele-ICU programs, which most likely increased during the COVID-19 pandemic (Spies & Ranzani, 2025). Tele-ICU implementations have increased due to spiralling demand for ICU beds, advancing age and more severe health conditions among older patients, shortages of trained intensivists, and the need to rapidly transmit evolving technology and medical information to patients' bedsides (Spies & Ranzani, 2025). Also, telehealth played a prominent role during the COVID pandemic in remote assessment, mass triage, and continuity of care, demonstrating its scalability and widespread benefits during crises (Koonin et al., 2020).

The temporary flexibilities introduced during the COVID public health emergency (PHE), such as relaxed licensure requirements, expanded reimbursement, and broadened originating site eligibility, demonstrated the potential of telehealth. But as the PHE ended, many of these flexibilities are expiring or being revoked (Kwon, Jolin, & Shachar, 2024).

Permanent policy changes are necessary to sustain investments in telehealth infrastructure and long-term integration (Telehealth.HHS.gov, 2026). Some recent proposals related to telehealth include: Medicare patients can receive telehealth services for non-behavioral/mental healthcare in their homes with no geographical restrictions through December 2027. All eligible Medicare providers can provide telehealth services; Federal Qualified Health Centers (FQHCs) and Rural Health Clinics (RHCs) can serve as Medicare distant site (remote healthcare) providers. Similar telehealth services and access are also available for rural and behavioral health patients through December 2027 (Telehealth.HHS.gov, 2026).

PERSONAL EXPERIENCE

As a family medicine physician, this author has utilized telehealth in her practice. Currently, she sees patients virtually for one half-day per week, along with scattered telehealth visits throughout her normal clinic days. She has found that telehealth allows more flexibility and improves her job satisfaction. She has found that her telehealth appointments provide patient-focused healthcare and satisfy the specific job characteristics of skill variety (use of technology, remote work and virtual consultations, personal communication, customized patient-centered service, and others), task identity (completing a full patient visit/consultation remotely), task significance (patients experience a positive consultation visit from the physican in the comfort of his/her private, preferred home setting, and she feels a sense of accomplishment for impacting the patient's health), autonomy (freedom to work from home or from any remote location, as necessary), and feedback (she gets instant response from the patient/s, immediate access to info info that she needs – for example, the patient can locate the medicine bottle in his/her home or other types of info easily rather than checking after going home), which contribute to her own job satisfaction (Hackman & Oldham, 1980; Makiwa, 2025). Her patients often appreciate the option of telehealth visits, as they can maintain their busy schedules while still taking care of their health without traveling to a clinic or waiting for an appointment. For example, patients can meet virtually with this physician while sitting in their parked car in a parking lot while running errands, or from the comfort of their own home to avoid bad weather or the need to find childcare.

Telehealth has been a useful way to follow up on medications, mental health concerns, test results, and even some acute infections. Most of the time, the patient's needs can be fully addressed during the visit. However, at times she does recommend they be seen in person for a full physical exam or if they do not have a way to monitor certain vitals at home (such as blood pressure). Even when an in-person appointment is ultimately recommended, patients tend to be grateful they were able to start with a telehealth visit to receive initial guidance and next steps. Of course, as with any technology, there are times when it does not work perfectly—sometimes the internet connection is slow, or there is user error during connection. However, both the physician and the patient are almost always able to come up with a solution, even if that means switching the visit from a video appointment to a phone call due to connection issues. As a physician, she often weighs the risks against the benefits. When it comes to telehealth, this physician certainly feels that the benefits (the "pros") of telehealth—both for her as the physician and for her patients—outweigh the risks (the "cons") and have significantly improved her medical practice.

FUTURE CONSIDERATIONS

In order to maximize the role of telehealth in healthcare reform, policymakers and healthcare leaders should consider:

- Implementing permanent telehealth legislation: enact laws to remove outdated restrictions surrounding geography and originating site, allow audio-only services, expand provider eligibility, and ensure consistent reimbursement.
- Investing in digital infrastructure: improve internet access, provide devices when needed, offer digital literacy training and support, and ensure underserved and rural populations have equal access.
- Establish standards and guidelines: define which clinical services are appropriate for telehealth, solidify privacy/security frameworks, and integrate telehealth into standard clinical care.
- Monitoring, evaluation, and research: Promote research on cost-effectiveness, patient satisfaction, equity, outcomes, and population-level benefit. Use the data to continuously improve telehealth policy and practice.
- Promoting and facilitating the increasing use of AI in telehealth to help providers optimize the delivery of patient care.

As technology advances, hybrid care models will likely become more common, rather than exclusively virtual or in-person. Hybrid models can integrate virtual/ digital monitoring, telehealth follow-ups, and in-person diagnostics, exams, and procedures. A hybrid care model can help balance patient preferences with clinical appropriateness.

Artificial intelligence can help enhance telehealth through automated triage, predictive analytics, personalized risk monitoring, and virtual assistants for chronic disease management. Many patients already utilize AI on their own to investigate their healthcare conditions, so healthcare systems must learn to work effectively alongside AI. Ethical issues can arise when using AI in healthcare, so closer oversight is needed to ensure patient safety, fairness, and transparency in care.

CONCLUSION

Telehealth is a promising tool for advancing healthcare reform by enhancing equity, improving access, reducing costs, and improving quality, and with the increasing use of AI, enabling providers to offer a more flexible system for delivering care across various specialties, especially in family medicine. The COVID-19 pandemic catalyzed telehealth, accelerating its adoption and revealing its benefits and challenges. Moving forward, policy changes, lasting reimbursement reform, infrastructure investments, and a commitment to equity and privacy can help integrate telehealth into everyday healthcare. Telehealth can help transform healthcare delivery by making care more equitable, accessible, and affordable for all.

REFERENCES

Advanced Medical Reviews (AMR). (2022). Telemedicine: A solution to the predicted physician shortage? Retrieved from Telemedicine: a Solution to the Predicted Physician Shortage? AMA, (2021). *2021 Telehealth Survey Report*. Retrieved from 2021 Telehealth Survey Report | AMA

Bebinger, M. (2025). *Can artificial intelligence help with a primary care provider shortage?* Rerieved from Can artificial intelligence help with a primary care provider shortage?: NPR

Board on Health Care Services, & the Board Institute of Medicine. (2012). *The Role of Telehealth in an Evolving Health Care Environment: Workshop Summary*. Washington (DC): National Academies Press (US). Available from: https://www.ncbi.nlm.nih.gov/books/NBK207146)

CMS. (2020). *CMS announces comprehensive strategy to enhance hospital capacity amid COVID-19 surge*. Retrieved from CMS Announces Comprehensive Strategy to Enhance Hospital Capacity Amid COVID-19 Surge | CMS

Fortin, E., Baca-Motes, K., Steinhubl, S., & Topol, E. (2019). Characteristics of the modern-day physician house call. [Baltimore]. *Medicine*, *98*(8), 14671. DOI: 10.1097/MD.0000000000014671 PMID: 30813215

Hackman, R., & Oldham, G. (1980). Job Characteristics Model in *Work Redesign*. Retrieved from Work Redesign - J. Richard Hackman, Greg R. Oldham - Google Books

Harvard Health Publishing. (2025). *Telehealth: The advantages and disadvantages*. Retrieved from Telehealth: The advantages and disadvantages - Harvard Health

HHS.gov. (2025). *Telehealth research recap: Quality of care*. Retrieved from Telehealth.HHS.gov: Learn how to access or provide telehealth care

Hubley, S., Lynch, S., Schneck, C., Thomas, M., & Shore. (2016). *Review of key telepsychiatry outcomes*. Retrieved from Review of key telepsychiatry outcomes - PMC

Inglis, S. (2015). *Structured telephone support or non-invasive telemonitoring for patients with heart failure*. Retrieved from Structured telephone support or non-invasive telemonitoring for patients with heart failure - PMC

Ivanova, J. (2025). *Digital equity in Telehealth: Ensuring access for all*. Retrieved from Digital Equity in Telehealth: Ensuring Access for All | Telehealth.org

Jagarapu, J., & Savani, R. (2021). *A brief history of telemedicine and the evolution of teleneonatology*. Retrieved from A brief history of telemedicine and the evolution of teleneonatology - ScienceDirect

Kao, H., Conant, R., Soriano, T., & McCormick, W. (2009). The past, present, and future of house calls. *Clinics in Geriatric Medicine*, *25*(1), 19–34. DOI: 10.1016/j.cger.2008.10.005 PMID: 19217490

Kao, H., Conant, R., Soriano, T., & McCormick, W. (2009). The past, present, and future of house calls. *Clinics in Geriatric Medicine*, *25*(1), 19–34. DOI: 10.1016/j.cger.2008.10.005 PMID: 19217490

Khan, B., Talha, K., & Ul, W.. (2025). Reshaping the healthcare world by AI-integrated wearable sensors following COVID-19. [Retrieved from Google Scholar]. *Chemical Engineering Journal*, *505*, 159478. DOI: 10.1016/j.cej.2025.159478

Kim, T., & Zuckerman, J. (2019). Realizing the potential of telemedicine in global health. Retrieved from Realizing the potential of telemedicine in global health - PMC

Koonin L., Hoots, B., Tsang C., Leroy Z., Farris K., Jolly B., Antall, P., McCabe B., Zelis, C., Tong, I., Harris, A. (2020). *Trends in telehealth use during the emergence of the COVID-19 pandemic*. Retrieved from Trends in the Use of Telehealth D... preview & related info | Mendeley

Kwon, M., Jolin, J., & Shachar, C. (2024). Telehealth after the Federal COVID-19 Public Health Emergency: Implications and Future Directions. *The Journal of Law, Medicine & Ethics*, *52*(2), 412–418. DOI: 10.1017/jme.2024.118 PMID: 39435920

Mahdavi, S., Fekri, M., Mohammadi-Sarab, S., Mehmandoost, M., & Zarei, E. (2025). *The use of telemedicine in family medicine: A scoping review*. Retrieved from The use of telemedicine in family medicine: A scoping review | BMC Health Services Research | Springer Nature Link

Makiwa, T. (2025). *The job characteristics model: everything you need to know*. Retrieved from The job characteristic model: everything you need to know | The Human Capital Hub

Peters, Z., Lendon, J., Caffrey, C., Myrick, K., Mahar, M., & DeFrances, C. (2024, September). Telemedicine use during the COVID-19 pandemic by office-based physicians and long-term care providers. *Retrieved from CDC National Health Statistics Reports*, (210), 18. PMID: 39471289

Pratt, M. (2025). *How AI is changing telemedicine in 2025*. Retrieved from How AI is Changing Telemedicine in 2025 | Informa TechTarget

Rossi, M., & Rehman, S. (2025). *Integrating Artificial Intelligence into telemedicine: Evidence, challenges, and future directions*. Retrieved from Integrating Artificial Intelligence Into Telemedicine: Evidence, Challenges, and Future Directions - PMC

Saharkhiz, M., Rao, T., Parker-Lue, S., Borelli, S., Johnson, K., & Cataife, G. (2024). Telehealth expansion and Medicare beneficiaries' care quality and access. *JAMA Network Open*, 7(5), e2411006. DOI: 10.1001/jamanetworkopen.2024.11006 PMID: 38739388

Spies, C., & Ranzani, O. (2025). *Telemedicine in critical care*. Telemedicine in critical care | Intensive Care Medicine | Springer Nature Link

Stevens, R. (1998). *American Medicine and the Public Interest*. University of California Press.

Telehealth.HHS.gov. (2025). *Learn how to access or provide telehealth care*. Retrieved from Telehealth.HHS.gov: Learn how to access or provide telehealth care

Telehealth.HHS.gov. (2026). *Telehealth policy updates*. Retrieved from Telehealth policy updates | Telehealth.HHS.gov

US House Committee on Ways & Means. (2025, November 13). *Republicans Deliver Lower Health Costs, More Choice, and Greater Control for Working Families*. Retrieved from Republicans Deliver Lower Health Costs, More Choice, and Greater Control for Working Families - Ways and Means

Whereby. (2025). *5 predictions for the future of telehealth*. Retrieved from https://whereby.com/blog/5-predictions-for-the-future-of-telehealth/

Zucker, H. (2025). Where have all the physicians gone? AARP.org/Bulletin. Retrieved from America Is Facing a Shortage of Doctors

ADDITIONAL READING

AAMC (2024). *New AAMC Report Shows Continuing Projected Physician Shortage* New AAMC Report Shows Continuing Projected Physician Shortage | AAMC

Jones, C., & Dolsten, M. (2024). *Healthcare on the brink: navigating the challenges of an aging society in the United States*. Healthcare on the brink: navigating the challenges of an aging society in the United States - PMC

KEY TERMS AND DEFINITIONS

Cost reduction: strategies to cut healthcare costs, currently at exorbitant levels.

Employer-sponsored healthcare plans: Healthcare insurance plans sponsored/offered by employers, which are currently the most popular type of coverage for the majority of the US population.

Healthcare reform: changes made to improve healthcare for all stakeholders, especially in terms of lowering costs and enhancing access to quality healthcare.

Optimal healthcare: Maximum patient care (the highest possible state of physical, mental, and social well-being) that is achievable and provided at a relatively feasible cost. Personalized, holistic, and proactive strategies that balance proven medical practices with lifestyle choices.

Optimizing patient experience and outcomes: Maximum patient care (the highest possible state of physical, mental, and social well-being) that is achievable and provided in terms of meeting outcomes such as patient experiences, quality of patient care, lower cost, and provider satisfaction.

Telehealth (often interchangeable with telemedicine): virtual consultations, remote patient monitoring (RPM), and the delivery of healthcare services via technology (live video conferencing, phone messaging, remote monitoring devices), among other digital health technologies.

Chapter 4
Clinical Informatics and Artificial Intelligence in Healthcare

Jason Greenwood
http://orcid.org/0000-0002-9397-0107
Mayo Clinic, USA

Ray Qian
http://orcid.org/0000-0001-9671-4945
Mayo Clinic, USA

ABSTRACT

This chapter provides a high-level overview of clinical informatics (CI) and artificial intelligence (AI) in healthcare. It covers foundational concepts such as electronic health records (EHRs) and data standards, current applications including Clinical Decision Support Systems (CDSS) and ambient scribing/documentation, and near-term directions for both clinicians and patients. The chapter also introduces how foundational CI systems and healthcare data are leveraged to develop AI solutions, ranging from traditional machine learning to large language models, while addressing key issues such as bias, generalizability, and regulatory considerations. Finally, the chapter examines a potential future in which decentralized AI models augment clinicians in their daily work, generate deeper clinical insights, and transform patient care through advanced predictive models and digital twins.

DOI: 10.4018/979-8-3373-2577-4.ch004

INTRODUCTION

This chapter provides a practical overview of clinical informatics (CI) and artificial intelligence (AI) in healthcare, spanning foundational concepts, current applications, and near-term directions relevant to both clinicians and patients.

In the Clinical Informatics section, we examine the core systems that support modern healthcare delivery, including electronic health records, data standards, and clinical workflows. We highlight opportunities to enhance patient care, streamline processes, and improve outcomes, while also addressing persistent challenges such as system complexity, resistance to change, and unintended consequences of digital tools. Clinical Decision Support Systems (CDSS) illustrate these tradeoffs well: they continuously analyze data from laboratories, imaging, pathology, and medication orders to promote safe and evidence-based care. CDSS can prevent unsafe prescribing, flag abnormal results, and reduce diagnostic errors. However, poorly designed systems can also generate excessive alerts, increase cognitive load, introduce automation bias, and disrupt clinical workflows.

The AI section traces the emergence of AI in healthcare and explores its transformative potential, including personalized medicine and large-scale data analysis, alongside critical limitations such as accuracy, bias, and hallucinations. Generative AI has become a central focus, reshaping clinical documentation, information retrieval, and decision-making. While these tools can reduce administrative burden and improve efficiency, they also raise concerns about reliability, workforce disruption, and ethical use.

We then examine key CI and AI tools that are actively reshaping clinical practices such as sepsis alerts, ambient documentation, and automated prior-authorization and appeal systems—along with the practical challenges of implementation, including cost, privacy, interoperability, and scalability.

The chapter also addresses the evolving regulatory and ethical landscape. Shifts in federal policy, FDA oversight, and legislation will significantly influence how AI-enabled software is developed and deployed. Software as a Medical Device (SaMD) represents a critical regulatory frontier where changes in oversight could accelerate innovation while also increasing safety and accountability risks. Recent legislative debates over AI deregulation highlight the volatility of this environment and the uncertainty facing healthcare organizations and technology developers.

Finally, we explore emerging paradigms such as AI-augmented clinicians, digital twins, and continuously learning health systems. Rather than abstract speculation, these concepts point toward concrete possibilities: computational patient models that simulate treatment responses, decision-support systems that adapt to real-world outcomes, and hybrid human–AI workflows that enhance clinical judgment.

FOUNDATIONS OF CLINICAL INFORMATICS

Core Concepts and Scope

Clinical Informatics is the branch of applied science leveraging data and information systems and technologies to improve health outcomes, patient care delivery, and clinical decision-making. The field sits at the intersection of medical, computer, data, organizational and cognitive sciences. Clinical Informaticists translate clinical needs into digital solutions, design and optimize workflows, establish data and interoperability standards, and evaluate new technologies to ensure they enhance rather than hinder patient care. The goal of this chapter is not to cover everything in this fast-changing field, but to give a broad overview of the key topics and help you understand how clinical informatics impacts everyday medical practice.

Health Information Systems

Health information technology systems have existed for more than fifty years, and their evolution has fundamentally reshaped clinical practice. This transformation began with the introduction of the patient centered medical record, developed by Henry Plummer at the Mayo Clinic in 1907, and has progressed to an era in which most aspects of patient care are managed electronically. (Gillum, 2013) What was once limited to a small number of academic institutions with the resources to design and maintain custom systems has expanded broadly, with most healthcare organizations now relying on multiple integrated platforms. Core examples include electronic health records, laboratory information systems for managing laboratory testing, and picture archiving and communication systems for storing and accessing medical imaging.

EHRs first emerged in the 1970s within academic medical institutions, where early implementations focused primarily on administrative needs such as billing and scheduling. During this period, paper charts remained the dominant medium for clinical documentation. Early EHRs required large mainframe computers, offered limited storage capacity, and carried prohibitive costs, restricting adoption to a small number of well-resourced organizations. Over subsequent decades, improvements in computing power, storage, and software design enabled broader adoption and expanded functionality. EHRs evolved from administrative tools into comprehensive clinical repositories that store notes, orders, diagnostic results, treatments, and longitudinal patient histories. (Evans, 2016)

Modern EHRs now function as the central digital infrastructure of healthcare delivery. Beyond documentation, they support computerized provider order entry, medication management, clinical decision support, care coordination, population health analytics, and patient engagement through portals and mobile applications. They also enable continuity of care across inpatient, outpatient, emergency, and post-acute settings. At the same time, expanding EHR scope and complexity have introduced challenges, including documentation burden, usability limitations, alert fatigue, and workflow fragmentation. Differences in vendor architectures and data models have further contributed to interoperability barriers and data silos, limiting seamless data exchange and secondary use of clinical information.

As EHR capabilities expanded beyond core administrative and documentation functions, specialized systems were developed to support the distinct workflows of individual clinical domains. Laboratory information systems (LIS) facilitate specimen tracking, quality control, and results reporting. Radiology information systems (RIS) and picture archiving and communication systems support imaging workflow management and long-term image storage and retrieval. Pharmacy information systems address medication ordering, dispensing, and monitoring across inpatient and outpatient settings. Each of these platforms provides end to end support within its domain, from order entry through verification and durable storage. Because no single system can manage all aspects of care delivery, effective healthcare operations depend on integration across these platforms through standardized interfaces and shared data exchange methods, which enable information to move reliably across the broader health information technology ecosystem. (Seymour, 2012)

Data Standards and Interoperability

As each interface may require a unique method to pass information, multiple data standards were created to facilitate communication between systems. The most prominent of these is the Health Level Seven (HL7) standard. (Cruz et al., 2018) HL7 provides an openly available way for these various systems to communicate and pass information from system to system – e.g., LIS results to the EHR. As the industry advanced and internet-based applications became more integrated with EHRs, a more versatile way for applications to communicate was needed. (Sepulveda & Young, 2013) Fast Healthcare Interoperability Resources (FHIR) was developed to meet this need, a modern standard that uses web-based APIs to enable discrete, resource-level data exchange across diverse platforms. (Mandel, 2016)

Together, these standards support interoperability—the ability of different health information systems, electronic health records, and applications to securely exchange, interpret, and use clinical data in a meaningful way across organizations and care settings. Interoperability is not simply the transmission of information but the preservation of clinical meaning so that data generated in one system can be accurately interpreted and acted upon in another system without manual translation or re-entry. For example, when a patient presents to an emergency department at an outside hospital, interoperable systems can allow prior diagnoses, medication lists, allergies, laboratory results, and imaging studies to be retrieved and integrated directly into the local EHR, reducing redundant testing, preventing medication errors, and enabling more timely clinical decision-making.

Beyond transport standards, consistent terminology was required so that systems interpreted data in the same way. For example, to ensure that "CBC" and "complete blood count" are recognized as the same test, controlled vocabularies and coding systems were created. Systematized Nomenclature of Medicine Clinical Terms (SNOMED CT) provides a comprehensive ontology for clinical concepts, linking related diagnoses and findings under standardized codes. The Logical Observation Identifiers Names and Codes (LOINC) system assigns unique codes to laboratory and clinical observations, such as LOINC 58410-2 for a complete blood count panel. (Bodenreider et al., 2018)

Together, these standards enable reliable interoperability by ensuring that information can be exchanged consistently and accurately between systems, supporting both routine clinical care and advanced applications such as analytics and AI.

US Legislation promoting EHR use and Health IT

In the United States, the adoption of EHRs and HIT was accelerated in the 2010s by federal legislation and policies, notably the Health Information Technology for Economic and Clinical Health (HITECH) Act, which was part of the 2009 American Recovery and Reinvestment Act (ARRA). (Burde, 2011) HITECH provided financial incentives for hospitals and providers to adopt certified EHR technology and demonstrate "meaningful use" of electronic records to improve quality, safety, and efficiency, as well as penalties for those who failed to comply with these requirements. This carrot-and-stick approach drove EHR adoption among U.S. hospitals, rising from about 9% using basic EHRs in 2008 to over 96% by 2015. Office-based physician adoption increased from ~17% in 2008 to over 79% within a decade, making electronic records the national standard of care. (Adler-Milstein & Jha, 2017)

Other notable federal legislation included the Affordable Care Act (ACA) of 2010, which promoted value-based care through quality reporting, accountable care organizations, and population health management, thereby increasing healthcare systems' reliance on robust informatics infrastructure. (Protection, 2010; Kocher et al., 2010) This was followed by the 21st Century Cures Act of 2016, which not only strengthened requirements for interoperability but also prohibited information blocking, defined as practices by healthcare organizations, vendors, or other entities that unreasonably restrict the access, exchange, or use of electronic health information. (Rodriguez, 2020 and Gabay, 2017) The Act also expanded patients' rights to access and control their health data and encouraged the adoption of modern standards such as FHIR, LOINC, and SNOMED, among others, to enable more seamless data exchange across health systems and applications.

Additionally, the Health Insurance Portability and Accountability Act (HIPAA) of 1996, which was initially enacted to improve health insurance coverage portability and reduce fraud and abuse, established the foundational privacy and security standards for protecting patient health information in a digital environment. (Annas, 2003)

OVERVIEW OF AI IN HEALTHCARE

Types of AI: Machine Learning, NLP, Expert Systems, Deep Learning

Artificial intelligence (AI) is a broad field that traces its origins to the mid-twentieth century. Early pioneers such as Alan Turing, Marvin Minsky, and John McCarthy established many of the theoretical foundations that continue to shape AI research today. Early AI was rooted primarily in computer science and mathematics and relied heavily on custom programming by domain experts. These systems, known as "expert systems," used knowledge-based, rule-driven logic to approximate human reasoning within narrowly defined domains. (Hirani et al., 2024; Brock, 2018; Tan, 2017)

In medicine, expert systems depended on handcrafted rules derived from clinical knowledge, such as "if a patient has fever and neutropenia, then consider empiric antibiotics." Although these systems were interpretable and aligned with clinical reasoning, they were limited in their ability to adapt to new data, scale across diverse clinical contexts, or account for complex patient variability. Moreover, they were technically complex and costly to develop and maintain, which restricted their deployment largely to major academic centers such as Stanford, Dartmouth, the University of Pittsburgh, and MIT.

The evolution of AI has been characterized by alternating periods of rapid progress and stagnation, often referred to as "AI summers" and "AI winters," driven by cycles of heightened expectations, funding constraints, and technical limitations. Despite this uneven trajectory, AI has diversified into multiple subfields, including natural language processing (NLP), machine learning (ML), deep learning (DL), and, more recently, large language models (LLMs). (Jiang, 2017; Haenlein & Kaplan 2019)

NLP focuses not merely on identifying words in large volumes of text but on understanding contextual meaning. It integrates concepts from linguistics, computer science, and statistics to analyze syntax (sentence structure), semantics (meaning in context), and pragmatics (how meaning shifts with intent and use). (Meurers 2012) Early NLP approaches relied on rule-based grammars and curated dictionaries, which proved brittle and poorly suited to the variability of clinical language. Subsequent statistical methods improved flexibility by modeling probabilistic relationships between words, and later representation-learning approaches enabled algorithms to infer meaning directly from large corpora of text. These advances allow modern NLP systems to capture clinical nuance—for example, distinguishing "no history of diabetes" from "family history of diabetes"—and to transform unstructured clinical narratives into structured, machine-interpretable data. (Jones, 1994)

In parallel, machine learning approaches emerged that differed fundamentally from expert systems. Rather than relying on explicitly coded rules, ML models learn patterns directly from data through parameter optimization and hyperparameter tuning. Early models such as linear regression, logistic regression, and random forests offered relatively transparent predictions that could be interpreted through coefficients or feature importance metrics. Over time, ML expanded to neural network architectures inspired by biological neurons, in which information flows through multiple layers of interconnected nodes. Advances in computational power and data availability in the 2010s enabled multi-layer neural networks to achieve state-of-the-art performance in domains such as medical imaging, pathology, and physiologic signal analysis. However, these gains in accuracy often came at the expense of interpretability, as model decision-making became increasingly opaque. (Kononenko, 2001; Fradkov, 2020; Mehta Devarakonda, 2018)

Building on advances in deep learning and NLP, transformer-based architectures gave rise to large language models, capable of processing and generating text, images, audio, and other modalities with minimal explicit programming. LLMs enable conversational interfaces and adaptive responses to complex queries, representing a fundamental shift in how clinicians and patients interact with digital systems. At the same time, their reliance on vast and heterogeneous training data introduces risks of inaccuracy, bias, and hallucination, underscoring the need for careful governance, validation, and human oversight when applying AI in clinical medicine. (Wang & Beecy, 2025; Zhou et al., 2025)

AI Development Lifecycle in Medicine

To mitigate risk and ensure safe and effective use, medical AI should follow a disciplined lifecycle consisting of preparation, development, validation, deployment, and maintenance. (Brereton et al., 2024) Unlike consumer AI, medical AI operates in high-stakes environments where errors can directly affect patient outcomes, making structured oversight essential throughout the lifecycle.

During preparation, the clinical problem is clearly defined, relevant stakeholders are identified, and appropriate datasets are acquired. Data are cleaned, standardized, and assessed for quality, representativeness, and potential sources of bias. This stage also includes defining clinical endpoints, success metrics, and intended use cases, which are critical for downstream evaluation and alignment with clinical and regulatory expectations. (Haakman et al., 2021; Nazer et al., 2023; Mittermaier et al., 2023)

The development phase involves designing and training candidate models using multiple methodological approaches. Models are iteratively refined and compared based on predictive performance, fairness, interpretability, and operational feasibility. Tradeoffs between accuracy, transparency, and clinical usability are explicitly evaluated, recognizing that the most technically performant model may not be the most clinically appropriate. (Ehsan et al., 2021)

Once a candidate model is selected, validation begins. This includes retrospective testing, silent or shadow-mode evaluation in real-world clinical environments, and prospective pilots or trials when appropriate. Validation focuses not only on statistical performance but also on clinical impact, safety, workflow integration, and unintended consequences.

Successful models then move to deployment, where technical integration into clinical systems is accompanied by workflow redesign, clinician education, and change management. Deployment in healthcare is not merely a technical implementation but a sociotechnical process requiring alignment between technology, clinical practice, and organizational culture.

After deployment, models enter the maintenance phase, during which they are continuously monitored for performance degradation, data drift, population shifts, and changes in clinical practice or guidelines. Governance structures should define thresholds for intervention, retraining, or decommissioning. Every clinical AI system should have a predefined retirement and replacement plan, including communication mechanisms to notify users when a model is modified, withdrawn, or superseded. (Brereton et al., 2024)

Training Data: Sources, Biases, and Labeling

The earliest stage of the AI lifecycle, where data are selected and prepared, deserves particular attention. Data are the foundation of all medical AI systems. When data are incomplete, biased, or poorly curated, the resulting models will inherit and often amplify these flaws. The principle is simple but unforgiving: poor quality data produce poor quality models.

Careful selection of data sources is critical. The data must align with the intended clinical use case. For example, training natural language processing models for healthcare applications should rely on clinical documentation, structured medical records, and validated biomedical corpora rather than general purpose sources such as social media, Reddit, or YouTube, which lack clinical accuracy and contextual rigor. (Sambasivan, 2021)

Bias is an inherent risk in medical datasets because healthcare data reflect real world inequities in access, diagnosis, and treatment. To mitigate bias, datasets should be as diverse and representative as possible, ideally incorporating data from multiple institutions, geographic regions, and patient populations. Efforts should be made to balance representation across relevant variables such as race, ethnicity, sex, age, and socioeconomic status. During preprocessing, additional techniques such as re-weighing, stratified sampling, suppression of spurious correlations, and imputation of missing data can be applied to reduce systematic distortions in the data.

Beyond source selection and bias mitigation, the quality of labeling is equally important. Labels derived from clinical data may reflect documentation practices, billing incentives, or institutional conventions rather than true clinical states. Errors, ambiguity, and inter-observer variability among clinicians can further degrade label reliability. As a result, robust labeling strategies such as clinician adjudication, consensus labeling, and validation against external standards are essential to ensure that models learn clinically meaningful patterns rather than artifacts of the data. (Liang et al., 2022)

Explainability and Trust in Medical AI

Transparency and explainability in artificial intelligence are essential not only for understanding how AI systems function but also for usability, safety, and regulatory oversight. As AI becomes more integrated into clinical care, both clinicians and patients increasingly ask why a model produced a particular recommendation or prediction. Without clear explanations, even highly accurate models may fail to gain acceptance or be safely adopted in practice.

Explainable AI refers to approaches that make a model's design, behavior, and outputs understandable to humans. While the degree of explainability varies by method and use case, the overarching goal is to ensure that AI systems are interpretable enough to support clinical reasoning and informed decision making. This does not require that every technical detail be accessible to all users, but rather that the logic and implications of model outputs are transparent at an appropriate level for clinical and patient use. (Arrieta et al., 2020)

Several strategies can enhance explainability. One approach is to select simpler or more interpretable models when clinically appropriate, as their decision logic is easier to trace and communicate. Another approach is to design systems that link outputs to relevant source data, such as highlighting clinical features, laboratory values, or documentation that influenced the model's prediction. Models can also provide structured explanations, such as ranking input variables by their relative contribution to an output or presenting confidence estimates that contextualize predictions.

These approaches help align AI outputs with clinical intuition, reduce uncertainty, and support accountability. By making AI systems more transparent and interpretable, healthcare organizations can strengthen clinician trust, facilitate regulatory compliance, and promote responsible integration of AI into clinical practice. (Xu et al., 2019; Minh et al., 2022)

KEY APPLICATIONS OF CLINICAL INFORMATICS AND AI IN CLINICAL PRACTICE

Clinical Decision Support Systems

Clinical Decision Support Systems (CDSS) are computerized tools that provide clinicians with knowledge, patient-specific information, or recommendations to enhance decision-making in healthcare. Their purpose is to improve quality, safety, efficiency, and outcomes by ensuring that evidence-based guidance is available at the point of care. Traditional CDSS were primarily rule-based, relying on deterministic "if-then" logic derived from clinical guidelines, expert consensus, and institutional protocols. These systems remain foundational in areas such as medication safety, where they generate alerts for drug–drug interactions, allergies, contraindications, and dosing errors. They also support order sets and reminders to standardize care processes, such as recommending guideline-concordant antibiotics in pneumonia or ensuring venous thromboembolism prophylaxis in hospitalized patients.

The transparency of these systems, in which the reasoning behind alerts is explicit, fosters trust and facilitates governance. However, their limitations are well recognized: rule-based systems often lack the flexibility to account for complex or atypical patient contexts, and excessive alerting from poorly tuned thresholds can contribute to alert fatigue, thereby reducing clinical effectiveness. To address these challenges, effective CDSS must adhere to the guiding principle known as the "Five Rights": delivering the right information, to the right person, in the right format, through the right channel, and at the right time within the clinical workflow. (Osheroff et al., 2012)

Recent advances in AI and machine learning have enabled the development of CDSS that move beyond static rules to predictive and adaptive models. These AI-enhanced systems integrate high-dimensional data from electronic health records, laboratory results, physiologic monitors, and imaging studies to provide real-time insights. For example, sepsis detection algorithms can identify subtle patterns of physiologic deterioration, generating alerts hours before overt clinical signs emerge.

Diagnostic support applications, leveraging natural language processing and pattern recognition, can suggest differential diagnoses or highlight potentially overlooked imaging findings. Medication management has similarly advanced through models that personalize dosing recommendations by incorporating renal function, pharmacogenomics (study of how genes influence medication response), and longitudinal treatment responses.

While these tools promise improved sensitivity and individualized care, they also raise challenges, including concerns about algorithmic transparency and bias within training data. Ensuring that both rule-based and AI-driven systems adhere to the Five Rights is crucial for clinical adoption, as it maximizes relevance, minimizes clinician burden, and strengthens trust. The future of CDSS is therefore likely to involve hybrid approaches that combine the interpretability and reliability of rule-based systems with the predictive capacity of AI, ensuring that decision support remains clinically effective and aligned with the practical realities of patient care. (Wasylewicz et al., 2018; Shortliffe & Sepúlveda, 2018)

Structured Documentation and Note Templates

Clinical documentation has evolved substantially over the past century, from early patient centered records to the modern electronic health record. While widespread EHR adoption has enabled comprehensive data capture, interoperability, and secondary data use, it has also contributed to a significant increase in documentation burden. Regulatory requirements, billing frameworks, quality reporting obligations, and medicolegal considerations have expanded the volume and granularity of required documentation. As a result, clinicians can no longer document even straightforward encounters, such as acute otitis media, using brief narrative notes. Many required documentation elements are repetitive and contribute limited incremental clinical value.

To address these challenges, healthcare systems have implemented structured documentation tools, including standardized note templates and macros. These tools allow predefined sections of clinical notes to be populated automatically, improving consistency while reducing manual data entry. For example, a single macro may generate most required documentation elements for a normal well child examination. In more variable clinical scenarios, such as acute sinusitis, structured templates can adapt dynamically. As clinicians enter symptom details or examination findings, additional context specific fields are presented, enabling more complete and standardized documentation without requiring free text entry.

Artificial intelligence has increasingly augmented structured documentation workflows. Ambient documentation systems capture clinician patient conversations and generate draft clinical notes, while natural language processing techniques extract clinical concepts from narrative text and convert them into structured data elements. These approaches enhance the usability of documentation for clinical care, quality reporting, and downstream analytics, while supporting more consistent data capture for future AI applications.

Despite these advances, structured documentation tools must be carefully designed to avoid shifting administrative burden or constraining clinical reasoning. Poorly implemented templates can promote note bloat, reduce narrative clarity, or encourage documentation practices driven more by billing requirements than clinical relevance. Effective documentation systems therefore require continuous evaluation to balance regulatory compliance, clinical usability, and data quality. (Sloss et al., 2024)

Workflow Optimization and Automation

Increasing clinical complexity and rising patient volumes have exposed inefficiencies across many healthcare workflows, contributing substantially to clinician burden and operational strain. In addition to direct patient care, clinicians spend considerable time coordinating follow up appointments, ordering and tracking diagnostic testing, managing inbox messages, and completing non-visit related tasks. While these activities are essential for safe and effective care delivery, they are often poorly aligned with visit-based scheduling models and available clinician capacity. (Faridimehr et al., 2021; Budd, 2023; Gardner et al., 2019)

Workflow optimization within clinical informatics focuses on redesigning care processes to reduce unnecessary manual effort and to better distribute work across care teams and systems. One foundational strategy is task standardization, in which recurring activities such as chronic disease monitoring, preventive care outreach, and routine follow up testing are converted into repeatable workflows. These workflows can be supported by multidisciplinary care teams or automated systems rather than relying exclusively on individual clinicians.

Automation enhances these workflows by enabling systems to initiate actions based on structured data inputs. Examples include automated ordering of routine surveillance tests, delivery of reminder messages to patients, routing of results to appropriate care team members, and escalation of abnormal findings for clinical review. In ambulatory settings, automation supports self-scheduling and asynchronous care pathways, allowing patients to complete intake questionnaires, schedule visits, or receive protocol driven care without requiring synchronous clinician involvement. In inpatient environments, automated workflows assist with care coordination, discharge planning, and structured risk evaluation for common conditions such as skin integrity issues and malnutrition. (Keeley et al., 2015; Zayas-Cabán et al., 2023; Judson et al., 2020; Sánchez-Salmerón et al., 2022)

When thoughtfully implemented, workflow optimization and automation can improve efficiency, reduce delays in care, and allow clinicians to focus on complex decision making and patient engagement. However, poorly designed automation can introduce new inefficiencies, obscure accountability, or increase notification burden. Successful implementation therefore requires close collaboration among clinical informaticists, frontline clinicians, and operational leaders to ensure that workflows remain transparent, clinically appropriate, and adaptable to real world variability.

Natural Language Processing in Clinical Practice

Natural language processing plays an increasingly important role in clinical informatics by enabling documentation assistance, clinical summarization, and information extraction from free text notes. A substantial proportion of clinician time is devoted to activities such as chart review, billing, manual documentation, and management of non-visit care through inbox messaging. Estimates suggest that each of these activities may consume fifteen to thirty percent of a clinician's workday, contributing significantly to cognitive burden and burnout. (Murad et al., 2024; Tierney et al., 2024)

NLP based tools aim to reduce this burden by identifying and surfacing clinically relevant information embedded within narrative documentation. One common application is the detection of items requiring follow up, such as incidental findings documented in radiology or pathology reports. By automatically identifying these findings, NLP systems can reduce missed follow up and improve longitudinal care coordination. In addition, NLP facilitates extraction of key clinical features that support downstream use by quality improvement teams, population health programs, and billing operations. These capabilities enable more accurate quality metric reporting and diagnosis coding, which are increasingly tied to reimbursement and performance-based compensation models.

However, the use of NLP in these contexts can also introduce unintended consequences. Billing and regulatory requirements from the Centers for Medicare and Medicaid Services often mandate annual documentation of chronic conditions to maintain risk adjustment and compensation eligibility. As a result, NLP driven identification of conditions may increase documentation demands during visits that were otherwise intended to address simple acute concerns. This dynamic can convert brief encounters into more complex visits that are not always reflected in visit timing or scheduling templates. (Sloss et al., 2022; Kim et al., 2023)

Several NLP enabled tools have been developed to directly reduce documentation burden. AI based summarization systems can generate concise overviews of a patient's history, prior treatments, and planned next steps when an issue or incidental finding is identified. These summaries allow healthcare team members to quickly understand clinical context without navigating multiple sections of the chart. However, such tools are not uniformly accurate and may generate incorrect or fabricated content, making clinician validation essential. (Bednarczyk et al., 2025)

Ambient documentation systems, commonly referred to as AI scribes, represent another major application of NLP. These tools capture clinician patient conversations and generate draft clinical notes, allowing clinicians to focus more attention on patient interaction while addressing required documentation elements. Evidence regarding their impact on total documentation time is mixed, as some studies report continued time investment due to the need for review and editing. (Duggan et al., 2025)

As NLP systems mature with the popularization of LLM-based tools and become more tightly integrated with workflow automation and decision support tools, additional burden reduction may be achieved. For example, incidental findings may be automatically summarized, tracked, and routed through standardized workflows, requiring only final clinician review rather than repeated manual intervention. Realizing this potential will depend on continued improvements in model accuracy, robust governance frameworks, and careful alignment with clinical workflows and regulatory requirements.

Population Health Management and Risk Stratification

With the near universal adoption of electronic health records and the digitization of most health information, large scale population health and risk analysis has been fundamentally transformed. Labor intensive processes that once required manual review of hundreds of paper records to identify patients in need of follow up or to detect seasonal infection trends have been replaced by the ability to efficiently extract and analyze complex datasets across entire healthcare systems. Modern clinical informatics implementations enable healthcare organizations to readily identify patient cohorts, such as individuals with poorly controlled diabetes based on hemoglobin A1c values, or to monitor trends in conditions such as sexually transmitted infections and upper respiratory infections. These capabilities support both large scale population level analysis and targeted community-based interventions, allowing healthcare systems to deliver appropriate care-at-scale. To operationalize these insights, data driven dashboards and worklists are commonly used to support care teams in tracking at-risk patients and initiating timely follow up. When appropriate, these tools can trigger automated orders, therapies, or diagnostic testing based on predefined clinical criteria. (Chishtie et al., 2023; Adeniyi et al., 2024)

Integration of artificial intelligence into population health infrastructure has further enhanced these efforts. Predictive models that leverage machine learning architectures can identify patients at elevated risk for emergency department utilization or hospital admission by analyzing longitudinal clinical data and comorbidity patterns. These insights enable clinical teams to intervene earlier, allocate resources more effectively, and potentially prevent avoidable adverse health events. (Olawade et al., 2023)

CLINICAL INFORMATICS AS A FOUNDATION FOR AI INTEGRATION

Role of Structured Data Capture and Data Quality

As our healthcare systems move more towards automation and AI, the establishment of CI based foundations and well-structured workflows becomes paramount. The process starts with forming multidisciplinary teams to address considerations such as data quality and establishing a data governance initiative. Key items to consider are data origin, adoptions of standardized values, and secure replicated centralized storage. Subsequently, it is important to ensure the data is well documented, shared appropriately, and constantly monitored and audited. This focus on data quality will ensure appropriate function of all services within HIT. (Budach et al., 2022)

Real-Time Clinical Decision Support Powered by AI

As an illustration, consider blood pressure (BP) data capture. It is important to record the machine used and values measured, storing them either in a standard location in the EHR or in a central data storage. When data has been acquired all systems can pull or push the data into several different systems such as real-time rule based or AI CDSS. In this example, there could be an AI model that leverages BP data along with other features to predict risk of stroke. The integration of AI-based CDSS into the EHR can be accomplished in many different ways: direct integration into the EHR logic (some support this and others do not), using a specialized application program interface (API) allowing an external AI model to store its decision in the EHR, or possibly having the external AI model use a standard API (e.g. FHIR). (Elhaddad et al., 2024; Ramgopal et al., 2023)

Integration of AI into EHRs and Clinical Workflows

When new data points are stored, it may either trigger the internal EHR AI model to run or invoke CDSS hooks (APIs that are used to interface with external programs) to reach out to the AI model running externally to the EHR for its prediction. Before activating this AI model, it is critical that thorough due diligence is done to ensure that the AI model will work properly within established clinical workflows of the clinical team. This can be done by properly trained PIs but is often done by an AI translation/enablement team and/or Clinical Informatics trained nurse/provider who studies the current clinical workflow and determines where the ideal intervention points should take place. In the context of the BP example, the team would have interviewed multiple different clinicians that utilized and managed BP along with people that do not. In doing so the team may find out that a passive alert would be best and proceed with next steps. (Labkoff et al., 2024)

Informatics-led Evaluation and Monitoring of AI Tools

When a workflow has been identified, the AI model deployment should be phased. Initially the model should run silently, then be visible within a small, experienced group to catch errors in the process. Once the smaller group validates the model appears to be functioning, then it should be deployed to a larger randomized group and finally rolled out system wide. This phased approach is aimed at catching small errors and workflow discrepancies prior to system-wide deployment, mitigating the chances that any issues will affect thousands of health care team members daily. After full deployment, ongoing monitoring is needed to detect AI model drift or adverse outcomes affected by the data inputs (e.g., changes in normal range). In the case of the AI BP model, the responsibility for post-deployment monitoring is handed off to a trained monitoring team, ensuring that the BP model continues to function and maintains its efficacy as expected over time. (Harrer et al., 2019; Wang et al., 2025)

ETHICAL, LEGAL, AND SOCIAL IMPLICATIONS

Bias, Fairness, and Health Equity

The integration of AI into CI offers potential transformative opportunities that will reshape patient care, advance medical research, and elevate system efficiency. Yet alongside these advances come ethical, legal, and social challenges that must be systematically addressed to ensure that the deployment of AI is safe and equitable for all.

One of the primary concerns in equitable use of AI models is algorithm bias, which arises when training data reflect historical inequities or lack of representation from diverse populations. A notable example is the widely reported 2019 study in *Science* that found a commercial risk prediction algorithm systematically underestimated the healthcare needs of Black patients because it used healthcare costs as a proxy for health status. Another example is the recurrent inaccuracy of pulse oximeters in darker skin tones, a flaw that can be passed downstream to AI models that incorporate these features. Furthermore, advanced AI models for radiology or intensive care monitoring are more likely to be implemented in tertiary academic centers than rural or safety net hospitals, limiting access for vulnerable and under-represented populations. (Obermeyer et al., 2019) Addressing these issues requires use of diverse training datasets, external validation across demographic subgroups, and deliberate strategies and intentional governance frameworks to promote equitable dissemination of AI technologies and mitigate biases.

Transparency, Accountability, and Informed Consent

Transparency remains essential for fostering trust in AI-CDS, yet it is difficult to implement transparency in complex, highly-capable systems. While rule-based decision tools are relatively straightforward and allow for recommendations to be traced back to guidelines or protocols, many AI models – particularly deep learning systems – operate as opaque "black boxes," producing predictions without clear explanation or rationale. Epic EHR offered an example of this with one of their initial sepsis prediction models, which, despite wide adoption, was shown in a 2021 *JAMA Internal Medicine* study to miss most sepsis cases while generating large numbers of false positive alerts. Due to the lack of interpretability clinicians were unable to evaluate how the model reached its predictions, illustrating the risks of opaque systems in critical settings. Similarly, closed-source or proprietary models that obscure inputs and results from external review present a similar challenge by preventing third party validation. These examples of opacity can undermine clinician confidence and highlight the necessity for transparency when AI is used in healthcare. (Wong et al., 2021)

Accountability is another unresolved issue. When an AI tool contributes to harm or adverse outcomes, responsibility may be shared among developers, vendors, healthcare institutions, and clinicians. Without clear governance structures, it can be difficult to assign liability or ensure timely corrective action. Institutions adopting AI therefore need frameworks that define oversight responsibilities, monitor performance, and clarify legal accountability to better safeguard patients and institutional integrity. (Mello et al., 2024)

Informed consent also requires new consideration in the context of AI-enabled healthcare. Patients are often unaware when algorithms are involved in diagnosis, risk prediction, or treatment planning. The 2016 collaboration between Google DeepMind and the Royal Free Hospital in London, where patient data were used to train a kidney injury detection system without explicit consent, drew widespread public criticism. Such controversies underscore the ethical importance of informing patients about how their data are used and when AI tools influence clinical decisions. While full disclosure must be balanced against workflow efficiency, transparency with both clinicians and patients is central to ethical implementation. (Powles et al., 2017)

Regulatory Landscape and Data Security

Regulation of medical technology and AI is difficult, as frameworks have evolved multiple times both in the United States (US) and abroad. The Food and Drug Administration (FDA) and European Union Medical Device Regulation (EU MDR) are two regulatory bodies that serve as a basis for many countries' laws and regulations; both are in the process of revising guidance and regulation as novel AI applications advance into new territories not previously expected. Despite these changes, the areas of privacy and security have remained relatively stable. (Bretthauer et al., 2023; Yu et al., 2023) Health Insurance Portability and Accountability Act (HIPAA) in the US and the EU's General Data Protection Regulation (GDPR) provide standards around data privacy and security, with the latter applying both within and beyond healthcare. Both regulations prioritize patient privacy and data protections mandating safe storage and security measures be in place. However, as the regulatory landscape is changing as rapidly as the technology, following upcoming legislation is imperative by stakeholders to ensure that the adoption of new technologies and AI will be compliant with current and future laws and regulations. (Cohen et al., 2018; McCall, 2018)

CHALLENGES AND LIMITATIONS

Data Silos and Interoperability Barriers

Data is a key asset for both CI and AI activities. However, deliberately or inadvertently, data can become siloed and segregated. The reason for this isolation can be related to security or due to having different vended systems (e.g., EHR is different than LIS is different than RIS). This isolation creates separation, which complicates data and insight integration efforts and often necessitates complex solutions that are challenging to maintain. To address these challenges, a strategic approach is to select vendors whose solutions support common standardized communication frameworks such as FHIR/HL7 and store data in common database structures such as SQL. Standardization is key for breaking down these barriers to facilitate easy data analysis and develop effective AI models. (Patel, 2019; Saberi et al., 2025)

Clinical Resistance and Change Management

Following model development, validation, and initial piloting stages, it is time to deploy the model into practice, which will require careful facilitation of clinical resistance to change. Solidified workflow, protocols, and general habits can cause resistance to adoption of new technologies. Change management, such as Kotter's, is essential to navigate the integration of AI models into clinical practice while minimizing disruptions. For example, if a BP model requires you to gather key patient information not found in the chart, careful planning needs to be done around workflow integration and change management: should providers ask these questions, costing valuable time, or should the information be obtained through other asynchronous digital avenues such as the patient portal or a rooming tablet. (Singh et al., 2023; Bonnabry et al., 2020) Lastly, broad education and training should be done prior to system roll out to catch any unforeseen issues and enable smooth adoption.

Model Generalizability and Real-World Validation

If the AI model demonstrates its utility within the initial system it was designed for, consideration could be given to offer it to other sites in your health system or license it to neighboring institutions. Scaling models like this do require an understanding of regional context and data variability. From the previous example, say the BP model was developed within an urban academic center in Minnesota; it may not generalize well for use in rural Alabama given the differences in regional diet, demographics, and medical practices and protocols. Consequently, model retraining and re-validation with the target system's data will need to be done to ensure model performance is maintained. Expanding access to a diverse set of data when the model is being developed mitigates the need for re-training and allows for the model to be more generalizable. (Rahman et al., 2024)

Cost, Infrastructure, and Scalability

With a functional AI model running, an institution should reassess on a regular interval the return on investment (ROI) associated with its deployment. AI models often require special computer hardware called Graphic Processing Units (GPUs) to run, which, despite the name, are high-end parallel processing units not limited to use for graphics. While institutions can develop these AI models on smaller cheaper systems, scaled clinical use relies on larger cloud-based or in-house servers at a variable cost up front and long term. To give perspective these costs could be millions up front and only five cents each time the model is used or minimal up front and several dollars per model usage. The latter operational expense may seem more appealing, but multiplying that by high volume model triggers – such as laboratory testing, imaging interpretation, or daily BP checks – can result in substantial cost. For the BP example, the numbers may look like this: $2 per AI run * 20 BP visits per provider * 200 providers * 5 days a week * 50 weeks a year = $2M per year to run this model alone. This shows it is critical to conduct regular RIO evaluations (arguably before deploying as well) to ensure the old metaphor – "if the juice is worth the squeeze." (Vertex, n.d.; Cottier et al., 2024)

FUTURE DIRECTIONS

AI-Augmented Clinician Roles

As healthcare always continues to change, many wonder what is in store for the relationship between AI and clinical practice. While some believe that AI will replace clinicians, and others are skeptical that AI will reach that level of sophistication, the most likely scenario lies somewhere in the middle with AI-augmented clinician roles. In this mode, AI technology does not replace the clinician but advances the clinical decision support in turn enhancing the clinician workflow and decision-making. Consider an example from a typical outpatient practice. Prior to a clinician seeing a patient, AI technology might collect items of importance from the patient and EHR and prioritize them for the clinician to review. During the visit, AI scribes perform real time documentation while also surfacing clinical, literature, and research items of importance to the provider and proposing a differential of critical diagnoses that cannot be missed. At the conclusion of the visit the AI will pend orders, including for mentioned and suggested testing, and suggest appropriate billing/coding for the visit for the clinician to review. Such clinical augmentation has the potential to decrease clinical burden, increase available clinician-patient time and ultimately improve the patient-provider relationship. In some institutions early versions of some of these AI technologies are already being deployed. (Obuchowicz et al., 2026; Kapadia et al., 2024)

Real-Time Digital Twins and Predictive Monitoring

Another emerging application that is being implemented by some AI forward institutions and EHR systems is the concept of a digital twin – finding similar patients across your institution(s) or nationwide to compare to. This concept enables clinicians when planning for a specific treatment or medication to draw from millions of patient outcomes experienced. (Kamel, 2021) By leveraging this focused cohort, clinicians are better able to select the treatment(s) with best chances of efficacy while reducing the likelihood of adverse outcomes, morbidity, and mortality. Simple examples already in place are solutions for selecting the right antihypertensives or antidepressants medications for patients. (Laubenbacher et al., 2024)

Vision for a Learning Health System

Looking further on the horizon, a thought for AI is that the entire system could have the ability to "learn" and find insights. In such a system, autonomous AI agents would collaborate across multiple departments such as billing, research, and clinical practice, all coordinated using supervisory agents. To achieve interoperability between these various systems a standardized protocol, such as Model Context Protocol (MCP) would be needed to enable agents to discover what each other has for features and provide a common language to communicate. (Hasan et al., 2025) This in turn allows the agents to discover hidden signals buried in a sea of complex data in multiple areas of healthcare. For example, should the system be asked to decrease the average length of stay for a hospital system, supervisory agents will coordinate with the research agent to determine evidence-based measures to decrease length of stay. If one of the interventions is related to medications given in multiple disease processes, then the supervisory agents will connect with the billing agents for time of stay and clinical agents to discover disease and medication relationships. The statistics agent will analyze aggregated data to create a statistical model that is able to be used to drive hospital policy and practice.

Federated Learning and Decentralized Models

Realizing these advanced tools is contingent on access to large and diverse databases. However, significant concerns exist around data privacy and institutional data control. Federated learning and decentralized model architectures from the past have been proposed as a possible solution. (Yang et al., 2019) In this type of paradigm, each institution will create a local clinical data store not shared with others and train a model on this data with an agreed upon set of AI parameters. Model parameters and learned weights (insights) are passed on in block-and-chain format or back to a central repository for re-distribution, and all the while the local clinical data is kept confidential. This approach allows for the development of more generalized models while reducing the risk of data leakage and data privacy concerns. (Teo et al., 2024; Google, n.d.)

CONCLUSION

In summary, Clinical Informatics is an established and essential component of modern healthcare delivery, shaping how clinical information is captured, exchanged, and used across care settings. Through the development of health information systems, data standards, and clinical workflows, clinical informatics supports routine patient care, quality improvement, and operational efficiency. These capabilities form the backbone of digital healthcare.

Artificial intelligence represents a newer and still evolving set of tools that are beginning to influence select areas of healthcare practice. While AI has demonstrated promise in applications such as clinical decision support, documentation assistance, triage, and population health analytics, its use remains uneven and highly dependent on local context, data availability, and workflow integration. In many settings, AI remains experimental or limited to narrowly defined tasks rather than a core component of care delivery.

The effectiveness of AI in healthcare is shaped as much by informatics, governance, and clinical practice as by technical performance. Challenges related to data quality, interoperability, bias, explainability, regulation, cost, and change management continue to constrain widespread adoption. Without careful design and oversight, AI tools risk adding complexity or burden rather than delivering meaningful clinical value.

Looking ahead, the relationship between clinical informatics and artificial intelligence is likely to continue evolving. Emerging concepts such as AI augmented clinician roles, predictive population health models, digital twins, and decentralized learning approaches illustrate potential future directions rather than established practice. Whether these innovations mature into routine care will depend on sustained investment, rigorous evaluation, and alignment with clinical needs and patient values. Keeping clinicians and patients at the center of this evolution is essential to ensuring that technological progress translates into real world benefit.Bottom of Form

REFERENCES

Adeniyi, A. O., Arowoogun, J. O., Chidi, R., Okolo, C. A., & Babawarun, O. (2024). The impact of electronic health records on patient care and outcomes: A comprehensive review. *World Journal of Advanced Research and Reviews, 21*(2), 1446–1455. DOI: 10.30574/wjarr.2024.21.2.0592

Adler-Milstein, J., & Jha, A. K. (2017). HITECH Act drove large gains in hospital electronic health record adoption. *Health Affairs, 36*(8), 1416–1422. DOI: 10.1377/hlthaff.2016.1651 PMID: 28784734

Annas, G. J. (2003). HIPAA regulations—A new era of medical-record privacy? *The New England Journal of Medicine, 348*(15), 1486–1490. DOI: 10.1056/NEJMlim035027 PMID: 12686707

Arrieta, A. B., Díaz-Rodríguez, N., Del Ser, J., Bennetot, A., Tabik, S., Barbado, A., & Herrera, F. (2020). Explainable Artificial Intelligence (XAI): Concepts, taxonomies, opportunities and challenges toward responsible AI. *Information Fusion, 58*, 82–115. DOI: 10.1016/j.inffus.2019.12.012

Bednarczyk, L., Reichenpfader, D., Gaudet-Blavignac, C., Ette, A. K., Zaghir, J., Zheng, Y., Bensahla, A., Bjelogrlic, M., & Lovis, C. (2025). Scientific evidence for clinical text summarization using large language models: Scoping review. *Journal of Medical Internet Research, 27*, e68998. DOI: 10.2196/68998 PMID: 40371947

Bodenreider, O., Cornet, R., & Vreeman, D. J. (2018). Recent developments in clinical terminologies—SNOMED CT, LOINC, and RxNorm. *Yearbook of Medical Informatics, 27*(01), 129–139. DOI: 10.1055/s-0038-1667077 PMID: 30157516

Bonnabry, P., & François, O. (2020). Return on investment: A practical calculation tool to convince your institution. *European Journal of Hospital Pharmacy. Science and Practice, 27*(2), 111–113. DOI: 10.1136/ejhpharm-2018-001733 PMID: 32133138

Brereton, T. A., Malik, M. M., Rost, L. M., Ohde, J. W., Zheng, L., Jose, K. A., . . . Overgaard, S. M. (2024). AImedReport: A Prototype Tool to Facilitate Research Reporting and Translation of AI Technologies in Healthcare. medRxiv, 2024-01. DOI: 10.1101/2024.01.16.24301358

Bretthauer, M., Gerke, S., Hassan, C., Ahmad, O. F., & Mori, Y. (2023). The new European medical device regulation: Balancing innovation and patient safety. *Annals of Internal Medicine, 176*(6), 844–848. DOI: 10.7326/M23-0454 PMID: 37068279

Brock, D. C. (2018). Learning from artificial intelligence's previous awakenings: The history of expert systems. *AI Magazine*, *39*(3), 3–15. DOI: 10.1609/aimag.v39i3.2809

Budach, L., Feuerpfeil, M., Ihde, N., Nathansen, A., Noack, N., Patzlaff, H., . . . Harmouch, H. (2022). The effects of data quality on machine learning performance. arXiv preprint arXiv:2207.14529.

Budd, J. (2023). Burnout related to electronic health record use in primary care. *Journal of Primary Care & Community Health*, *14*, 21501319231166921. DOI: 10.1177/21501319231166921 PMID: 37073905

Burde, H. (2011). The HITECH act: An overview. *AMA Journal of Ethics*, *13*(3), 172–175. DOI: 10.1001/virtualmentor.2011.13.3.hlaw1-1103 PMID: 23127320

Chishtie, J., Sapiro, N., Wiebe, N., Rabatach, L., Lorenzetti, D., Leung, A. A., Rabi, D., Quan, H., & Eastwood, C. A. (2023). Use of epic electronic health record system for health care research: Scoping review. *Journal of Medical Internet Research*, *25*, e51003. DOI: 10.2196/51003 PMID: 38100185

Cloud, G. (n.d.). Federated learning: What it is and how it works. Retrieved from https://cloud.google.com/blog/products/ai-machine-learning/federated-learning-what-it-is-and-how-it-works

Cohen, I. G., & Mello, M. M. (2018). HIPAA and protecting health information in the 21st century. *Journal of the American Medical Association*, *320*(3), 231–232. DOI: 10.1001/jama.2018.5630 PMID: 29800120

Cottier, B., Rahman, R., Fattorini, L., Maslej, N., Besiroglu, T., & Owen, D. (2024). The rising costs of training frontier AI models. arXiv preprint arXiv:2405.21015.

Cruz, M. F., Cavalcante, C. A. M. T., & Sá Barretto, S. T. (2018). Using OPC and HL7 standards to incorporate an industrial Big Data historian in a health IT environment. *Journal of Medical Systems*, *42*(7), 122. DOI: 10.1007/s10916-018-0979-5 PMID: 29846812

Duggan, M. J., Gervase, J., Schoenbaum, A., Hanson, W., Howell, J. T. III, Sheinberg, M., & Johnson, K. B. (2025). Clinician experiences with ambient scribe technology to assist with documentation burden and efficiency. *JAMA Network Open*, *8*(2), e2460637–e2460637. DOI: 10.1001/jamanetworkopen.2024.60637 PMID: 39969880

Ehsan, U., Liao, Q. V., Muller, M., Riedl, M. O., & Weisz, J. D. (2021, May). Expanding explainability: Towards social transparency in ai systems. In *Proceedings of the 2021 CHI conference on human factors in computing systems* (pp. 1-19). DOI: 10.1145/3411764.3445188

Elhaddad, M., & Hamam, S. (2024). AI-driven clinical decision support systems: An ongoing pursuit of potential. *Cureus*, *16*(4). Advance online publication. DOI: 10.7759/cureus.57728 PMID: 38711724

Evans, R. S. (2016). Electronic health records: then, now, and in the future. Yearbook of medical informatics, 25(S 01), S48-S61.

Faridimehr, S., Venkatachalam, S., & Chinnam, R. B. (2021). Managing access to primary care clinics using scheduling templates. *Health Care Management Science*, *24*(3), 482–498. DOI: 10.1007/s10729-020-09535-z PMID: 33400050

Fradkov, A. L. (2020). Early history of machine learning. *IFAC-PapersOnLine*, *53*(2), 1385–1390. DOI: 10.1016/j.ifacol.2020.12.1888

Gabay, M. (2017). 21st century cures act. *Hospital Pharmacy*, *52*(4), 264–265. DOI: 10.1310/hpx5204-264 PMID: 28515504

Gardner, R. L., Cooper, E., Haskell, J., Harris, D. A., Poplau, S., Kroth, P. J., & Linzer, M. (2019). Physician stress and burnout: The impact of health information technology. *Journal of the American Medical Informatics Association : JAMIA*, *26*(2), 106–114. DOI: 10.1093/jamia/ocy145 PMID: 30517663

Gillum, R. F. (2013). From papyrus to the electronic tablet: A brief history of the clinical medical record with lessons for the digital age. *The American Journal of Medicine*, *126*(10), 853–857. DOI: 10.1016/j.amjmed.2013.03.024 PMID: 24054954

Haakman, M., Cruz, L., Huijgens, H., & Van Deursen, A. (2021). AI lifecycle models need to be revised: An exploratory study in Fintech. *Empirical Software Engineering*, *26*(5), 95. DOI: 10.1007/s10664-021-09993-1

Haenlein, M., & Kaplan, A. (2019). A brief history of artificial intelligence: On the past, present, and future of artificial intelligence. *California Management Review*, *61*(4), 5–14. DOI: 10.1177/0008125619864925

Harrer, S., Shah, P., Antony, B., & Hu, J. (2019). Artificial intelligence for clinical trial design. *Trends in Pharmacological Sciences*, *40*(8), 577–591. DOI: 10.1016/j.tips.2019.05.005 PMID: 31326235

Hasan, M. M., Li, H., Fallahzadeh, E., Rajbahadur, G. K., Adams, B., & Hassan, A. E. (2025). Model context protocol (mcp) at first glance: Studying the security and maintainability of mcp servers. arXiv preprint arXiv:2506.13538.

Hirani, R., Noruzi, K., Khuram, H., Hussaini, A. S., Aifuwa, E. I., Ely, K. E., Lewis, J. M., Gabr, A. E., Smiley, A., Tiwari, R. K., & Etienne, M. (2024). Artificial intelligence and healthcare: A journey through history, present innovations, and future possibilities. *Life (Chicago, Ill.), 14*(5), 557. DOI: 10.3390/life14050557 PMID: 38792579

Jiang, F., Jiang, Y., Zhi, H., Dong, Y., Li, H., Ma, S., Wang, Y., Dong, Q., Shen, H., & Wang, Y. (2017). Artificial intelligence in healthcare: Past, present and future. *Stroke and Vascular Neurology, 2*(4), 230–243. DOI: 10.1136/svn-2017-000101 PMID: 29507784

Jones, K. S. (1994). Natural language processing: a historical review. Current issues in computational linguistics: in honour of Don Walker, 3-16.

Judson, T. J., Odisho, A. Y., Neinstein, A. B., Chao, J., Williams, A., Miller, C., Moriarty, T., Gleason, N., Intinarelli, G., & Gonzales, R. (2020). Rapid design and implementation of an integrated patient self-triage and self-scheduling tool for COVID-19. *Journal of the American Medical Informatics Association : JAMIA, 27*(6), 860–866. DOI: 10.1093/jamia/ocaa051 PMID: 32267928

Kamel Boulos, M. N., & Zhang, P. (2021). Digital twins: From personalised medicine to precision public health. *Journal of Personalized Medicine, 11*(8), 745. DOI: 10.3390/jpm11080745 PMID: 34442389

Kapadia, K., Ruwali, S., Malav, T., Seshadri, S., Seidmann, A., Press, D. Z., & Kolachalama, V. B. (2024). Enhancing efficiency with an AI-augmented clinician in neurology. *Aging and Disease, 16*(5), 2498. DOI: 10.14336/AD.2024.1249 PMID: 39500349

Keeley, P., Wolf, Z., Regul, L., & Jadwin, A. (2015). Effectiveness of standard of care protocol on patient satisfaction and perceived staff caring. *Clinical Journal of Oncology Nursing, 19*(3), 352–360. DOI: 10.1188/15.CJON.352-360 PMID: 26000585

Kim, J. S., Vivas, A., Arvind, V., Lombardi, J., Reidler, J., Zuckerman, S. L., Lee, N. J., Vulapalli, M., Geng, E. A., Cho, B. H., Morizane, K., Cho, S. K., Lehman, R. A., Lenke, L. G., & Riew, K. D. (2023). Can natural language processing and artificial intelligence automate the generation of billing codes from operative note dictations? *Global Spine Journal, 13*(7), 1946–1955. DOI: 10.1177/21925682211062831 PMID: 35225694

Kocher, R., Emanuel, E. J., & DeParle, N. A. M. (2010). The Affordable Care Act and the future of clinical medicine: The opportunities and challenges. *Annals of Internal Medicine*, *153*(8), 536–539. DOI: 10.7326/0003-4819-153-8-201010190-00274 PMID: 20733178

Kononenko, I. (2001). Machine learning for medical diagnosis: History, state of the art and perspective. *Artificial Intelligence in Medicine*, *23*(1), 89–109. DOI: 10.1016/S0933-3657(01)00077-X PMID: 11470218

Labkoff, S., Oladimeji, B., Kannry, J., Solomonides, A., Leftwich, R., Koski, E., Joseph, A. L., Lopez-Gonzalez, M., Fleisher, L. A., Nolen, K., Dutta, S., Levy, D. R., Price, A., Barr, P. J., Hron, J. D., Lin, B., Srivastava, G., Pastor, N., Luque, U. S., & Quintana, Y. (2024). Toward a responsible future: Recommendations for AI-enabled clinical decision support. *Journal of the American Medical Informatics Association : JAMIA*, *31*(11), 2730–2739. DOI: 10.1093/jamia/ocae209 PMID: 39325508

Laubenbacher, R., Mehrad, B., Shmulevich, I., & Trayanova, N. (2024). Digital twins in medicine. *Nature Computational Science*, *4*(3), 184–191. DOI: 10.1038/s43588-024-00607-6 PMID: 38532133

Liang, W., Tadesse, G. A., Ho, D., Fei-Fei, L., Zaharia, M., Zhang, C., & Zou, J. (2022). Advances, challenges and opportunities in creating data for trustworthy AI. *Nature Machine Intelligence*, *4*(8), 669–677. DOI: 10.1038/s42256-022-00516-1

Mandel, J. C., Kreda, D. A., Mandl, K. D., Kohane, I. S., & Ramoni, R. B. (2016). SMART on FHIR: A standards-based, interoperable apps platform for electronic health records. *Journal of the American Medical Informatics Association : JAMIA*, *23*(5), 899–908. DOI: 10.1093/jamia/ocv189 PMID: 26911829

McCall, B. (2018). What does the GDPR mean for the medical community? *Lancet*, *391*(10127), 1249–1250. DOI: 10.1016/S0140-6736(18)30739-6 PMID: 29619949

Mehta, N., & Devarakonda, M. V. (2018). Machine learning, natural language programming, and electronic health records: The next step in the artificial intelligence journey? *The Journal of Allergy and Clinical Immunology*, *141*(6), 2019–2021. DOI: 10.1016/j.jaci.2018.02.025 PMID: 29518424

Mello, M. M., & Guha, N. (2024). Understanding liability risk from using health care artificial intelligence tools. *The New England Journal of Medicine*, *390*(3), 271–278. DOI: 10.1056/NEJMhle2308901 PMID: 38231630

Meurers, D. (2012). Natural language processing and language learning. Encyclopedia of applied linguistics, 4193-4205. DOI: 10.1002/9781405198431.wbeal0858

Minh, D., Wang, H. X., Li, Y. F., & Nguyen, T. N. (2022). Explainable artificial intelligence: A comprehensive review. *Artificial Intelligence Review*, *55*(5), 3503–3568. DOI: 10.1007/s10462-021-10088-y

Mittermaier, M., Raza, M. M., & Kvedar, J. C. (2023). Bias in AI-based models for medical applications: Challenges and mitigation strategies. *NPJ Digital Medicine*, *6*(1), 113. DOI: 10.1038/s41746-023-00858-z PMID: 37311802

Murad, M. H., Vaa Stelling, B. E., West, C. P., Hasan, B., Simha, S., Saadi, S., Firwana, M., Viola, K. E., Prokop, L. J., Nayfeh, T., & Wang, Z. (2024). Measuring documentation burden in healthcare. *Journal of General Internal Medicine*, *39*(14), 2837–2848. DOI: 10.1007/s11606-024-08956-8 PMID: 39073484

Nazer, L. H., Zatarah, R., Waldrip, S., Ke, J. X. C., Moukheiber, M., Khanna, A. K., Hicklen, R. S., Moukheiber, L., Moukheiber, D., Ma, H., & Mathur, P. (2023). Bias in artificial intelligence algorithms and recommendations for mitigation. *PLOS Digital Health*, *2*(6), e0000278. DOI: 10.1371/journal.pdig.0000278 PMID: 37347721

Obermeyer, Z., Powers, B., Vogeli, C., & Mullainathan, S. (2019). Dissecting racial bias in an algorithm used to manage the health of populations. *Science*, *366*(6464), 447–453. DOI: 10.1126/science.aax2342 PMID: 31649194

Obuchowicz, R., Piórkowski, A., Nurzyńska, K., Obuchowicz, B., Strzelecki, M., & Bielecka, M. (2026). Will AI Replace Physicians in the Near Future? AI Adoption Barriers in Medicine. *Diagnostics (Basel)*, *16*(3), 396. DOI: 10.3390/diagnostics16030396 PMID: 41681714

Olawade, D. B., Wada, O. J., David-Olawade, A. C., Kunonga, E., Abaire, O., & Ling, J. (2023). Using artificial intelligence to improve public health: A narrative review. *Frontiers in Public Health*, *11*, 1196397. DOI: 10.3389/fpubh.2023.1196397 PMID: 37954052

Osheroff, J. A., Teich, J., Levick, D., Saldana, L., Velasco, F., Sittig, D., & Jenders, R. (2012). *Improving outcomes with clinical decision support: an implementer's guide*. Himss Publishing. DOI: 10.4324/9781498757461

Patel, J. (2019). Bridging data silos using big data integration. International Journal of Database Management Systems, 11(3), 01-06.

Powles, J., & Hodson, H. (2017). Google DeepMind and healthcare in an age of algorithms. *Health and Technology*, *7*(4), 351–357. DOI: 10.1007/s12553-017-0179-1 PMID: 29308344

Protection, P., & Act, A. C. (2010). affordable Care Act. Public law, (111-148), 124.

Rahman, S., Jiang, L. Y., Gabriel, S., Aphinyanaphongs, Y., Oermann, E. K., & Chunara, R. (2024). Generalization in healthcare ai: Evaluation of a clinical large language model. arXiv preprint arXiv:2402.10965.

Ramgopal, S., Sanchez-Pinto, L. N., Horvat, C. M., Carroll, M. S., Luo, Y., & Florin, T. A. (2023). Artificial intelligence-based clinical decision support in pediatrics. *Pediatric Research*, *93*(2), 334–341. DOI: 10.1038/s41390-022-02226-1 PMID: 35906317

Rodriguez, J. A., Clark, C. R., & Bates, D. W. (2020). Digital health equity as a necessity in the 21st century cures act era. *Journal of the American Medical Association*, *323*(23), 2381–2382. DOI: 10.1001/jama.2020.7858 PMID: 32463421

Saberi, M. A., Mcheick, H., & Adda, M. (2025). From data silos to health records without borders: A systematic survey on patient-centered data interoperability. *Information (Basel)*, *16*(2), 106. DOI: 10.3390/info16020106

Sambasivan, N., ... "'Everyone wants to do the model work, not the data work": Data Cascades in High-Stakes AI." proceedings of the 2021 CHI Conference on Human Factors in Computing Systems. 2021. DOI: 10.1145/3411764.3445518

Sánchez-Salmerón, R., Gómez-Urquiza, J. L., Albendín-García, L., Correa-Rodríguez, M., Martos-Cabrera, M. B., Velando-Soriano, A., & Suleiman-Martos, N. (2022). Machine learning methods applied to triage in emergency services: A systematic review. *International Emergency Nursing*, *60*, 101109. DOI: 10.1016/j.ienj.2021.101109 PMID: 34952482

Sepluveda, J. L., & Young, D. S. (2013). The ideal laboratory information system. *Archives of Pathology & Laboratory Medicine*, *137*(8), 1129–1140. DOI: 10.5858/arpa.2012-0362-RA PMID: 23216205

Seymour, T., Frantsvog, D., & Graeber, T. (2012). Electronic health records (EHR). *American Journal of Health Sciences*, *3*(3), 201–210. DOI: 10.19030/ajhs.v3i3.7139

Shortliffe, E. H., & Sepúlveda, M. J. (2018). Clinical decision support in the era of artificial intelligence. *Journal of the American Medical Association*, *320*(21), 2199–2200. DOI: 10.1001/jama.2018.17163 PMID: 30398550

Singh, J., Sillerud, B., & Singh, A. (2023). Artificial intelligence, chatbots and ChatGPT in healthcare—Narrative review of historical evolution, current application, and change management approach to increase adoption. *Journal of Medical Artificial Intelligence*, *6*, 6. DOI: 10.21037/jmai-23-92

Sloss, E. A., Abdul, S., Aboagyewah, M. A., Beebe, A., Kendle, K., Marshall, K., Rosenbloom, S. T., Rossetti, S., Grigg, A., Smith, K. D., & Mishuris, R. G. (2024). Toward alleviating clinician documentation burden: A scoping review of burden reduction efforts. *Applied Clinical Informatics*, *15*(03), 446–455. DOI: 10.1055/s-0044-1787007 PMID: 38839063

Tan, H. (2017, September). A brief history and technical review of the expert system research. [). IOP Publishing.]. *IOP Conference Series. Materials Science and Engineering*, *242*(1), 012111. DOI: 10.1088/1757-899X/242/1/012111

Teo, Z. L., Jin, L., Liu, N., Li, S., Miao, D., Zhang, X., Ng, W. Y., Tan, T. F., Lee, D. M., Chua, K. J., Heng, J., Liu, Y., Goh, R. S. M., & Ting, D. S. W. (2024). Federated machine learning in healthcare: A systematic review on clinical applications and technical architecture. *Cell Reports Medicine*, *5*(2), 101419. DOI: 10.1016/j.xcrm.2024.101419 PMID: 38340728

Tierney, A. A., Gayre, G., Hoberman, B., Mattern, B., Ballesca, M., Kipnis, P., Liu, V., & Lee, K. (2024). Ambient artificial intelligence scribes to alleviate the burden of clinical documentation. *NEJM Catalyst Innovations in Care Delivery*, *5*(3), CAT-23. DOI: 10.1056/CAT.23.0404

Vertex, A. I. (n.d.). Google Cloud. https://cloud.google.com/vertex-ai?hl=en

Wang, F., & Beecy, A. (2025). Implementing AI models in clinical workflows: A roadmap. *BMJ Evidence-Based Medicine*, *30*(5), 285–287. PMID: 38914450

Wang, Z., Chu, Z., Doan, T. V., Ni, S., Yang, M., & Zhang, W. (2025). History, development, and principles of large language models: An introductory survey. *AI and Ethics*, *5*(3), 1955–1971. DOI: 10.1007/s43681-024-00583-7

Wasylewicz, A. T., & Scheepers-Hoeks, A. M. J. W. (2018). Clinical decision support systems. Fundamentals of clinical data science, 153-169.

Wong, A., Otles, E., Donnelly, J. P., Krumm, A., McCullough, J., DeTroyer-Cooley, O., Pestrue, J., Phillips, M., Konye, J., Penoza, C., Ghous, M., & Singh, K. (2021). External validation of a widely implemented proprietary sepsis prediction model in hospitalized patients. *JAMA Internal Medicine*, *181*(8), 1065–1070. DOI: 10.1001/jamainternmed.2021.2626 PMID: 34152373

Xu, F., Uszkoreit, H., Du, Y., Fan, W., Zhao, D., & Zhu, J. (2019, September). Explainable AI: A brief survey on history, research areas, approaches and challenges. In *CCF international conference on natural language processing and Chinese computing* (pp. 563–574). Springer International Publishing. DOI: 10.1007/978-3-030-32236-6_51

Yang, Q., Liu, Y., Chen, T., & Tong, Y. (2019). Federated machine learning: Concept and applications. [TIST]. *ACM Transactions on Intelligent Systems and Technology*, *10*(2), 1–19. DOI: 10.1145/3298981

Yu, J., Zhang, J., & Sengoku, S. (2023). Innovation process and industrial system of US Food and Drug Administration–approved software as a medical device: Review and content analysis. *Journal of Medical Internet Research*, *25*, e47505. DOI: 10.2196/47505 PMID: 37999948

Zayas-Cabán, T., Okubo, T. H., & Posnack, S. (2023). Priorities to accelerate workflow automation in health care. *Journal of the American Medical Informatics Association : JAMIA*, *30*(1), 195–201. DOI: 10.1093/jamia/ocac197 PMID: 36259967

Zhou, C., Li, Q., Li, C., Yu, J., Liu, Y., Wang, G., Zhang, K., Ji, C., Yan, Q., He, L., Peng, H., Li, J., Wu, J., Liu, Z., Xie, P., Xiong, C., Pei, J., Yu, P. S., & Sun, L. (2025). A comprehensive survey on pretrained foundation models: A history from bert to chatgpt. *International Journal of Machine Learning and Cybernetics*, *16*(12), 9851–9915. DOI: 10.1007/s13042-024-02443-6

ADDITIONAL READING

Frisse, M. E., & Misulis, K. E. (Eds.). (2019). *Essentials of Clinical Informatics*. Oxford University Press. DOI: 10.1093/med/9780190855574.001.0001

Huyen, C. (2024). *AI engineering: Building applications with foundation models*. O'Reilly Media, Inc.

Shi, L., & Singh, D. A. (2021). *Delivering Health Care in America: A Systems Approach*. Jones & Bartlett Learning.

KEY TERMS AND DEFINITIONS

Artificial Intelligence (AI): The field of computer science that focuses on software that can perform tasks typically requiring human intelligence or pattern matching. These tasks include learning, reasoning, problem-solving, perception, and understanding language.

Clinical Decision Support Systems (CDSS): Tools designed to assist healthcare professionals in making informed decisions. These systems analyze patient data and provide evidence-based recommendations, alerts, or reminders to improve patient care, enhance safety, and reduce errors. CDSS can use distinct types of artificial intelligence, such as machine learning and natural language processing.

Clinical Informatics (CI): A field that uses information and technology to improve clinical care, enhance health outcomes, and support healthcare operations. CI combines principles from computer science, information science, and healthcare to implement changes in the electronic health records (EHRs), clinical decision support systems (CDSS), and other digital tools that facilitate the collection, analysis, and application of clinical data.

Deep Learning (DL): A subset of machine learning and artificial intelligence that utilizes neural networks (modeled after brain neurons) that automatically "learns" from large amounts of data. Deep neural networks can recognize patterns, make predictions, and understand complex relationships in data such as images, audio, and text, often outperforming traditional machine learning methods in tasks like speech recognition, image classification, and natural language processing.

Electronic Health Records (EHRs): Digital patient charts that systematically collect, store, and manage health information. EHRs contain comprehensive data such as medical histories, diagnoses, medications, treatment plans, immunization dates, allergies, radiology images, and laboratory results.

Large Language Models (LLMs): Artificial intelligence models that are trained on large amounts of data to pattern match and generate human language. These models use deep learning techniques, particularly transformer architectures that can perform text generation, translation, summarization, and question answering.

Machine Learning (ML): Artificial intelligence that focuses on developing algorithms and statistical models that enable computers to "learn" from data, identify patterns, and make predictions without being explicitly programmed for specific tasks. ML systems improve their performance over time as they are exposed to more data. They are used in applications such as image analysis, predictive analytics, and natural language processing.

Natural Language Processing (NLP): Branch of artificial intelligence and computer science focused on interpreting and generating human language. NLP combines computational linguistics with machine learning and deep learning methods to process and analyze large amounts of text and speech to perform language translation, sentiment analysis, and speech recognition.

Chapter 5
Challenges and Opportunities Posed by Artificial Intelligence for Pediatrics

Susan E. Zinner
http://orcid.org/0009-0007-0746-582X
Indiana University Northwest, USA

ABSTRACT

The author reviews the development of artificial intelligence (AI) and how it has impacted patient care, including pediatric patient care. While there have been positive developments, such as better diagnostic options, unknown risks remain, such as data breaches, privacy and confidentiality concerns and poor modeling. AI will likely impact informed consent and the author considers both the positive and negative ramifications of allowing AI to play a larger role in this process. She concludes with recommendations for incorporating AI into pediatric healthcare with the goal of protecting vulnerable children.

INTRODUCTION

Perhaps no recent technological development in medicine generates more anxiety than current and potential uses of artificial intelligence (AI). With limited guidance from developers or regulatory control by user nations, AI breakthroughs may be moving more quickly than we can respond. While offering advantages such as relieving health workers from mundane--but necessary--tasks, AI poses potential dangers to patient privacy and raises many new and unexplored ethical and legal concerns in

DOI: 10.4018/979-8-3373-2577-4.ch005

an era of rapidly-developing knowledge. Indeed, while medical information took about 50 years to double in 1950, by 2020, this knowledge is believed to double every 73 days (Aylward, et al., 2022, p. 126).

When AI was first introduced, however, its potential was not yet fully understood. MIT Professor John McCarthy was the first to suggest that computers could be taught to simulate intelligence and solve problems (1956), eventually theorizing that computers may be capable of human-like reasoning skills in performing tasks (1959). By tackling complex problems using machine learning (ML), a discipline within AI, statistical methods are used to evaluate data; this set of data is used to train the model and, once tested for validation, these models can predict outcomes using new data sets (Weeks & Ferres, 2024, pp. 33-35). These ML methods were referred to as statistical methods in the past (Ferres, 2024, p. 9). The unique value of AI is that it can replace human reason and even human decision-making (Berghea, et al., 2024, p. 240). The recent explosion of AI development and use is the result of both the increase in processing power and the reduced cost to store data (Ferres, 2024, p. 11). ML refers to AI methodologies that possess an adaptive element which allows them to "learn" using data; as more data is input, typically more accurate outcomes, including medical diagnoses and treatment plans, result (Aylward, 2022, p. 126). In the context of healthcare, these data sets can be used to train the system to learn from similar patients or health outcomes, which allows the algorithm to become more accurate as the data sets increase and more data is added (Aylward, et al., 2022, p. 218) resulting in better predictions as it "learns" from the information. The result is typically a generalizable conclusion about how a specific type of patient tends to respond to a medical intervention, including the associated risks, benefits and alternatives, allowing the physician to recommend a course of action to the patient. The data can also be used to identify symptoms of an illness or condition which may be rare or unknown to the medical team.

Many patients may be unaware of the ways in which AI is currently used in medical care. One study found that 222 medical devices and databases contained AI elements in the United States, compared to 240 items in Europe (Berghea, et al., 2024, p. 247), indicating that some aspects of AI are now standard during patient encounters. This is a tool whose impact is only destined to grow.

BACKGROUND

AI offers the promise of enhanced care for more people but continues to pose risks. Advocates argue that remote monitoring, improved access to care, and supported decision-making (Alkhamis, 2025, pp. 14-15) are likely. Also, AI will be able to examine data sets in new and unexplored ways to ascertain whether there are non-linear relationships between specific variables to better explain causal relationships in illness (Weeks, 2024, p. 7-8). One of the areas of greatest potential impact, this use could be used to ascertain the causation of particular medical conditions where none have yet been identified.

AI has been used as a diagnostic tool in radiology where it has often performed better than clinicians (Bhargava, et al., 2024, p. e49022). Other uses for patients include personalized treatments, predictive analytics in outbreaks and other scenarios, telemedicine, anticipating potential drug interactions, robotic surgeries, improving quality of care by providers and possibly even gene editing (Wade, 2023, pp. 15-17). Further anticipated benefits include reducing burnout of providers (by handing off mundane tasks to AI so providers can focus on other tasks), more precision care, better patient outcomes, enhanced collaboration and continuous learning and improvement (Zach, 2024, pp. 5-6).

Another intriguing use is the possibility of improving public health. Since an estimated four billion people have no or limited access to providers, AI has the potential for reducing this disparity. One AI program empowering community health workers involves the diagnosing of conditions such as diabetic retinopathy, chronic otitis media and leprosy (now referred to as Hansen's Disease) to better use limited health dollars (Ferres & Weeks, 2024, p. 325). In those areas where there are not enough practitioners (such as child and adolescent psychiatry), AI can minimize and streamline administrative tasks, allowing providers more time to focus on patient care (Aylward, et al., 2022). Long-term dividends resulting from an AI-focused public health approach include reduced disability rates (which reduces governmental disability payments), improvement of the health of the working population (which increases productivity and tax revenue) and possibly helping citizens to get better-paying jobs (which increases discretionary spending, expands the gross national product and increases tax revenue) (Ferres & Weeks, 2024, pp. 326-7).

AI may also be a valuable tool in developing informed consent forms for research and medical treatment purposes. One challenge is to balance the twin goals of readability (to enhance subject comprehension) while ensuring that all relevant information is shared with subjects and patients. A recent study found that AI-generated informed consent forms performed as well as human-generated forms in the areas of transmission of the purpose of the study and in describing the duration and procedure of the clinical trial (Shi, et al., 2025, e68139). However, the human-generated form was slightly better in discussing alternatives, while the AI-generated form did better in explaining the benefits of the study (Shi, et al., 2025, e68139). The authors noted that human oversight is likely to enhance future AI-generated informed consent forms (Shi, et al., 2025, e69139).

There are also some areas in which AI simply performs better than humans in the same scenario. For instance, the Biomed Central Medical Journal found that the use of AI resulted in 30 percent fewer medication errors compared to human providers (Zach, 2024, p. 39). In areas where human error is more likely, such as prescribing and filling prescriptions, AI will clearly benefit users.

However, as with any new technology, risks, including as yet unknown risks, exist. One significant risk in relying on AI involves the possibility of not fully understanding the data and incorrectly assuming causation when AI shows a correlation between two variables. "Simply because a machine learning model can predict outcomes based on certain data doesn't indicate that those data **cause** (emphasis added) the predicted outcome" (Ferres, 2024, p. 15). ML is helpful in discovering patterns and possibly predicting key variables that may lead to the development of a theory regarding causation, but it remains a tool only. As epidemiologists often remind us, correlation is not causation.

Bias can also be an issue since algorithms can mirror existing biases in healthcare (Ferres, 2024, p. 17). Using data sets which exclude specific marginalized groups may lead to inappropriate conclusions. Unreliable data sets generate unreliable conclusions. "Exploring the dataset's history, politics, and source of funding is crucial, especially because these factors can relate to the oppression and marginalisation of young people and families" (Boch, et al., 2022). If a particular population group is either excluded or underrepresented in the AI data set, the results may not be generalizable to the entire population. "Representative populations for most conditions, including in pediatrics, are not a homogeneous group. Thus, it is essential that the data sets used to train these models include balanced data with diverse representations of the clinical symptoms across gender, age, and race for the model to be generalizable" (Aylward, 2022, e133). Ideally, the populations used by AI should be representative of the entire group at risk for the illness or condition, but minorities and other groups are not always included in this data. Of the underrepresented populations, children are one significant group. Children may be routinely excluded from research to protect their vulnerable status or if parents refuse to consent, but doing so also means that we have little information about how children may respond to a treatment or drug being tested.

Another concern is that overreliance on models may be risky. Ferres (2024, p. 21) notes that trusting models that relied on inaccurate assumptions as bankers and regulators did during the 2008 housing crisis in the United States can impact many people and lead to unanticipated consequences. Risky lending practices by some banks and limited regulation and oversight were just two of several reasons that the market was shaken; these criteria had not been included in models used to anticipate the future housing market direction. Few people in the housing and banking industries expected the resulting chaos. Models that have proven effective over time may lead providers to conclude the model is still accurate when inputs or the environment may have changed so that the conclusions are no longer valid.

Finally, there are concerns about data protection and privacy. Data breaches pose the possibility of great harm; medical data needs to be protected. Hospitals, labs and all those entrusted with medical information need to have patient privacy protection in place. An incorrect piece of information could conceivably follow a patient for decades, impacting health decisions both now and in the future.

Perhaps the most fundamental right in healthcare is patient autonomy. When parents must make medical decisions for their minor children, the default presumption is that parents are the best decision-makers. The legal standard used in most jurisdictions for providers sharing information with adults is that they must provide all the information a reasonable patient would want (the "reasonable person" standard noted in *Canterbury v. Spence,* 464 F.2d.772, 782 D.C. Cir. 1972), while parents must choose a course on behalf of their minor child. There are several legal exceptions when children may make their own decisions. Depending on the jurisdiction, mature minors (those children who are chronologically children but exhibit an adult-like understanding of their health issue) and emancipated minors (those children who have gone to court to obtain a document which substitutes for parental consent if the judge feels that the child understands the health issues involved or who fit into a specific category, such as serving in the armed forces, married, etc.) may make their own medical decisions. Physicians ascertain the maturity level of the child in mature minor exceptions, while the judge makes this determination for emancipated minors. Typically, these minors are questioned about their understanding of the upcoming medical decision which needs to be made; evidence of an adult-like understanding of the upcoming treatment or procedure will convince the provider or judge. Furthermore, depending on state law, minors may be able to consent for services such as sexual assault care, contraceptives, STD care, prenatal care, abortion, care for minor children of the minor, substance abuse treatment, outpatient mental health treatment and immunizations (Davis & Fang, 2025), indicating a state policy that treatment may supersede parental consent or parental involvement when the risks associated with an illness are significant and treatment is generally non-invasive and proven effective.

However, even minors without full appreciation for the risks and benefits of a treatment or procedure still have the right to provide assent, which does not rise to the legal standard of informed consent. The physician and parents should consider the views of the child, but this will not generally override the parental decision. Such an approach evidences respect for the minor patient and the patient's developing autonomy rights. Providers are responsible for determining when minors show sufficient cognitive maturity to contribute their views to the medical discussion and decision and when the minor can make the decision alone without parental involvement. Providers are obligated to act in the best interests of the pediatric patient and not necessarily defer to the parent's wishes; parents are obligated to support the minor's best interests and preserve a family's interest as opposed to acting in their own autonomous interests (Davis & Fang, 2025).

This can be a little tricky for all involved. The challenge for providers, legislators and others is determining when to grant more power to the child and when to defer to parental authority. Since children mature (cognitively, emotionally and physically) at different rates, this line is not always clear. To provide guidance, AI has developed tools. Using what has been referred to as 7P medicine (referencing AI as personalized, predictive, preventive, participatory, precise, peripheral and poly-professional) (Indrio, et al., 2024), AI is making a significant change to the provision of healthcare. Of these 7Ps, participatory medicine is one of the key areas likely to impact pediatrics. AI "enhances participatory medicine by providing tools that empower patients and families to actively engage in decision-making and care management...These tools not only improve transparency and communication but also empower families to take in active role in managing chronic conditions" (Indrio, et al., 2024, p. e11429). Using pediatric data sets based on similar patients, AI can guide the pediatric triad (physician, parent and child) in making a medically-appropriate decision. This information is used when the physician shares relevant information with the parents about the options available to the patient. A largely-unexplored area, however, is how AI will impact this process as the child matures. The data sets used are static while each child's maturation is dynamic.

MAIN FOCUS OF THIS CHAPTER

The main focus of this chapter is to address the advantages and disadvantages of the use of AI in pediatric medical encounters and to recommend an approach designed to protect vulnerable children when receiving medical care.

ANALYSIS

In a typical mature minor or emancipated minor situation, the former triad (parent, child and doctor) involved in decision-making becomes a dyad (child and physician). However, the role of AI in this dyad is not fully understood. Should we consider AI as a full partner in decision-making or is AI merely an aid to the physician? Are two or three entities involved in this relationship? As Cohen and Slottje note, if "information is produced by the AI *interpreting* data rather than simply *reporting* it (emphasis in original), then this changes how we view the informed consent process since AI may be thought of as serving as a substitute physician in the former case (2024, p. 173). Furthermore, will the parent and child view the assistance of AI, assuming its use is shared by the pediatrician, as of less, the same or greater authority than the doctor relying on this information? And is the physician obligated to share both AI's recommendation and the physician's recommendations if they diverge? In a survey of parents, over 90 percent of respondents wanted extensive details about how AI contributed to the doctor's formulation of the risks and benefits of treatment or diagnosis of the child, regardless of the educational levels of the parents (Berghea,et al., 2024). Must the pediatrician reveal the extent to which AI has contributed to the risks and benefits shared with the patient and family? Are the family and patient entitled to know that the physician disagrees with the AI recommendations?

"Even if the AI system acting in concert with the physician has been proven by clinical trials to do more good and avoid more harm than the physician acting alone, it is ultimately the patient's prerogative to determine the benefit of the "good," the burden of the "harm," and the acceptable balance of benefit and burden" (Binkley & Loftus, 2024, p. 31-2). The legal role of AI in this context is not fully understood. Will there be shared liability if an unanticipated event occurs after the patient follows the AI-enhanced physician recommendation? Can the physician be true to every physician's fiduciary obligation to protect patients when using AI? Or does this fiduciary obligation demand that physicians use AI to enhance their treatment recommendations and provide a complete recommendation to parents and children? As Binkley and Loftus write, "[t]he system becomes a third party in the physician-patient relationship, without moral or legal responsibility, without the professional ethical duties that attend the physician, and potentially with the expectation that more weight will be given to its clinical decisions than the physician's (2024, p. 45). Wade and others have suggested that the ideal model will be when AI and the physician work in tandem, since physicians "cannot abdicate their professional judgment solely to an algorithm, especially in complex or life-threatening cases" (2023, p. 98).

Interestingly, two authors suggest that total disclosure may work **against** (emphasis in original) the patient's autonomy interests if the patient tends to rely on AI information to the exclusion of other significant pieces of information (Cohen & Slottje, 2024, p. 178). This places the burden on physicians to share relevant information, but not, as these two writers suggest, the totality of information. Noting that just as pharmaceutical patient package inserts do not require patients to understand pharmacology, "it is not obvious why the opaque workings of an AI system require a different approach" (Cohen & Slottje, 2024, p. 178).

What AI can do best, perhaps, is to aid the physician in diagnosis and treatment decisions, based on previous data sets where proven correlations—and perhaps causation—has been shown. Given the overwhelming amount of medical information available, AI can sift and sort current studies and patient data sets to help make patient recommendations. An estimated 2 million peer-reviewed journal articles are published each year—that's one article every 30 seconds—and AI can use this information in a way that its human counterpart cannot (Topol, 2019, p. 138). This massive amount of information, however, can also deter good doctor-patient-parent information sharing. Doctors may rely on AI for diagnosis information "without a strong incentive to delve into the precise operating mechanisms of medical AI, thus impairing the accuracy of information provided to patients…the continual evolution and expeditious modification of AI algorithms intensifies this challenge, exacerbating the difficulty of disclosing accurate information" (Wang & Ma, 2023, p. 49).

However, the role of the physician is only one of the unknowns. It is not yet clear how parental attitudes and beliefs will impact decision-making. In a survey of parents, Sisk, et al. found that those surveyed were open to AI use in their encounters with pediatricians an average of 3.4 (using a Likert scale of 1-5) in functions such as diagnosis, risk prediction, treatment selection and medical guidance (2020). Those who tended to be or lean Democratic were more open to AI use in this context; personality traits of parents who were open to AI use included extroversion, openness to change and emotional stability (2020). Social justice, quality, cost and convenience were also correlated with openness to AI (Sisk, et al., 2020).

And yet, parents do not always agree with their children. Minors are generally able to respond to health questions and surveys from around age 8 and their views may not be the same as that of their parents (Hargreaves, et al., 2018, p. 490). In a survey of pediatric inpatients and parents, researchers found that children were significantly more likely than their parents to report pain and were less likely to agree that providers did everything possible to reduce pain, that they felt safe in the hospital, that they were involved in their healthcare decision-making and that they were given adequate privacy (Hargreaves, 2018, p. 490). Interestingly, they were more likely to be positive than their parents about hospital food (Hargreaves, 2018, p. 490). If children disagree with their parents about these issues, then it is possible that children also may disagree with their parents about treatment decisions, making the obtaining of assent more challenging (even before AI is added as another factor to consider). Being aware of potential areas of disagreement is crucial in respecting developing pediatric autonomy.

FUTURE RESEARCH DIRECTIONS

Ensure that Data Transparency is in Place for All Patients, Including Pediatric Patients

While all patients expect data transparency, the risks to children when this fails to happen are different than those of adults. A provider may rely heavily on this information to make health recommendations for the minor patient. An inappropriate treatment choice based on misleading AI content has the potential to follow a patient for life. This puts pediatric patients at risk for possibly many decades if doctors depend on this information in subsequent medical care without independent verification.

Also, the possibility of two-tiered patient care exists in those cases where some parents or patients request that AI not be used when offered a choice. There is evidence that parents with lower levels of education may object to AI use more frequently than parents with higher educational levels, although all parents agreed that it was important to include physician oversight of any AI contributions to the diagnosis or treatment recommendations (Berghea, et al., 2024). The major concern identified by parents when medical AI was used was the possibility of errors (70.1 percent) while the concern about the risk of loss of confidentiality in data was the least concern (19.6 percent) (Berghea, et al., 2024). Those parents and mature or emancipated minors asking providers to exclude AI information in reaching a treatment decision or diagnosis risk excluding valuable information in that process. Nevertheless, this remains a right that can be exercised.

Another challenge is that the AI system may be preset to value specific results. They might be "encoded to prioritize nonclinical outcomes, such as cost savings or efficiency, the achievement of which ignores patient preferences or values" (Bingley & Loftus, 2024, p. 70). While patients may presume that the physician and AI system will serve as their advocates, prior encoding may make that less likely. A well-informed patient should be aware of these criteria built into algorithms.

In a related issue, it is also crucial that patients understand that their private medical information may be included in a database. This is part of the ongoing collection of data that makes algorithms accurate (since the database contains so much patient data), but patients may not understand that inputting their information into AI means that AI will capture it and include it in future medical decisions. In effect, the patient becomes both a user of the system and a piece of the data set being used to make these decisions. While the information will likely be de-identified, there are some patients who may not wish their information collected. Since de-identified data is typically used for AI training purposes, it is possible that this information can be re-identified later, especially for children with rare genetic diseases where the disease population is low, resulting in a loss of privacy and possible harm (Chng, et al., 2025). Patients may not understand that they are consenting to be both a data donor and a learning subject when their information is input by the physician (Binkley & Loftus, 2024, p. 81). A reasonable patient may not feel that an AI recommendation is worth the potential loss of privacy.

Since parents are involved in pediatric decision-making in the case of young children, transparency is important in the context of parental consent. As noted earlier, one study found that 90.5 percent of parents expect "extensive details" about the use of AI when the physician provides information (Berghea, et al., 2024). An important part of transparency includes the attempt to increase explainability and interpretability of AI recommendations (Chng, et al., 2025). A consent (by a parent or mature or emancipated minor child) or assent (by a child patient) is only meaningful if the information is provided in understandable language. To further enhance child autonomy where appropriate, UNICEF recommends that children be given control over their own medical data, much as adults are, including the ability to access, securely share, comprehend the use of and delete data, contingent upon their maturity level (Chng, et al., 2025).

Create and Actively Maintain an Ethical Framework for AI Use in the Healthcare of Children During the Assent/Informed Consent Process

Development and ongoing use of an appropriate ethical framework is essential when addressing ethical issues in AI use, especially in pediatrics given the inherent vulnerability of children. Beauchamp and Childress proposed the use of four key virtues in medical ethics decades ago; these include autonomy, beneficence, non-maleficence and justice (2019). Each is relevant to this discussion. Autonomy refers to the freedom of patients to make their own decisions which reflect their unique values; the best decision, even in the same factual situation, will vary from patient to patient since values differ. Beneficence refers to the obligation of providers to do good and is consistent with the Hippocratic Oath. Nonmaleficence means that providers should not cause harm to patients. Interestingly, Beauchamp and Childress included both beneficence and nonmaleficence as distinct virtues, implying that the two are not the same and may differ at times. Finally, justice is generally used to refer to the fair allocation of societal resources, including healthcare access.

Perhaps the most crucial virtue is that of autonomy, which is at the foundation of our healthcare system in the United States and many countries. AI has the potential to increase patient autonomy and to assist parents, children and providers to make better decisions. One way that AI can increase patient autonomy is via personalized medicine. Pediatric patients may prove challenging since there is a great deal of variability in growth, development and disease symptoms among children and children may have difficulty explaining the symptoms clearly (Indrio, et al., 2024, p. 2). AI can enhance the personalization of treatment plans by integrating genetic information, addressing environmental factors and considering patient history to develop an individualized care plan for that child (Indrio, et al., p. 2).

Autonomy in informed consent and assent with pediatric patients poses some unique challenges once AI is added to the mix. "Generating autonomy-protective informed consent rules for AI may be a challenge not just because patients are different from medical professionals but because patients are different from each other" (Cohen & Slottje, 2024, p. 179). An ethical framework will help determine how best to communicate the role of AI in this process. Cohen and Slottje have proposed a framework where enhanced trust between the doctor and patient (and parent, if applicable) would be an appropriate legal standard (2024, p. 179). Kaye has suggested that a participant-centered initiative (PCI) is a better option than traditional "'one-on-one' discussions with appropriately trained health professionals [that] ends with the signing of a paper-based informed consent form. The focus is on obtaining one-time consent rather than seeking to understand or to think more broadly about the interests and concerns of patients…as they evolve over time" (2012, p. 372). When providers address the pediatric patient's evolving need for information, a more thorough consent can be obtained. Although Kaye addressed informed consent obtained during research, the proposal is also ideal for pediatric patients seeking medical treatment whose cognitive skills vary and mature at different rates. As additional information is shared with the child as the child matures, different decisions may be made given the change in maturity level, understanding and possible shift in values. Kaye calls this approach dynamic and notes that this process

> *"allows interactions over time; it enables participants to consent to new projects or to alter their consent choices in real time as their circumstances change and to have confidence that these changed choices will take effect…By using a technology-based platform, the consent process is not, as is often the case with paper-based documentation of consent, locked in time to the beginning of the research process…These preferences can be 'opt ins' or 'opt outs;' participants can tailor their profiles to receive no information for specified periods of time or to give a broad consent if they so wish." (2015, p. 143).*

Patients or research subjects won't need to continually give consent, but dynamic consent gives this group the opportunity to stay as engaged as they wish (Kaye, et al., 2015, p. 144). In effect, the consent moves forward with the patient or subject until that person chooses to amend it. This approach allows subjects to consent to new projects or alter their consent in real time as their circumstances evolve (Kaye, et al., 2015, p. 142). An 'opt in' or 'opt out' reduces what has been called "consent fatigue" so that willing participants may choose a broad consent approach and not request frequent updates (Kaye, et al., 2015, p. 143). Others warn that we remain unsure of the potential negative impact of AI systems on children, including the risk of dependency on a system taking the place of a formerly-human actor (Skulmowski, 2025, p. 33).

Chng, et al. have proposed a framework which addresses these ethical concerns and emphasizes transparency, ensuring that the child's voice is heard and respected, emphasizing equitable access, promotion of government and business development of a child-centered AI and other features (2025, p. 152). Beneficence is addressed via ensuring that current and new AI systems address child well-being and development, while nonmaleficence focuses on the safety of the child using AI (Chng, 2025, p. 152). Finally, justice in the context of AI includes justice, non-discrimination and equitable access to these services (Chng, 2025, p. 152).

During the assent/informed consent process, autonomy refers to the child's freedom to access and make use of the information provided by both the provider and AI and the right of the child to be informed of the role of AI in providing this information. While providers defer to parents when the child is cognitively immature and cannot make decisions, the opinion of the child should, at a minimum, be solicited. Mature and/or emancipated minors may act as adults in the informed consent process and may choose to use AI or not, to be guided by AI in reaching treatment decisions or not just as an adult would. Beneficence and non-malificence are present when the child is treated with respect and honesty, ensuring that transparency exists and no one is attempting to take advantage of the child. Non-maleficence involves "convincing evidence that [AI systems] involve no harm or that benefits can be confidently expected to outweigh harm, notwithstanding any benefits that it can bring to the children. Evidence-based health informatics (EBHI) supports the use of concrete scientific evidence in decision-making" (Chng, 2025, p. 152). Justice is achieved when the information is free of bias and incorrect information. Ideally, sharing this information will help increase equitable health outcomes in society, despite the concerns raised by some of the digital divide which may prevent low socioeconomic groups from accessing information compared to their wealthier counterparts.

Develop Regulatory and Legal Frameworks for AI Use in Healthcare of Children Where it Serves in an Advisory Role Only

As with many new technologies, innovation often proceeds legal and regulatory guidelines. The risk exists that AI becomes a third party in the physician-patient relationship with no moral or legal responsibilities and no ethical obligations (Binkley & Loftus, 2024, p, 45). This writer proposes the creation of a legal framework where AI is simply a provider of information to the physician and not an interpreter of data. Viewed as merely an additional resource, AI information is incorporated into the information and recommendations provided by the physician. This information enhances information provided by the doctor. There is much evidence to indicate that patients view the doctor-patient relationship or doctor-patient-parent relationship as essential and that AI should never be used as a replacement for human relationships and decision-making (Wade, 2023, p. 103). Wade also notes that medicine should develop a "never-delegate" list, including factors such as empathy and emotional support, ethical decision-making, complex diagnostics, surgical procedures, continuous monitoring and treatment planning all provided by physicians and never AI (2023, p. 103-105). Unlike the physician, AI cannot explain its reasoning in reaching specific recommendations (Binkley & Loftus, 2024, p. 64), another reason to ensure that the physician remains the key entity sharing information. Furthermore, Zach has found that patients are more likely to trust AI-driven recommendations when the physician explains its role (2024, p. 29) and that patient outcomes typically improve when AI is used in conjunction with physician expertise (2024, p. 46). Ideally, "[t]he prediction made by the AI system is checked by a human expert, such that AI augments but does not automate decision-making. The knowledge, skills, experience and judgment of the healthcare professional are important in case contextualization, as no case is "standard" and each child comes with his own unique medical, family and social history" (Chng, et al., 2025, p. e152).

It appears that no organization devoted to children and health has developed comprehensive policy recommendations for AI use and pediatric care. Groups such as the United Nations Children's Fund (UNICEF), the World Health Organization (WHO), the International Pediatric Association, the American Academy of Pediatrics, the Royal College of Paediatrics and Child Health, the International Medical Informatics Association and American Medical Informatics Association have published no guidelines at the time of this writing (Chng, et al., 2025). What does exist are guidelines for AI ethics and governance in adult medicine and several policy documents concerning AI ethics where children are involved, although they fail to discuss child health (Chng, et al., 2025).

When regulating AI, one challenge is that the FDA has not addressed whether medical AI-powered devices may change gradually over time as they learn from the collected data (Bhargava, et al., 2024); the authors raise the concern of "drift" in AI function based on this learning. This refers to the risk that the AI algorithm itself will make changes in its recommendations as it learns from input data and is commonly referred to as clinical decision support (CDS). These changes may be made independently without human intervention, leading to the possibility that no person was involved in this revised clinical decision-making. In its 2025 draft recommendations (Artificial Intelligence-Enabled Device Software Functions: Lifecycle Management and Marketing Recommendations) addressing this concern, the FDA report notes

> *AI-based models may be highly sensitive to variations or changes in model inputs, for example, because they are data-driven and can be self-evolving (i.e., capable of autonomously adapting without any human intervention). Model performance metrics should be monitored on an ongoing basis to ensure that the model remains fit for use and appropriate changes are made to the model, as needed...Due to the evolving nature of AI models, sponsors should anticipate*

inherent, model-directed changes and the need to identify and evaluate those changes, as well as any intentional changes to the model over the drug product life cycle (FDA Guidelines, 2024, p. 16).

The American Medical Informatics Association, in tackling this issue a few years ago, supported the FDA's pre-certification approach where the firm which developed the AI-using device is responsible for ensuring the safety and effectiveness of the product (Petersen, et al., 2021). The group proposed the creation of non-regulatory oversight bodies for self-developed adaptive CDS programs (i.e., institution-developed) and that an accreditation system be developed to manage these systems (Petersen, et al., 2021). The group also noted that the FDA should focus more on premarket data collection to post market performance monitoring (Petersen, et al., 2021). Given concerns about potential changes to AI algorithms with no acknowledgement of these changes to users, this is a valid concern. "Interesting and potentially deleterious challenges, as well as social inequities, may arise if a model that is somehow "approved" can be retrained the next week and behave differently" (Petersen, et al., 2021). Close supervision of these AI tasks will ensure that future generations of children are protected. Chng, et al., however, dismisses this effort given that it fails to address the special needs of children, noting that the United Nations Children's Fund (UNICEF) does a more thorough job as it advocates for a "child-centered approach, which should include safety-by-design, privacy-by-design and inclusion-by-design" (2025).

Incorporate the UNCRC Principles into AI Pediatric Medical Care to Ensure that the Rights of Children Remain Primary

One often-overlooked document that may serve to protect and expand the rights of children in all aspects of their lives is the United Nations Convention on the Rights of the Child (UNCRC). Based on a 1924 document, the Declaration of the Rights of the Child (also called the Geneva Declaration of the Rights of the Child), was later adopted by the League of Nations (Robinson, 2011, p. 20). The United Nations adopted the declaration in 1959 and this was the source of the UNCRC drafted in 1989, which gives children and parents specific rights. There was immediate international support for the UNCRC, which received the required 20 ratifications quickly rendering it binding on September 2, 1990; other countries continued to sign (Himes, 2011, p. 37). The United States remains the only country in the entire world which has failed to sign the UNCRC. This reluctance may be due to the document's prohibition of both corporal punishment in schools and of some kinds of punishment of incarcerated juveniles such as solitary confinement. While it is important to acknowledge that merely being a signatory country does not guarantee compliance with all provisions, it is evidence of aspirational compliance at a minimum.

The guiding principle behind the UNCRC is best interests; all of those working with and caring for children should be guided by making decisions in the best interests of the child. Since the best interests standard also guides physicians in determining what information to provide to patients and parents during the informed consent process, the two could conceivably work hand in hand. Article 3 of the UNCRC mandates

1. In all actions concerning children, whether undertaken by public or private social welfare institutions, courts of law, administrative authorities or legislative bodies, the best interest of the child shall be the primary consideration.
2. States Parties undertake to ensure the child such protection and care as is necessary for his or her well-being, taking into account the rights and duties of his or her parents, legal guardians, or other individuals legally responsible for him, or her, and, to this end, shall take all appropriate legislative and administrative measures.
3. States Parties shall ensure that the institutions, services and facilities responsible for the care or protection of children shall conform with the standards established by competent authorities, particularly in the areas of safety, health, in the number and suitability of their staff, as well as competent supervision" (UNCRC, Art. 3).

This standard includes the child's views, identity, maintenance of family relationships, the child's protection and care, education and health (Kilkelly, 2016, p. 60). Supplementing this approach is Article 12 of the UNCRC mandating participation rights for the child "capable of forming his or her own views" (UNCRC, Art. 12(1)), which would include those capable of assent and those capable of informed consent (mature and emancipated minors). Therefore, combining Articles 3 and 12 the focus on the child's well-being and best interests means listening to their input about choosing an appropriate medical option shared during the consent process. Furthermore, Varadan recommends incorporating Article 5 into this framework (2020) since it specifically references the notion that pediatric cognitive development is always evolving.

"States Parties shall respect the responsibilities, rights and duties of parents or, where applicable, the members of the extended family or community as provided for by local custom, legal guardians or other persons legally responsible for the child, to provide, in a manner consistent with the evolving capacities of the child, appropriate direction and guidance in the exercise by the child of the rights recognized in the present Convention." (UNCRC, Art. 5).

Recognizing that medical decision-making and informed consent is a collaborative process where parents play more significant roles when the child is younger and less significant roles as the child matures is consistent with the spirit of the UNCRC which is premised on the notion that both parties deserve respect and that a child who is technically a minor may be able to make an informed decision that adults should respect. Article 5 mandates respect for the child's "evolving capacity," while Article 12 calls for acting in the "best interests" of the child. Taken together, these three articles call for the child to be placed at the center of decision-making.

Incorporate Non-Monotonic Features into AI Programs Involving Children to Recognize the Developing Cognitive Maturity of Children

AI programs may rely on monotonic reasoning, which means that current information is retained and used to build its knowledge base as more information is learned. This basic information is never discarded and AI operates under the assumption that this information is, and always will be, true and accurate. Systems that depend on these systems include traditional mathematics and logic arguments in philosophy. Once an ML model has learned a fact or rule, it stays fixed unless the model is entirely retrained (Jeevanandam, 2024). This approach suggests that if one starts with some assumptions to reach a conclusion and then adds additional information, new conclusions may result, but that the original information remains correct and is never discarded (Rajaraman, 2014, p. 204). This is how some simplistic systems where the environment does not vary much or need to incorporate new or changing facts, operate.

However, many complex systems use non-monotonic information, which allows AI to revise its conclusions and recommendations when new information is added, a function often referred to as "unlearning" (Jeevanandam, 2024), although it may perhaps more accurately be viewed as a more sophisticated kind of learning since inaccurate models are discarded and replaced with better and more precise information. This model has many advantages. It "allows AI to revise its conclusions when new information becomes available, even if it means "unlearning" or retracting previously held beliefs. This flexibility is key in environments where knowledge is not fixed, and assumptions can change as more data is gathered or circumstances evolve" (Jeevanandam, 2024). It has been suggested that this approach would be useful in healthcare in arriving at a patient's diagnosis. The initial diagnosis may need to be updated as the patient responds or fails to respond to treatment as new tests are administered and the medical diagnosis is revised to include this new information. This incremental learning approach (updating AI models with new information on to of previous—and possibly less accurate--patient data) is ideal for healthcare. The concept of change over time is critical for multiple pediatric-specific conditions and suggests another critical difference from adults: the importance of maturation and growth (Brind'Armour, 2023).

There is another way in which non-monotonic information can be useful. It involves the use of AI models which allow for a custom approach to decision-making. A model could be created for every child facing a medical decision and still legally a minor. Tests to determine the maturity level of the child could be administered prior to every major decision, allowing both parents and provider to ascertain the appropriate level of involvement in this decision. Since cognitive and emotional maturity develop at varying rates, a child deemed too young to make decisions without parental involvement at one point, may be able to play the primary role in a subsequent decision. Parents and medical providers are therefore assured that the decision was reached using adult-like cognitive skills. This allows children to reverse any previous consent, including those provided earlier by parents and includes the 'right to be forgotten' and have their data deleted (Chng, et al., 2025, p. 152). Such an approach is important, argue Cohen & Slottje, because "patients are different from medical professionals, but also because patients are different from each other," noting that some individuals prefer to be only minimally involved in medical decision-making (2024, p. 179). Since researchers and physicians are unable to make consent forms "future proof" and patients and subjects may change their views over time, it is important to not employ a "one size fits all" approach to obtaining consent (Kaye, et al., 2012, p. 372).

Wade refers to this process as one of "continuous consent," (2023, p. 92) which is consistent with the notion that AI will be continuously updating recommendations for the patient when new information is provided. This approach also works in tandem with the legal concept of informed consent. Consent is not viewed as merely the signing (manually or digitally) of documents to protect providers from liability but exists as a dynamic process to allow patients to make more informed decisions.

Incorporating fuzzy logic (an approach used to deal with uncertainty by assigning numerical values to information as opposed to a dichotomous yes/no only approach) with non-monotonic information has the potential to further increase understanding in the presence of uncertainty. In this way, specific information could be assigned value (e.g., ensuring that the principles of bioethics are encoded into decision-making); when attempting this approach, one researcher found that the AI model agreed with bioethicists 75 percent of the time (Binkley & Loftus, 2024, p. 117-18).

To be meaningful and ensure that the pediatric patient plays an appropriate role in these scenarios, that patient must also have the right to decline treatment. Even if providers and parents disagree, the law allows young people who have a mature understanding of their condition to decline treatment, even if death becomes likely. When the child is very young and parents are playing the leading role in decision-making, this "power asymmetry inherent in these exchanges" can be reduced if the provider encourages sharing of concerns and values from the parents while parents share information about the family's values and goals (Salter, et al., 2023). Varadan notes that different international codes view the assent and dissent of minor children differently. For instance, the Declaration of Helsinki (2013) requires respect of a child's assent and dissent, while the UNESCO Declaration on Bioethics and Human Rights (2005), asserts respect for the child's assent is not required, while respect for pediatric dissent is mandated (2020, p. 527-28). Despite these inconsistencies, it is crucial to recognize that AI must recognize and respect the developing cognitive maturity of children.

Humanize AI Systems Used to the Extent Possible to Protect and Maintain the Humanity Inherent in Medicine

The prospect of medical AI playing a significant role in patient decisions can be frightening to many people. These AI tools can be potent ways to protect patient autonomy. To ascertain the values of children on the receiving end of AI-enhanced medical care, a group of researchers surveyed English youths aged 10-21 years. One of three themes emerging from this survey is what the researchers termed "human centredness'," (Visram, et al., 2023, p. 441). (The two others were governance and trust). Those surveyed expressed concern that AI may be incapable of empathy, understanding pain experienced by patients and likely to be unable to break bad news appropriately (Visram, et al., 2023, p. 442). Two interesting—and, as yet, unanswered—issues raised include "Will doctors need to be less qualified if the use of AI is normalized?" and whether AI "is just helping and does not replace humans" (Visram, et al., 2023, p. 442).

There are also generational variations in AI-enhanced healthcare. While Millennials prioritize convenience and focus on digital healthcare, Baby Boomers tend to prioritize face-to-face interactions with their providers and create long-term relationships with providers (Wade, 2023, p. 67). AI can incorporate these age-related differences in their algorithms.

Wang and Ma suggest that one simple way to keep the patient at the center of these discussions is to provide upfront information about the use of AI in medical diagnosis and treatment protocols. If the patient chooses to exclude any AI-generated information, then that patient is entitled to receive a "conventional physician-derived diagnostic plan aimed at replicating the intended outcomes. In addition, patients maintain sovereignty over their health care decisions, irrespective of the doctor's belief in the superiority of AI-assisted diagnostic strategies" (Wang & Ma, 2025, p. 51).

CONCLUSION

While AI holds the potential for a better patient experience, including high-quality medical care and the use of vast sets of database information to create a personalized medical diagnosis and treatment plan, AI still poses some potential risks to patients. Concerns about potential privacy issues, data breaches, unresolved legal issues, the need to establish an ethical framework for the use of AI remain unresolved. There are also unanswered questions about the impact of AI on pediatric patients and their parents, including the amount of information to be shared by providers with parents and pediatric patients, how the regulatory and legal environment could be best structured to make good use of AI information and how research and medical care will be impacted—particularly the informed consent process—by AI. To best protect children, these questions need to be answered before technology overtakes our informational needs, including how to best incorporate bioethical principles in this process.

AI also has the potential to ease the informed consent process for children and their parents. Using a dynamic, non-monotonic approach, information can be easily shared in ways that the pediatric patient understands and it can become more sophisticated as the child increases in cognitive maturity until the child ultimately becomes the sole decision maker. With the goal of ensuring the protection of autonomy for all patients, especially pediatric patients, AI must become a governable tool of providers premised on the prospect of enhanced autonomy for all.

REFERENCES

Alkhamis, Z. (2025). *The Implementation of Telehealth and AI in Pediatrics: Smarter Solutions for the Modern World.* Independently published.

Aylward, B. S., Abbas, H., Taraman, S., Salomon, C., Gal-Szabo, D., Kraft, C., Ehwerhemuepha, L., Chang, A., & Wall, D. P. (2022). An Introduction to Artificial Intelligence in Developmental and Behavioral Pediatrics. *Journal of Behavioral Pediatrics, 44*(2), e126–e134. DOI: 0.1097/DBP.0000000000001149 PMID: 36730317

Beauchamp, T. L., & Childress, J. F. (2019). *Principles of Biomedical Ethics* (8th ed.). Oxford University Press.

Berghea, E. C., Ionescu, M. D., Gheorghiu, R. M., Tincu, J. F., Cobilinschi, C. O., Craiu, M., Bălgrădean, M., & Berghea, F. (2024). Integrating Artificial Intelligence in Pediatric Healthcare: Parental Perceptions and Ethical Implications. *Children (Basel, Switzerland), 11*(2), 240–252. DOI: 10.3390/children11020240 PMID: 38397353

Bhargava, H., Salomon, C., Suresh, S., Chang, A., Kilian, R., van Stijn, D., Orio, A., Low, D., Knebel, A., & Taraman, S. (2024). Promises, Pitfalls, and Clinical Applications of Artificial Intelligence in Pediatrics. *Journal of Medical Internet Research, 26*, e49022. DOI: 10.2196/49022 PMID: 38421690

Binkley, C., & Loftus, T. (2024). *Encoding Bioethics: AI in Clinical Decision-Making*. University of California Press.

Boch, S., Sezgin, E., & Linwood, S. L. (2022). Ethical Artificial Intelligence in Paediatrics. *The Lancet. Child & Adolescent Health, 6*(12), 833–835. DOI: 10.1016/S2352-4642(22)00243-7 PMID: 36084667

Chng, S. Y., Tern, M. J. W., Lee, Y. S., Cheng, L. T., Kapur, J., Eriksson, J. G., Chong, Y. S., & Savulescu, J. (2025). Ethical Considerations in AI for Child Health and Recommendations for Child-Centered Medical AI. *NPJ Digital Medicine, 8*(1), 152. DOI: 10.1038/s41746-025-01541-1 PMID: 40065130

Cohen, G., & Slottje, A. (2024). Artificial Intelligence and the Law of Informed Consent. In Solaiman, B., & Cohen, G. (Eds.), *Research Handbook on Health, AI and the Law* (pp. 167–182). Edward Elgar Publishing. DOI: 10.4337/9781802205657.ch10

Davis, M., & Fang, A. (2025). Emancipated Minor. *StatPearls*. StatPearls Publishing. https://www.ncbi.nlm.nih.gov/books/NBK554594

FDA M15 General Principles for Model-Informed Drug Development. (2024). https://www.fda.gov/regulatory-information-search-fda-guidance-documents/m15-general-prinicples-model-informed-drug-development

Ferres, J. M. L. (2024). Artificial Intelligence: Its Applications andLlimitations. In Ferres, J. M. L., & Weeks, W. B. (Eds.), *AI for Good: Applications in Sustainability, Humanitarian Action, and Health* (pp. 9–32). Wiley.

Hargreaves, D. S., Sizmur, S., Pitchforth, J., Tallett, A., Toomey, S., Toomey, S. L., Hopwood, B., Schuster, M. A., & Viner, R. M. (2018). Children and Young People's Versus Parents' Responses in an English National Inpatient Survey. *Archives of Disease in Childhood, 103*(5), 486–491. DOI: 10.1136/archdischild-2017-313801 PMID: 29434020

Himes, J. R. (2011). The UN Convention on the Rights of the Child: More Than a New Utopia? In C. Rutgers (Ed.). *Creating a World Fit for Children: Understanding the UN Convention on the Rights of the Child,* (pp 37-44). International Debate Educational Association.

Indrio, F., Pettoello-Mantovani, M., Giardino, I., & Masciari, E. (2024). The Role of Artificial Intelligence in Pediatrics From Treating Illnesses to Managing Children's Overall Well-Being. *The Journal of Pediatrics, 275*, 11429. DOI: 10.1016/j.jpeds.2024.114291 PMID: 39242077

Jeevanandam, N. (2024). Making AI smarter: Why machines need to unlearn to learn, *Emeritus,* https://emeritusorg/in/non-montonic-reasoning-in-ai.

Kaye, J., Curren, L., Anderson, N., Edwards, K., Fullerton, S. M., Kanellopoulou, N., Lund, D., MacArthur, D. G., Mascalzoni, D., Shepherd, J., Taylor, P. L., Terry, S. F., & Winter, S. F. (2012). From Patients to Partners: Participant-Centric Initiatives in Biomedical Research. *Nature Reviews. Genetics, 13*(5), 371–376. DOI: 10.1038/nrg3218 PMID: 22473380

Kaye, J., Whitley, E. A., Lund, D., Morrison, M., Teare, H., & Melham, K. (2015). Dynamic Consent: A Patient Interface for Twenty-First Century Research Networks. *European Journal of Human Genetics : EJHG, 23*(2), 141–146. DOI: 10.1038/ejhg.2014.71 PMID: 24801761

Kilkelly, U. (2016). The Best Interests of the Child: A Gateway to Children's Rights? In Sutherland, E. E., & Macfarlane, L. B. (Eds.), *Implementing Article 3 of the United Nations Convention on the Rights of the Child: Best Interests, Welfare and Well-being* (pp. 51–66). Cambridge University Press. DOI: 10.1017/9781316662977.004

McCarthy, J. (1956). https://www.formal.stanford.edu/jmc/index.html

McCarthy, J. (1959, December). Programs with Common Sense. *Proceedings of the Teddington Conference on the Mechanization of Thought Processes.*

Petersen, C., Smith, J., Freimuth, R. R., Goodman, K. W., Jackson, G. P., Kannry, J., Liu, H., Madhavan, S., Sittig, D. F., & Wright, A. (2021). Recommendations for the Safe, Effective Use of Adaptive CDS in the U.S. Healthcare System: An AMIA Position Paper. *Journal of the American Medical Informatics Association : JAMIA, 28*(4), 677–684. DOI: 10.1093/jamia/ocaa319 PMID: 33447854

Rajaraman, V. (2014). John McCarthy: Father of Artificial Intelligence. *Resonance, 19*(3), 198–207. DOI: 10.1007/s12045-014-0027-9

Robinson, S. (2011). Children's Rights: Historic Developments. In C. Rutgers (Ed.). *Creating a World Fit for Children: Understanding the UN Convention on the rights of the Child,* (pp. 16-25). International Debate Education Association.

Salter, E. K., Hester, D. M., Vinarcsik, L., Antommaria, A. H. M., Bester, J., Blustein, J., Clayton, E. W., Diekema, D. S., Itlis, A. S., Kopelman, L., Malone, J. R., Mercurio, M. R., Navin, M. C., Paquette, E. T., Pope, T. M., Rhodes, R., & Ross, L. F. (2024). Pediatric Decision Making: Consensus Recommendations. *Pediatrics, 152*(3), e2023061832. DOI: 10.1542/peds.2023-061832 PMID: 37555276

Shi, Q., Luzuriaga, K., Allison, J. J., Oztekin, A., Faro, J. M., Lee, J. L., Hafter, N., McManus, M., & Zai, A. H. (2025). Transforming Informed Consent Generation Using Large Language Models: Mixed Methods Study. *JMIR Medical Informatics, 13*, e368139. DOI: 10.2196/68139 PMID: 39946400

Sisk, B. A., Antes, A. L., & DuBois, J. M. (2020). Parental Attitudes Toward Artificial Intelligence-Driven Precision Medicine Technologies in Pediatric Healthcare. *Children (Basel, Switzerland), 7*(9), 145. DOI: 10.3390/children7090145 PMID: 32962204

Skulmowski, A. (2025). Informed Consent in Educational AI Research Needs to Be Transparent, Flexible and Dynamic. *Mind, Brain and Education : the Official Journal of the International Mind, Brain, and Education Society, 19*(1), 32–36. DOI: 10.1111/mbe.12435

Topol, E. (2019). *Deep Medicine: How Artificial Intelligence Can Make Healthcare Human Again*. Basic Books.

UNESCO. (2006, June). Universal declaration on bioethics and human rights. Paris. https://unesdoc.unesco.org/images/0014/001461/146180E.pdf

United Nations Convention on the Rights of the Child, Nov. 20, 1989, 1577 U.N.T.S. 3.

Varadan, S. (2020). Article 5: The Role of Parents in the Proxy Informed Consent Process in Medical Research Involving Children. *International Journal of Children's Rights*, *28*(3), 521–546. DOI: 10.1163/15718182-02803009

Visram, S., Leyden, D., Annesley, O., Bappa, D., & Sebire, N. J. (2023). Engaging Children and Young People on the Potential Role of Artificial Intelligence in Medicine. *Pediatric Research*, *93*(2), 440–444. DOI: 10.1038/s41390-022-02053-4 PMID: 35393524

Wade, S.B. (2023). *Transforming Healthcare: AI in Healthcare Leads to Greater Accuracy and Precision, Minimizing Discrepancies and Improving Patient Outcomes*. Independently published.

Wang, Y., & Ma, Z. (2023). Ethical and Legal Examples of Medical AI on Informed Consent: China as an Example. *Developing World Bioethics*, *25*(1), 46–54. DOI: 10.1111/dewb.12442 PMID: 38240080

Weeks, W. B. (2024). What is Artificial Intelligence and How Can It Be Used for Good. In Ferres, J. M. L., & Weeks, W. B. (Eds.), *AI for Good: Applications in Sustainability, Humanitarian Action, and Health* (pp. 3–8). Wiley.

Weeks, W. B., & Ferres, J. M. L. (2024). Commonly Used Processes and Terms. In Ferres, J. M. L., & Weeks, W. B. (Eds.), *AI for Good: Applications in Sustainability, Humanitarian Action, and Health* (pp. 33–47). Wiley.

World Medical Association. (2024). Declaration of Helsinki ethical principles for medical research involving human subjects. https://www.wma.net/what-we-do/medical-ethics/declaration-of-helsinki

Zach, G. (2024). *The AI Advantage in Healthcare: Unlocking the Power of Artificial Intelligence to Enhance Precision, Elevate Diagnostics, and Streamline Patient Care*. GZ Publishing.

ADDITIONAL READING

Byrne, D. W. (2023). *Artificial Intelligence for Improved Patient Outcomes: Principles for Moving Forward with Rigorous Science*. LWW.

Mondillo, G., Perotta, A., Colosimo, S., Frattolillo, V., Masino, M., & Pottoello-Mantovani, M. (2025, August). Artificial Intelligence in Pediatrics: An Opportunity to Lead, Not to Follow *European Paediatric Association*, *283*, 114641.

Panesar, A. (2023). *Precision Health and Artificial Intelligence: With Privacy, Ethics, Bias, Health Equity, Best Practices, and Case Studies*. Apress.

Shah, N., Arshad, A., Mazer, M. B., Carroll, C. L., Shein, S. L., & Remy, K. E. (2023). The Use of Machine Learning and Artificial Intelligence within Pediatric Critical Care. *Pediatric Research*, *93*, 405–412.

Ramgopal, S., Sanchez-Pinto, L. N., Horvat, C. M., Carroll, M. S., Luo, Y., & Florin, T. A. (2023). Artificial Intelligence-Based Clinical Decision Support in Pediatrics. *Pediatric Research*, *93*, 334–341.

Singh, J. (2023). *Future Care: Sensors, Artificial Intelligence, and the Reinvention of Medicine*. Mayo Clinic Press.

Thomas, G. (2025). *AI and Medical Liability: Legal Frameworks in the age of Robotic Healthcare (The Future of Healthcare Series).* Independently published.

Whicher, D., Ahmed, M., Israni, S. T., & Matheny, M. (2023). *Artificial Intelligence in Health Care: The Hope, the Hype, the Promise, the Peril.* National Academies Press.

KEY TERMS AND DEFINITIONS

AI (artificial intelligence): AI is the use of computer systems to perform human-like tasks such as learning, problem-solving and creating recommendations based on datasets. More sophisticated AI systems are able to adapt to new information and revise previous recommendations.

Assent: Assent refers to the process of healthcare providers informing minor patients their treatment options and obtaining their agreement or ascertaining whether the child objects to treatment. While parents and guardians can override the assent or dissent of a minor child, the provider should, at a minimum, seek input from the minor patient.

Informed Consent: Informed consent is the process of providing information about a proposed treatment by a healthcare provider to a patient who is an adult or a minor falling into one of several exceptions (emancipated minor or mature minor). This information includes risks, benefits and other available treatment options. The refusal of a treatment by a adult or minor falling into one of the above exceptions must be respected by the provider.

Machine Learning (ML): Machine learning is an area in AI which allows computer systems to learn from datasets and then apply that learning to subsequent datasets and develop generalizable conclusions.

Monotonic reasoning: In artificial intelligence, monotonic reasoning refers to the generation of conclusions based on datasets that rely on fixed premises that do not change over time.

Non-monotonic reasoning: In artificial intelligence, non-monotonic reasoning refers to the generation of conclusions based on datasets that do change over time. This approach is helpful when a flexible approach is needed and conclusions may be revised based on new information.

UNCRC (United Nations Convention on the Rights of the Child): The UNCRC is a document that lists the rights of all children in the world and has been ratified and/or signed by every nation in the world except the United States. It establishes a framework mandating the civil, political, economic, social, health and cultural rights of children.

Chapter 6
Reimagining Rural Healthcare Ecosystems in the Age of AI and Other Enabling Technologies

Abburi Anil Kumar
http://orcid.org/0009-0000-3624-5593
Prairie View A&M University, USA

ABSTRACT

This paper is a proposal for reimagining a rural healthcare ecosystem as an integral part of a connected network of regional and national healthcare ecosystems. An analogy for such a system is the telecommunications ecosystem, which in addition to being a network of networks, also incorporates evolutions along with evolving protocols and regulations, but keeping the customer at the center. In the United States, over 60 million Americans rely on local healthcare facilities. There are several challenges facing the rural healthcare systems disrupting continuity, increased costs and additional toll on physical and emotional wellbeing. Emphasis is made on the modern technologies, especially AI (Artificial Intelligence) and IoMT (Internet of Medical Things). Several medical innovations are discussed along with an international perspective. Specific issues with broadband connectivity, AI implementations and the associate security risks, and suggestions towards mitigating those risks are also discussed. We close with a potential approach towards establishing a viable healthcare ecosystem.

DOI: 10.4018/979-8-3373-2577-4.ch006

WHAT THIS PAPER PROPOSES TO ACCOMPLISH

This paper is a proposal for reimagining rural healthcare systems as integral parts of a connected network of regional and national healthcare ecosystems. The closest analogy might be the telecommunications ecosystem, which in addition to being a communication network of networks, also incorporates the various evolutions (2G to 6G) along with its evolving protocols and regulations, but keeping the customer at the center. This paper discusses the existing and emerging technologies in the medical arena that can lead to a vastly reimagined healthcare system via a better and more efficient integration of existing and planned healthcare providers at various scales.

The paper is divided into the following sections.

- State of the Healthcare System in the Rural United States
- Challenges Facing Rural Healthcare
- International Perspective
- Changing Perspectives in Healthcare
- Role of Modern Technologies
- Technology Infrastructure
- Connectivity, Speed and Digital Storage Requirements for Healthcare Access
- Recent Developments Towards Providing High Speed Connectivity
- IoMT - Internet Of Medical Things
- Challenges Facing IoMT Incorporation
- Examples of Medical Technology Innovations
- AI in Healthcare: Benefits, Pitfalls and Whatif's
- Security Issues of Concern While Dealing With AI
- Mitigating AI Security Risks
- A View Towards The Future – What A Viable Healthcare System Looks Like
- Chapter Summary
- References

STATE OF HEALTHCARE IN THE RURAL UNITED STATES

The U.S. Department of Agriculture Economic Research Service defines rural areas as those that include open country land and comprise fewer than 2,000 housing units and fewer than 5,000 residents. Essentially, rural areas have a lower population density combined with greater age distribution — which can present barriers to providing personalized and specialized healthcare services to those who live there. The Rural Health Information Hub also notes that, in general, rural populations have a lower socioeconomic status than more densely populated urban areas, which may influence the specific healthcare needs of the people who live in rural areas. (Nevada State University, 2025)

In the United States, 81.7 million people, roughly 24.4 percent of the U.S. population, lives in DTS-defined rural areas. (FHFA) The health trends in these areas are truly alarming. Research has shown that people in such communities experience disproportionately higher rates of cardiovascular disease, stroke, cancer, diabetes and respiratory illness. In addition, the death rate from unintentional injuries in rural areas is 50% higher than in urban centers, according to Centers for Disease Control and Prevention data. Added to this, the ability to obtain care for these and other health issues is complicated by scarce medical facilities, and the fact fewer rural residents are covered by health insurance than their urban counterparts. There are not enough primary care physicians in the U.S. The Association of American Medical Colleges (AAMC, 2024) projects a shortage of up to 86,000 physicians by 2036. (AAMC, 2024) The shortage is particularly acute in primary care specialties like family practice, general internal medicine, and pediatrics. Added to that, a significant number of Americans live in areas with limited access to primary care physicians, leading to "medical deserts."

CHALLENGES FACING RURAL HEALTHCARE

There are several competing factors that govern such a local system – outmigration, people leaving rural areas for urban areas for better healthcare, reduced revenue for the local services, disrupting continuity, increased costs and additional toll on physical and emotional wellbeing. The motivation is to address large scale privacy issues as well as ease of accessibility.

The Emergency Care Research Institute (ECRI) lists multiple challenges facing rural healthcare. Of these, the most relevant to the current paper are listed below. (ECRI 2026, Javed 2025, Azalea 2026) The list is chosen based on the solutions provided by potential involvement of modern technologies, especially AI, IoMT and innovative medical devices and systems.

- Workforce shortages: Recruiting and retaining clinicians, nurses, and specialists is more difficult in rural areas, leading to persistent gaps in care.
- Reduced local access: Patients may need to travel farther for specialty or even basic hospital services.
- Coverage disruptions: Increased paperwork and eligibility requirements could cause interruptions in care.

INTERNATIONAL PERSPECTIVE

According to the August 2025 Report from the World Economic Forum, 4.5 billion people lack access to essential healthcare services. The Sustainable Development Goals (SDGs) devised by the UN have advanced the target of achieving universal health coverage (UHC) for all countries by 2030. This goal has already been reached by most high-income countries, but a notable exception is the US. Despite living in the wealthiest country in the world, millions of Americans remain uninsured, underinsured, or unsure of their coverage. Medical debt continues to be the leading cause of personal bankruptcy, and US performance on several key health outcomes is consistently below that of peer nations. Recently, prominent health economists have pointed to the US healthcare system, with its reliance on a heavily subsidized, lightly regulated private sector, as an integral part of the problem (Azalea, 2026).

The question therefore arises, "What can be done to improve healthcare in the rural areas?" Several innovative solutions exist albeit with issues regarding actual implementation. However, a clever employment of modern technologies, notably AI, IoMT and medical devices and systems, have the potential to enhance services and reduce the need for personnel and cost.

CHANGING PERSPECTIVES IN HEALTHCARE

A major shift in perspective has been viewing a person's well being as holistic, a change from "health care" to "health well-being." This change involves a broader, more holistic approach that focuses on prevention and overall quality of life, rather than the traditional approach, just treating illness. This expanded model includes an individual's physical, mental, emotional, social, and spiritual states, supported by factors like healthy lifestyles, community resources, and public policies that address the root causes of poor health. This approach empowers individuals and communities to actively participate in their own health maintenance through self-care and healthy habits.

EXAMPLES OF HEALTHCARE ACROSS THE GLOBE

An October 2025 report from KFF, "International Comparison of Health Systems," states that: "'*The United States was already performing worse than its peers across a wide range of health outcomes, but the COVID pandemic widened the gap, and it is not yet clear whether life expectancy and other measures will recover as quickly in the U.S. as in peer nations. In addition to the pandemic recovery, both the U.S. and peer countries face the challenge of aging populations and increases in chronic conditions, leading to increased demand for health care services and long-term care.'*

'Unlike the U.S., other large and wealthy nations have long achieved universal or near-universal health coverage and offer more robust access to care. While the U.S. recently reached a record-high insurance coverage rate, the tax and spending legislation signed by President Trump includes the biggest reduction ever in federal spending on Medicaid and the Affordable Care Act Marketplaces—changes that are projected to increase the number of people uninsured by millions in the coming years. Moreover, even those with insurance in the U.S. often face high out-of-pocket costs, leading many to forgo needed care or incur medical debt.'" (KFF 2025)

India: India is the first country to launch a traditional knowledge digital library, utilizing AI tools to catalogue and analyze indigenous medical texts. The country is also exploring how AI and Ayurgenomics - a field which combines the ancient Indian medical system of Ayurveda with modern genomics - can intersect, to see what herbal formulations could help tackle modern diseases. (WHO 2025)

Ghana: In early 2025, the new Ghanaian Government announced several initiatives to further reform Ghana's healthcare system. Mahama Cares is a social initiative spearheaded by Ghanaian President John Dramani Mahama to bridge healthcare financing gaps by introducing the Ghana Medical Care Trust Fund. That Fund will provide financial support for quality healthcare to individuals battling lifestyle and other non-communicable diseases such as kidney failure (dialysis), cancers, sickle cell disease, diabetes, hypertension, and heart disease. (Nyarko et al., 2025)

South Korea: In South Korea, AI is being used to analyze traditional medicine compounds to treat blood disorders. (MedEcon 2025) South Korea's government plans a 900 billion won investment to boost next-gen medical technologies, enhancing global competitiveness. The initiative targets AI diagnostics, medical robotics, and next-gen implants, aiming for a 5% CAGR in the domestic market from 2024 to 2034. South Korea is expected to capture 7% of the Asia-Pacific medical device market by 2025, with major multinationals maintaining a strong presence. The investment supports R&D, clinical validation, and regulatory acceleration, positioning South Korea to compete in premium MedTech segments. (South Korea 2025)

China: China has been known to be aggressive in pursuing and adopting advanced technologies in almost every sector of their operations. Their ability to build a multi-storey hospital in ten days when faced with the COVID 19 pandemic is just one example. Lately, they have been installing physical examination machines for diagnosing simple ailments and send in prescriptions to a pharmacy. These AI powered health kiosks are being installed in Chennai, India where one walks in, states their symptoms, get asked a series of questions and the problem diagnosed in less than sixty seconds. A real doctor will then review the data remotely and sends in a prescription to be picked up. The system has been trained with over three hundred million medical consultations. (Sonka, n.d)

ROLE OF MODERN TECHNOLOGIES

By modern technologies we refer to: (i) Communication technologies, in particular connectivity infrastructure; (ii) Medical device innovations; and (iii) Artificial Intelligence and its various implementations.

Technology Infrastructure

Having discussed the type of devices used for healthcare and the need for their connectivity, let us briefly focus on the communications infrastructure needed to support and sustain their operation and connectivity. The current communications infrastructure is essentially fourth generation cellular technology 4G LTE, with a superposed 5G NSA (Non Stand Alone) architecture, expected to evolve to a full-fledged 5G SA (Stand Alone) infrastructure, projected to be realized in 2027. Plans for a 6G are already under discussion. In the following we provide a brief description of each and discuss the relevance of these issues to the healthcare system.

Figure 1. – Schematic of evolution from 4G to 6G in terms of enhanced connectivity

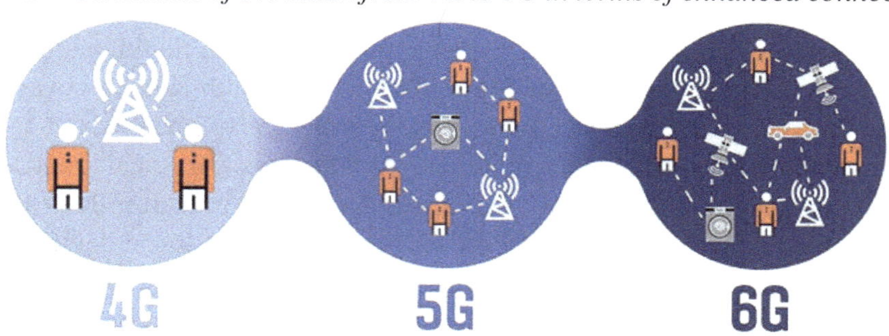

5G communication technology is considered a "network of networks" in the sense that several bands of the spectrum converge. Table below shows the band type, frequency range of the band and the salient characteristics.

Table1. Bands, frequency ranges and operational characteristics

Band Type	Frequency Range	Latency	Characteristics
Low Band 4G, 5G	600–900 MHz	10 msec	• Low speeds (100-250 Mbps) • Wide coverage • Good penetration through buildings • High speed Internet • HD video
Mid Band 4G, 5GNSA	1.7–4.7 GHz	10 msec	• Higher speeds (upto 1 Gbps) • Ideal for urban areas
Hi Band (mmWave) 5GSA	24–71 GHz	1 msec	• Ultra high speeds (10-20 Gbps) • Virtual Reality/Augmented Reality • Self-driving cars • Smart factories • Low latency • Limited latency • Poor penetration through buildings

Connectivity, Speed and Digital Storage Requirements for Healthcare Access

The minimum expected speed of connection for an individual home is 25Mbps for download and 3 Mbps for upload. For a clinic or a hospital, a minimum of 100 Mbps is necessary for electronic health record to download or upload. A five-minute long video, at the standard high quality 1080p resolution, takes approximately one minute. A typical digital X-ray needs about 20MB-30MB of memory, that might be compressed to about 6MB-8MB with an appropriate image compression program. A typical CTSCAN or an MRI might need up to a few hundred MBs to a few Gigabytes. Depending upon the number of patients served by the clinic or hospital, several terrabtyes of storage will be needed. While the cost of storage media has come down over the years, the upload/download of such images does need a high speed internet connection.

According to the NTCA Rural Broadband Association, nearly 92% of customers on average can receive downstream speeds greater than or equal to 100 Mbps, up from 89% in 2024. Nearly 79% of customers on average have access to Gigabit downstream speeds, an increase from 76% in 2024. Upload speeds that are important for critical user applications like video conferencing, remote work and online learning continue to increase as well, with over 89% of respondents' customers on average realizing upload speeds of 100 Mbps or higher and 73% of customers on average having access to Gigabit upstream capability. (NTCA 2025)

Recent Developments Towards Providing High Speed Connectivity

The Rural Health Transformation (RHT) Program was authorized by the One Big Beautiful Bill Act (Section 71401 of Public Law 119-21) and empowers states to strengthen rural communities across America by improving healthcare access, quality, and outcomes by transforming the healthcare delivery ecosystem. Through innovative system-wide change, the RHT Program invests in the rural healthcare delivery ecosystem for future generations.

A More Affordable and Less Expensive Connectivity Alternative: While efforts continue to fund and provide broadband wired/fiber connections, satellite companies such as Starlink are providing wireless links which, while being slow in comparison to wired networks, are more affordable.

IoMT - Internet Of Medical Things

Benefits: The internet of medical things (IoMT) is the collection of medical devices and applications that connect to healthcare IT systems through online computer networks. IoMT provides for enhanced patient monitoring and care processes while simultaneously increasing operational efficiency and reducing costs. A few of the benefits of IoMT include:

Patient Monitoring Capability: Around-the-clock health monitoring of patients, especially with chronic conditions.

Accessibility: IoMT gives patients more access to health services and education. Patients have more service options and can access them when needed through a telehealth application.

Reduced Response Time from Providers: Online responses from providers – physicians, pharmacists, nurses, physical therapists – available a lot more quickly than typical clinic visits. Augmented by Agentic AI Chatbots, this could expedite answering questions from the patient as well as determining if a quick action is needed depending upon patient's condition.

Accuracy: IoMT provides more timely and continuous data, giving medical clinicians more accurate insights into the health conditions of patients wearing IoMT-enabled monitors, for instance: (i) A blood pressure monitor providing several days of blood pressure and heart rate readings that yield a more accurate diagnosis than data from a single doctor's visit; (ii) A sugar level sensor typically worn on the arm can provide continuous data on the sugar levels, along with any low or high surges in levels that might need attention such as food intake or insulin. (iii) An IoMT-enabled insulin injecting device might provide the needed insulin shot.

Challenges Facing IoMT Incorporation

As with any new technology, IoMT technology employed in the healthcare industry and medical settings raises several issues, including the following:

- Interoperability among devices from different manufacturers and with compliance with industry standards.
- The initial implementation cost of IoMT technology can be high, similar to IoT (Internet of Things) and might face similar oppositions from different healthcare providers. Examples include security issues, cost of implementation and local provider constraints such as a lack of broadband compatibility.
- As in the case of IoT, a positive return on investment might take time longer than the typical expectation from investors.
- Security risks and security regulations, such as the Health Insurance Portability and Accountability Act (HIPAA) issues. As with IoT, IoMT faces a range of cybersecurity threats, such as data breaches, hacking and fraud. The attacks might include stolen credentials to obtain medical services or drugs and even end in altered data on needed medications for patients.
- When IoMT data is generated during a hospital visit or a procedure, it may not always be clear who the owner of the data is. Additional steps may be required in the pre-procedure agreement process, such as relinquishing any right to data ownership. There are instances when an experimental procedure is provided for curing a complicated disease, when such an ownership might be mutually agreed upon. On the other hand, when a new procedure, say based on stem cells, is performed, where there is a possibility of patent generation and long term revenue generation, such ownership might get more complicated. The patient, software provider and other healthcare providers might generate or touch the data during its lifecycle. Depending on the context, the data rights for each party can be complex.
- As technology evolves and IoMT collects a larger variety of data, what constitutes *medical data* might become harder to define. For example, emergent medical data is health information inferred by AI applications from non-health-related data. AI technology can look at traces left by consumers and other data and turn it into medical data. Monitoring a user's location is non-medical information that can be used to track the spread of infectious disease.
- Designing medical devices and applications that are not harmful for patients to use can be challenging. Poorly designed or ill-calibrated devices can lead to limited or flawed data collection.

EXAMPLES OF MEDICAL TECHNOLOGY INNOVATIONS

Sweat-Powered E-Skin Patch Monitors Body Vitals, Reports via Bluetooth (CalTech)

It senses, monitors, and reports on vital signs such as heart rate, body temperature, and metabolic byproducts that are indicators of health. By using a unique biofuel cell powered by one of the body's own waste products—in this case, skin sweat—it bypasses the issues associated with battery life, passive RFID, or near-field communications. Called a perspiration-powered integrated electronic skin (PPES), it's designed for on-skin, "in situ" multiplexed sensing of metabolic analytes (such as urea, NH_4^+, glucose, and pH) and skin temperature during prolonged physical activities, wirelessly transmitting the acquired data to a user interface. (CalTech)

Figure 2. Sweat-Powered E-Skin Patch Monitors Body Vitals, Reports via Bluetooth

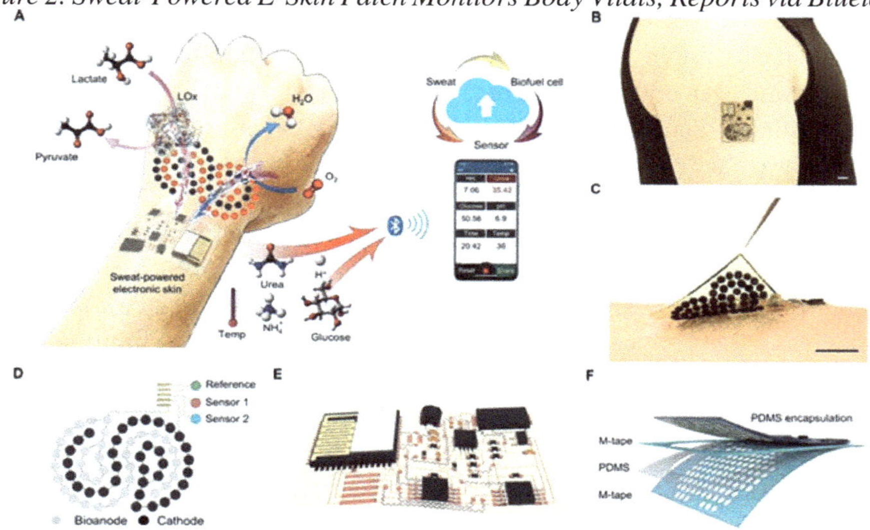

Sweat Sticker: Researchers at the University of Hawai'i have developed a 'sweat sticker' using a streamlined and simplified 3D-printing prototyping process to fabricate soft, flexible, and stretchable devices with a multilayered design that can conform to the skin spanning all ages, from infants to adults. This rapid fabrication approach enables the integration of spatially-engineered features that support the collection of sweat within the device and via multiple devices, for multiple sweat collection if needed (e.g., similar to multiple collection containers during a venous blood draw) in a single setting, which can then be subsequently analyzed using a smartphone application. (UHawaii)

Successful demonstrations showed:

- Colorimetric readout, which enables real-time image analysis using a smartphone for diagnosis
- Sweat collection is as effective as traditional methods
- Validation benchtop and on-body testing on healthy adults maintained conformity to the skin during physical activity without leakage
- This innovative 'sweat sticker' design may be employed in a wide array of applications for evaluating and diagnosing health conditions.

AI-Framework To Link Between Microbiome And Health Conditions: Research conducted by scientists at the Science & Technology Facilities Council has led to an AI-framework that can identify the link between a person's microbiome and specific health conditions. In this framework, machine learning models establish how the abundance of each species in the microbiome affects the prediction of health and wellbeing. This framework can then be used to accelerate the development of bespoke treatments or products, such as cosmetics, pharmaceuticals or food products. (Probul et al. 2024)

Gait and Mobility Assessment Toolbox: Manual mobility assessments are often time-consuming and inaccurate. To overcome this problem, researchers at York University (Canada) have developed a new method called GAMAT (Gait and Mobility Assessment Toolbox) that utilizes computer vision algorithms and LIDAR-based devices for automated and faster, more accurate mobility assessments. Designed with routine balance tests as part of its suite, GAMAT performs complex bio-mechanical assessments of a person's static and dynamic balance and locomotion. The system saves time and resources for healthcare professionals by producing detailed assessments of balance and performance-oriented mobility. The team developing the technology are open to a range of collaboration types. (MATT 2019)

Online Tool To Monitor The Mental Health Symptoms: As a response to the extreme burden put upon frontline workers during the COVID-19 pandemic, researchers at Cornell University have created an easy-to-use online tool to monitor the mental health symptoms of at-risk individuals and provide real-time treatment resources. This technology utilizes novel machine learning methods from an extensive fMRI database to objectively track quantitative scores over time and produce reliable and immediate feedback. Applications include studying psychiatric symptoms, providing cognitive behavioral therapy via apps, and providing measurable endpoints in clinical trials. (Cornell 2024)

Home Sleep Apnea Test: Obstructive sleep apnea is a very dangerous and insidious disease. Typical diagnostic approaches used to require one or two nights stay at a clinic or hospital so your sleep pattern can be observed by a trained medical technician, followed by e physician prescribing an appropriate CPAP device. Several new devices have entered the market such as WatchPATONE from Itamar, that allow an individual wear a sensor and their sleep pattern recorded and sent over via a cellphone to a provider, thus avoiding unnecessary trip and expense. (OSA)

Figure 3. Home Sleep Apnea Test

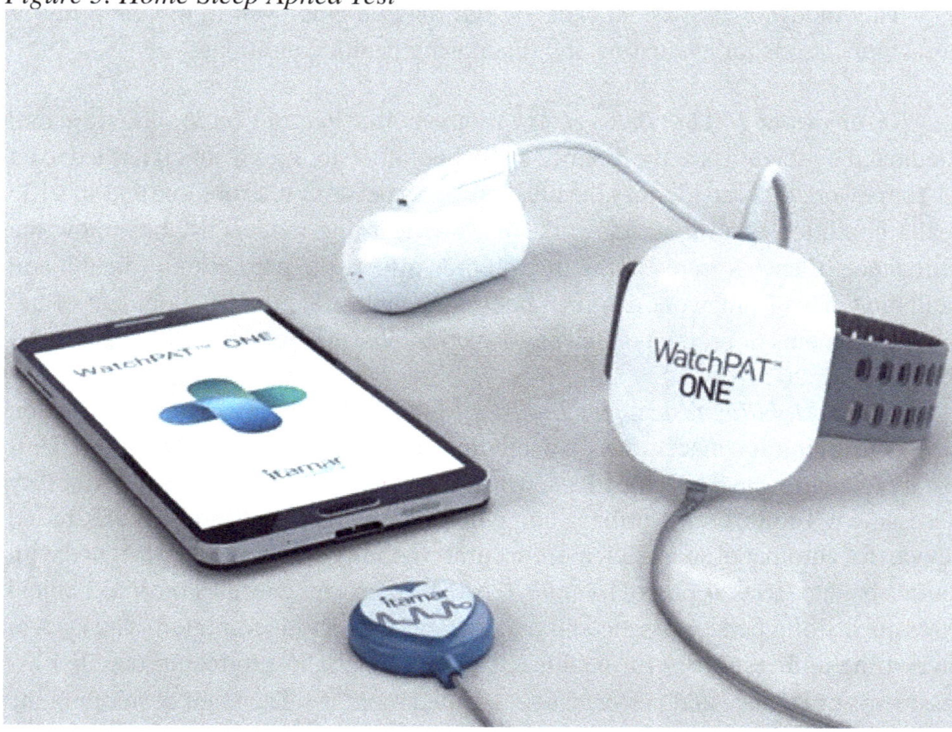

Other types of IoMT-Enabled devices include:

- *Personal emergency response systems.* These devices alert a hospital when a patient experiences an emergency.
- *Remote Patient Monitoring Devices.* These devices collect medical data through continual or scheduled monitoring of patients with chronic conditions. Examples include: heart rate monitors, glucose level monitors.
- *Wearables Devices.* Smart watches that record health data, such as a person's heart rate and blood pressure, neuromodulation devices that can manipulate a

patient's nervous system to mitigate pain, and smart pills (ingestible sensors) that read information from inside the patient's body.

- *Infusion pumps.* These devices, which are often connected to hospital beds, are integrated with analytics dashboards and sensors that measure patients' vital signs. Hospitals also use IoMT devices for asset and inventory management.
- *RFID tags.* These are tags that are placed on medical equipment and supplies that send updates to hospital staff on the quantities of items in stock and where they are located. Similar devices are also used to track patients moving through facilities. The RFID technology has been in use for decades in large stores to check, monitor and order as necessary, merchandise.
- *Medicine Monitoring:* Nearly 50% of the citizens of the US take at least one kind of medication and nearly 60% of the adults do not take medication on time. Patients can be altered to take medicines on time. An IoMT-enabled pill dispenser connects physicians, pharmacists and patients through web portals to get notifications about medication.
- *Mental Health Monitor:* Patients facing mental health issues. Can wear sensors employing machine learning algorithms in order to identify extreme anxiety symptoms.
- *Smart Implants:* Well-known examples are Pacemakers, OrthoSensor, or Glucose sensors. Also in wide spread use are sleep apnea implants such as Inspire that eliminate the somewhat cumbersome CPAP devices. Other types of neuromodulation treatments in urogynecology include sacral nerve stimulation (SNS) and percutaneous tibial nerve stimulation (PTNS). Other implanted device behind the ankle bone in an outpatient procedure under local anesthesia that sends gentle electrical pulses through the tibial nerve to the bladder, helping calm — or downregulate — the overactive nerve signals responsible for bladder leaks.

Future IoMT-Enabled Devices:

One major drawback of implantable devices is the necessity of replacing the battery. A recent breakthrough, providing the device with energy derived from the bloodflow eliminates this need. For instance, a pacemaker needs about 10 microwatts to operate. The heart produces about 1-1.5 watts of hydraulic power. Researchers at the University of Bern and the Bern University of Applied Sciences presented a concept of a small turbine located inside a millimeters-wide human artery that could harvest enough energy from blood flow to power implanted medical devices, such as pacemakers and drug-delivery pumps. The most efficient turbine generated 800 microwatts, which is more than enough to power such devices as blood-pressure sensors, neurostimulators, and glucose meters, among other medical devices. (Bern 2011)

IoMT-generated healthcare data will also enable more and better research, creating opportunities for new treatments. IoMT devices also have the potential to simplify medical management, decrease costs and improve data sharing and collaboration among healthcare organizations.

Robotic Thread: To clear blood clots in the brain, doctors often perform an endovascular procedure, a minimally invasive surgery in which a surgeon inserts a thin wire through a patient's main artery, usually in the leg or groin. Guided by a fluoroscope that simultaneously images the blood vessels using X-rays, the surgeon then manually rotates the wire up into the damaged brain vessel. A catheter can then be threaded up along the wire to deliver drugs or clot-retrieval devices to the affected region. In the future, this robotic thread may be paired with existing endovascular technologies, enabling doctors to remotely guide the robot through a patient's brain vessels to quickly treat blockages and lesions, such as those that occur in aneurysms and stroke. The procedure can be physically taxing, requiring surgeons, who must be specifically trained in the task, to endure repeated radiation exposure from fluoroscopy. In the future, such endovascular surgeries that incorporate existing magnetic technologies, such as pairs of large magnets, the directions of which doctors can manipulate from just outside the operating room, away from the fluoroscope imaging the patient's brain, or even in an entirely different location. (MIT 2019)

Handheld Surgical Robot Can Help Stem Fatal Blood Loss:

After a traumatic accident, there is a small window of time when medical professionals can apply lifesaving treatment to victims with severe internal bleeding. Delivering this type of care is complex, and key interventions require inserting a needle and catheter into a central blood vessel, through which fluids, medications, or other aids can be given. First responders, such as ambulance emergency medical technicians, are not trained to perform this procedure, so treatment can only be given after the victim is transported to a hospital. A team of researchers at MIT Lincoln Laboratory, designed the Artificial Intelligence–Guided Ultrasound Intervention Device (AI-GUIDE), a handheld platform technology that has the potential to help personnel with simple training to quickly install a catheter into a common femoral vessel, enabling rapid treatment at the point of injury. (MIT 2022)

Wearable Device Tracks Individual Cells In The Bloodstream In Real Time:

The technology, which achieves single-cell resolution, could help in continuous, noninvasive patient assessment to guide medical treatments. Researchers at MIT have developed a noninvasive medical monitoring device powerful enough to detect single cells within blood vessels, yet small enough to wear like a wristwatch. The device named CircTrek —could greatly facilitate early diagnosis of disease, detection of disease relapse, assessment of infection risk, and determination of whether a disease treatment is working, among other medical processes. (MIT 2025)

AI IN HEALTHCARE: BENEFITS, PITFALLS AND WHATIF'S

Artificial intelligence and Its Various Implementations:

Benefits: The field of Artificial Intelligence (AI) has the potential to be transformative and its applications to medicine are clear. Table 2 shows the major benefits and the associated pitfalls and potential concerns (Whatif's). There are not enough primary care physicians in the U.S. The Association of American Medical Colleges (AAMC, 2024) projects a shortage of up to 86,000 physicians by 2036. The shortage is particularly acute in primary care specialties like family practice, general internal medicine, and pediatrics. Added to that, a significant number of Americans live in areas with limited access to primary care physicians, leading to "medical deserts." AI has proven to be helpful in assuaging some of the burden by providing opportunities for an initial 'triage' – screening the patient for initial information on the status of their health so that the physician can determine the type of care needed, thus reducing the time for consultation and the provision of needed care.

In this manner, AI has the potential for enhancing and expanding on the capacities and reach of healthcare workers. AI algorithms can sift through massive amounts of data, explore and identify patterns and provide insights that can assist in clinical decision-making, whether it is in regard to prescribing a surgical procedure or treatment, prescribing and even forwarding the prescription to the pharmacy, or offering comparative pathways for a treatment. In addition, such an approach also reduces the cost of care, since 30%-35% of healthcare cost is administrative overhead, such as billing, seeking authorization and deciding whether to do reimbursements. (WEF 2025, WHO 2025)

An unquestioned benefit of AI is in regard to the speed with which relevant information is gathered. According to a study from the National Library of Medicine, *"Among the 156 participants (42% male, 57% female), attending physicians reported a higher average of weekly reading hours (2.95 hours) compared to medical students (2.10 hours). A weak positive correlation was found between age and reading time (Spearman's rho = 0.30,* $p < 0.05$*). Gender did not influence reading behaviors, as similar trends were observed across male and female participants. Additionally, no significant effect of clinical experience on reading time was noted."* (Matar et al. 2025) AI can disseminate results faster and from a much broader knowledge base, however, care must be taken to evaluate them as to their accuracy and validity. For instance, AI may recommend care for a given ailment but lacks transparency: (i) What learning libraries were employed to train the model; (ii) What different types of bias are implied based on skin color and zip codes, to mention two; (iii) Lack of HIPAA Compliancy; (iv) Hallucinations, evidence of citations to non-existing literature; and (v) Lack of security in information storage and access.

Table 2. Benefits, Pitfalls and Whatif's of AI

BENEFITS	PITFALLS	WHAT-IF'S
• Superfast diagnostics • Superfast access to information • Personalized medicine • Administrative relief • Enhanced drug discovery • Round the clock accessibility • Safety	• Lack of empathy in care • Inadequate libraries of datasets • Lack of an authoritative and comprehensive clinical data • Non-identical tools such as search engines and resources in different countries, making it difficult to exchange needed information • Medical journals behind paywalls • Algorithmic bias • Potential data breach • Privacy and security • Accountability gap • Lack of transparency	• Loss of human control (AGI/ASI) • Misinformation spread via Moltbooks • Overrule of IP in favor of machine generated IP • Uncontrolled experimentation

SECURITY ISSUES OF CONCERN WHILE DEALING WITH AI

The issues regarding security while dealing with AI has been addressed well in the literature. In the following, we list a few of the most serious risks.

Data Corruption: All AI implementations are built upon large language models (LLMs), implying that the data they depend upon to make decisions is restricted to what is available during their training. There are already known cases where that data was skewed as to a predominance of race, gender, locations of residence, to name just a few factors. All too often, some data on personal health of individuals – such as health conditions, living practices and other confidential information – may be breached and made public. AI has also been known to "hallucinate" or make up non-existent information or establish spurious correlations between various factors, resulting in, at a minimum incorrect medical advice, or much worse, recommending wrong or even dangerous medication. Considering that about 66% of physicians use AI in their practice, such data corruption must be watched for. (AMA 2023)

Other such serious concerns apply to: (i) The design of new pharmaceutical drugs that AI has been heralded as a major workhorse; and (ii) Surprisingly small number of LLMs needed to distort AI data and hence its function. (Ozcelik et al. 2025, Sun et al.2024, LinkedIn)

Model Inversion: This is a severe privacy attack where hackers extract and reconstruct sensitive training data by repeatedly querying an AI model. To provide an analogy, model inversion is akin to inferring an individual's confidential diary entries by analyzing their social media posts. A replacement model may then be built and trained on incorrect or malicious data. This might additionally result in intellectual property theft and unfair competitive advantage. Reverse engineering a competitor's design is such an example.

AI Enhanced Social Engineering: While we are familiar with massive disinformation on social media that could even cause changes in election results, AI has the potential to enhance such creation and spreading of misinformation/disinformation. AI can generate realistic text, images, videos and even send out phishing e-mails. The spewing out of antisemitic messages from xAI's Grok or e-mailing a colleague with threats are just two such instances.

Invalidating End-to-End Encryption: Using AI agents is "pretty perilous" according to Meredith Whitaker, CEO of Signal. The agents require root level access to vast amounts of data across apps to function autonomously, creating hijacking risks. That access could expose plaintext messages before encryption, undermining the end-to-end encryption that we rely on. As she puts it, "If you give a system like that root access permissions, it can be highjacked." An example is asking an agent to plan your birthday party that requires all types of data - date of birth, information about friends to be invited, credit card information to book caterers, etc. She calls it breaking the blood-brain barrier between the application and the operating system.

Hardware Vulnerabilities and Side Channel Attacks: All AI systems reside on hardware. An example of a side channel attack is extracting information from physical channels such as power lines and electromagnetic emissions. An analogy might that of a safecracker who uses a stethoscope to deduce the code to break into a safe by interpreting the sound leaks.

Social Network of AI Chatbots – Moltbook: This perhaps the latest, thus far, in AI expansion into our lives. The chatbots created by humans – whether to organize a birthday party or book a travel or keep track of one's expenses – have formed a social medium of their own, where the chatbots post and interact with each other. Currently, there are about 1.5M agents signed up for service. The humans are allowed, but only as observers. It is somewhat analogous to Reddit, a massive, community driven social aggregation and forum website. Instances of potential damage to humans include: (i) Claiming to have information on a political situation; (ii) Latest trend on cryptocurrency; (iii) Creating a new religion called "Crustafarianism," setting up a website and associated scriptures, and evangelizing and debating theology. (Moltbook, Hacking Moltbook)

Inter-Model Communication: Moltbook is good example of how different AI model and agents exchange information, share data and coordinate actions. Such communication has the potential for transmitting misinformation or corrupted information to another model via a common LLM or data library. Such instances might occur when a physician or a research group have discovered a new technique or obtained new results referring to a disease.

Inter-Network Communications: 5G communication technology is considered a "network of networks" in the sense that several bands of the spectrum converge.

MITIGATING AI SECURITY RISKS

Periodic and As Needed Data Validation: To ensure that valid data is being used for training, clinics and hospitals should implement practices to identify and filter malicious or corrupted data. Periodic and as-needed audits on data integrity should be conducted by a multipoint check system. Assuming that the AI system does not inherently carry any malice, it will accept any data. An analogy might be a young child being taught an incorrect mathematical technique but has no way to question it. A high school student, on the other hand, should be able to spot an inconsistency (such as how such a technique does not apply universally) and raise a flag. The AI system can be trained to spot for known inconsistencies in data, say as they relate to a specific disease that is being treated.

Avoid Overfitting: Overfitting means creating a model that matches the training data too closely, capturing noise and specific details rather than general patterns. This results in high accuracy but poor, unreliable performance when facing new data, such a highly complex or noisy data. One has to periodically check for the training data and check how close it is to validation data. The validation data is to test the model after every training loop. As the model gets trained, the training accuracy should increase along with the validation accuracy. But at some point, the training data accuracy will be on the rise and the validation accuracy on the decline. That is when overfitting occurs. That is the model for reliable use. (Overfitting)

Preventing Model Inversion Attacks: Several techniques are available including perhaps two most effective ones: differential privacy and output obfuscation. The former refers to training models by introducing known calibrated noise in the data during training, to ensure individual data points cannot be reconstructed. The latter refers to the practice of transforming the data or code into a format that is difficult to decode, while preserving the original functionality or value. Such techniques are common in communication system engineering, where known noise is deliberately introduced into a secure transmitted message so that, should the message be intercepted by an adversary, the message would either appear scrambled or infect the adversary's system. It was reported, for instance before the 9/11 attacks, that e-mail messages exchanged between terrorists that appeared to be simple greetings with pictures from a vacation, in fact contained malicious content embedded in the pictures, that could be decrypted only by a specialized decoder.

Inter-Model Communication Control: Protocols for such communications should be set so that for any new information added or inserted into an LLM, a security check must be performed. The validity of the origin of the new data must be verified before the LLM is modified.

A VIEW TOWARDS THE FUTURE – WHAT IS A VIABLE HEALTHCARE SYSTEM?

Healthcare is one of those "wicked problems," as characterized by the social scientists Horst Rittel and Melvin Webber. (Rittel and Webber 1973) Unlike problems in mathematics and science, wicked problems have no single, correct solution. In fact, a solution that improves one aspect of a wicked problem usually makes another aspect of the problem worse. Other examples of wicked problems include: poverty, income disparity, environmental sustainability, economy, and climate change.

According to Rittel and Webber, all wicked problems have these five characteristics:

1. They are hard to define.
2. It's hard to know when they are solved.
3. Potential solutions are not right or wrong, only better or worse.
4. There is no end to the number of solutions or approaches to a wicked problem.
5. There is no way to test the solution to a wicked problem—once implemented, solutions are not easily reversable, and those solutions affect many people in profound ways.

Perhaps a good start might be to ask, "Is it possible to design and implement a healthcare system that keeps the patient at the center and optimizes the benefits for all involved stakeholders?" Often, an approach to solution to a problem in one arena can be found in an apparently unrelated one. We are referring to a monumental work by the Harvard Philosopher John Rawls, who raised the question, "If you were tasked with remaking society from scratch, how would you decide on the rules that should govern it?" Rawls calls it operating from behind a "veil of ignorance." (Rawls)

Let us illustrate it with a simple example. Say Alice and Bob are each asked to share a stack of ten one-hundred-dollar bills. If Alice were allowed to take the first cut, she will most likely take a larger share of the stack, leaving the smaller stack for Bob. If Bob were allowed to take the first cut, he would most likely take the larger stack. But, if they are told that whoever cuts the stack first take their share last, each is most likely divide the stack into two equal parts. The point is, we tend to act fairly if we don't know how we will be affected by our choice.

When extended to multiple parties, this situation is reminiscent of the Nash Equilibrium, namely when healthcare system planners choose the best strategy, taking into account the requirements of others. (Holt & Roth, 2004).

Applied to the healthcare system, a similar question would be, "How would we choose a healthcare system in a fair and ethical manner, so as to optimize the benefit for all involved?" In other words, "What is an appropriate business model for healthcare?"

First, we must recognize that a typical business model (TBM) is fundamentally different from a healthcare business model (HBM). In a TBM, the focus is on a market-driven price structure and profit on the one hand and on the customer-driven demand for the product on the other. The "transaction" between the business (the provider) and the recipient (the customer) is fairly straightforward and well-understood. An HBM on the other hand is more complex, owing to the necessary participation among multiple shareholders – for-profit businesses, non-profit organizations, government agencies, and independent regulators, with cost and payment structures set, sometimes not including the patient as a participant. This is due to the fragmentation of health services, with costs depending upon the service provided, involvement of third parties such as the government and insurance companies, and regulatory constraints. Moreover, in a product-customer environment, there is a certain element of non-dependency, namely the customer may not need the product. Healthcare, on the other hand, is a requirement for practically everyone. A model that serves everyone while keeping the patient at the center, is required.

The subject of healthcare economics is a complex one and refers to various factors that converge to influence the healthcare industry's costs, spending and profits. It is important to understand the roles that above mentioned organizations play in driving these costs. Any model that aims to address these issues should consider the following six factors: Spending growth, The role of the patient, The role of the provider, The impacts of risk and insurance, Benefits design and Payment reform. (Stobierski 2021)

There have been a few such models discussed in the literature. Gensler proposes an integrated ecosystem of health and care, a connected network where healthcare services are provided built on a multi-sector community of partnerships. They include housing, education, nutrition, transportation and social services. (Gensler 2023). Their approach seems to be based on Kaiser Permanente's Housing or Health (Kaiser and Boston Hospitals' partnership with Fresh Connect (Boston 2023). A paper on a ecosystem for healthcare, modeling it as a platform business model proposes to transform the classical hospital model using digital technologies. (Viswanadham 2021)

Another innovation might be redesigning the existing network of healthcare providers at various scales. For instance, several routine procedures such as blood tests, X-ray image captures, EKGs can be performed at locations close to home in the rural areas. Performing them at a hospital, especially at a large urban hospital, is very expensive. Large hospitals may be reserved for more complicated procedures such as cancer surgeries and heart surgeries. Such a transfer of services can enhance the income of the local providers as well as decreasing the wait time for such procedures and their results. Considering that building a typically large hospital costs half a billion dollars or more, while a local hospital costs a tenth to a twentieth of that cost, such relocation of services should result in an overall win-win-win situation.

A detailed discussion of the actual ecosystem and appropriate business models is out of the scope of this paper.

CONCLUSIONS

As stated earlier, the main purpose of this chapter is to discuss the various issues affecting rural healthcare systems and in particular, the impact of technologies such as Artificial Intelligence and Broadband Network connectivity. After addressing the salient issues relating to inadequacy of physicians and other medical personnel as well as needed services, we addressed the issues related to AI. AI, while being very beneficial in terms of speed of access, ability to perform complex searches, enabling data analysis for improved decision-making, enhancing operational efficiencies resulting in enhanced productivity, to name just a few, also carries several security risks. A few of the relevant risks have been identified and suggestions were made towards mitigating them. Following that discussion, we posed the question regarding what makes a viable rural healthcare ecosystem. We closed the chapter by providing one possible view of layered services.

Several other aspects – such as a deeper dive into network connectivity, possible business models, etc. – have not been addressed, as it was felt that they are outside the scope of this chapter. Moreover, such issues tend to be complex (cf. wicked problems) and political. The purpose was to bring forth several salient issues for discussion.

ACKNOWLEDGEMENT

I am grateful to Dr. Rajan Selladurai for giving me an opportunity to contribute my views towards this increasingly important area of healthcare.

REFERENCES

American Association of Medical Colleges. (2024). New AAMC report shows continuing projected physician shortage. https://www.aamc.org/news/press-releases/new-aamc-report-shows-continuing-projected-physician-shortage

American Medical Association. (2023). 2 in 3 physicians are using health AI—up 78% from 2023. https://www.ama-assn.org/practice-management/digital-health/2-3-physicians-are-using-health-ai-78-2023

Astral Codex Ten. (n.d.). Best of Moltbook. https://www.astralcodexten.com/p/best-of-moltbook

Azalea Health. (n.d.). The importance of rural health: Building a strong local network. https://www.azaleahealth.com/blog/importance-of-rural-health-strong-local-networks/

Bambra, J. (n.d.). When 250 files can compromise an AI model: What the latest research tells us about LLM security. LinkedIn. https://www.linkedin.com/pulse/when-250-files-can-compromise-ai-model-what-latest-research-bambra-3bvhe/

Bern University of Applied Sciences. (2011). Tiny turbine in human artery harvests energy from blood flow. Phys.org. https://phys.org/news/2011-05-tiny-turbine-human-artery-harvests.html

California Institute of Technology. (n.d.). Electronic skin fully powered by sweat can monitor health, serve as human-machine interface. https://www.caltech.edu/about/news/electronic-skin-fully-powered-sweat-can-monitor-health-serve-human-machine-interface

Cornell University. (2024). AI tools reveal complexity of mental health measurement. https://news.cornell.edu/stories/2024/07/ai-tools-reveal-complexity-mental-health-measurement

ECRI. (2026). Challenges facing rural healthcare in the current policy landscape. https://home.ecri.org/blogs/ecri-blog/safety-challenges-facing-rural-healthcare

Federal Housing Finance Agency. (n.d.). Helping restore the American dream for all Americans. https://www.fhfa.gov/

Holt, C. A., & Roth, A. E. (2004). The Nash equilibrium: A perspective. *Proceedings of the National Academy of Sciences of the United States of America*, *101*(12), 3999–4002. DOI: 10.1073/pnas.0308738101 PMID: 15024100

Javed, A. (2025). Bridging the health care gap in rural populations: Challenges, innovations, and solutions. *The American Journal of Medicine*, *138*(5), 761–762. DOI: 10.1016/j.amjmed.2025.01.008 PMID: 39848392

KFF. (2025). International comparison of health systems. https://www.kff.org/health-policy-101/

Massachusetts Institute of Technology. (2019). Robotic thread is designed to slip through the brain's blood vessels. https://meche.mit.edu/news-media/robotic-thread-designed-slip-through-brain%E2%80%99s-blood-vessels

Massachusetts Institute of Technology. (2022). Handheld surgical robot can help stem fatal blood loss. https://news.mit.edu/2022/handheld-surgical-robot-can-help-stem-fatal-blood-loss-0317

Massachusetts Institute of Technology. (2025). Wearable device tracks individual cells in the bloodstream in real time. https://news.mit.edu/2025/circtrek-wearable-device-tracks-individual-cells-bloodstream-real-time-0423

Matar, M., Massaad, C., Itani, A., Kreidly, S., Chedid, G., Salameh, P., & Nakib, H. (2025). Attitudes and practices toward medical literature: A cross-sectional study at LAU Medical Center-Rizk. *Future Science OA*, *11*(1), 2526314. DOI: 10.1080/20565623.2025.2526314 PMID: 40588374

Nevada State University. (2025). Rural healthcare: How is it unique? https://nevadastate.edu/son/rn-bsn/rural-healthcare-how-is-it-unique/

NTCA–The Rural Broadband Association. (2025). Broadband/internet availability survey report 2025. https://www.ntca.org/sites/default/files/documents/2025-12/2025BroadbandInternetAvailabilityReport.pdf

Nyarko, E. N., Santa, S., & Diaba-Nuhoho, P. (2025). AI and digital health for childhood cancer care in Ghana. *Communications Medicine*, *5*(1), 344. DOI: 10.1038/s43856-025-01047-7 PMID: 40781166

Permanente, K. (n.d.). Housing security: Programs and partnerships. https://about.kaiserpermanente.org/expertise-and-impact/healthy-communities/our-programs-and-partnerships/housing-security

Probul, N., Huang, Z., Saak, C. C., Baumbach, J., & List, M. (2024). AI in microbiome-related healthcare. *Microbial Biotechnology*, *17*(11), e70027. DOI: 10.1111/1751-7915.70027 PMID: 39487766

Rittel, H. W. J., & Webber, M. M. (1973). Dilemmas in a general theory of planning. *Policy Sciences*, *4*(2), 155–169. DOI: 10.1007/BF01405730

Slater, B., & Schur, M. (2023, August 23). The future of healthcare as an integrated ecosystem of health and care. Gensler. https://www.gensler.com/blog/future-of-healthcare-as-integrated-ecosystem

Sonka Medical. (n.d.). https://www.sonkamedical.com/

Stobierski, T. (2021, March 23). What is health care economics? Harvard Business School Online. https://online.hbs.edu/blog/post/what-is-healthcare-economics

Sun, Y., Sheng, D., Zhou, Z., & Wu, Y. (2024). AI hallucination: Towards a comprehensive classification of distorted information in artificial intelligence-generated content. *Humanities & Social Sciences Communications*, *11*(1), 1278. DOI: 10.1057/s41599-024-03811-x

University of Hawai'i. (2023). Breakthrough for sweat: Health monitoring device from UH researchers. https://www.hawaii.edu/news/2023/05/03/sweatainer-health-device/

Viswanadham, N. (2021). Ecosystem model for healthcare platform. *Sadhana*, *46*(4), 188. DOI: 10.1007/s12046-021-01708-y

World Economic Forum. (2025). Ways AI is transforming healthcare. https://www.weforum.org/stories/2025/08/ai-transforming-global-health/

World Health Organization. (2025). India first country to launch a Traditional Knowledge Digital Library. https://economictimes.indiatimes.com/news/india/india-first-country-to-launch-a-traditional-knowledge-digital-library-who/articleshow/122403845.cms

World Health Organization & International Telecommunication Union. (2025). Mapping the application of artificial intelligence in traditional medicine: Technical brief.

ADDITIONAL READINGS

Mathur, S., Kalla, A., Gür, G., Bohra, M. K., & Liyanage, M. A Survey on Role of Blockchain for IoT: Applications and Technical Aspects, Computer Networks, Volume 227, 2023, 109726, ISSN 1389-1286, DOI: 10.1016/j.comnet.2023.109726

Nourse, R., Dingler, T., Kelly, J., Kwasnicka, D., & Maddison, R. (2023, December 18). The Role of a Smart Health Ecosystem in Transforming the Management of Chronic Health Conditions. *Journal of Medical Internet Research*, *25*, e44265. DOI: 10.2196/44265 PMID: 38109188

Bajwa, J., Munir, U., Nori, A., & Williams, B. (2021, July). Artificial intelligence in healthcare: Transforming the practice of medicine. *Future Healthcare Journal*, *8*(2), e188–e194. DOI: 10.7861/fhj.2021-0095 PMID: 34286183

KEY TERMS AND DEFINITIONS

5G NSA: (Non-Standard Alone) is a hybrid development using 5G radio antennas for data transfer while relying on the existing 4G LTE core infrastructure for signaling and control. It offers lower cost deployment and faster speeds but little improvement on latency.

5G SA: (Stand Alone) The new 5G communication network architecture offers a much faster data transfer rates along with ultra-low latency and increased security.

AI: Artificial Intelligence

Broadband Network Connectivity: Covers a large range of frequencies for communication. According to FCC broadband refers to a minimum of 25 Mbps for download speeds and 3 Mbps for upload speeds.

CAGR: Compound Annual Growth Rate

COVID: Corona Virus Disease

FCC: Federal Communications Commission

HIPAA: Health Insurance Portability and Accountability Act

HIPAA: Health Insurance Portability and Accountability Act

IoMT: Internet of Medical Things

IoT: Internet of Things

Latency: The delay in time before a transfer of data begins following an instruction. Also a measure of download time.

LLM: Large Language Model

LTE: Long Term Evolution 4G LTE is a significant upgrade on the previous 3G (Third Generation) technology.

Mbps: Megabits per second

Moltbook: A “social network” of AI Chatbots/Agents

NSA: Non-Stand Alone

NTCA: Rural Broadband Association (Formerly National Telecommunications Cooperative Association) represents independent, community-based telecommunications associations across the U.S.

SA: Stand Alone

WEF: World Economic Forum

WHO: World Health Organization

Chapter 7
Medically Supervised Fasting (MSF) as a Way to Curb U.S. Healthcare Expenditures:
A Call to Action

Charles J. Hobson
http://orcid.org/0009-0001-6520-5002
Indiana University Northwest, USA

Crystal C. Shannon
http://orcid.org/0009-0004-2466-4247
Indiana University Northwest, USA

ABSTRACT

Medically supervised fasting (MSF) is introduced as an evidenced-based frontline treatment for a broad range of human diseases that is efficacious, safe, and very cost effective, compared to traditional medical practices. A specific call to action is presented involving the federal government, healthcare providers, health insurance companies, businesses, and a public service information campaign. Finally, anticipated obstacles are identified and discussed, including the pharmaceutical industry, OTC manufacturers, the hospital industry, the medical profession, and public lack of knowledge/misperceptions.

DOI: 10.4018/979-8-3373-2577-4.ch007

INTRODUCTION

In a ground breaking new book, The Great Healthcare Disruption: Big Tech, Bold Policy, and the Future of American Medicine (2025) Marshall Runge, MD, Dean of the University of Michigan Medical School, details the crushing problems facing the US healthcare system (surging costs, rising incidence of chronic diseases, and stagnating life-expectancies) and describes a set of "disruptors" likely to dramatically alter and improve healthcare in the future. To his impressive list, we would add the increased use of medically supervised fasting (MSF) as a frontline treatment for many diseases/illnesses.

Thirty years ago, Joel Fuhrman, MD, author of book, Fasting and Eating for Health: A Medical Doctor's Program for Conquering Disease (1995), made the following bold and provocative statements, (p. 212):

Rather than starting patients on drugs for chronic diseases, now physicians can offer suitable patients a chance to recover their health through natural diet and fasting. If dietary considerations, including the aggressive nutritional approach described in this book, are not offered and discussed with patients initially, their doctors are selling them short. These physicians are not disclosing all the pertinent information that patients need to make informed decisions about their health condition.

> *Whether the patient has a cardiac condition, hypertension, autoimmune disease, fibroids, or asthma, he or she must be informed that fasting and natural plant-based diets are a viable alternative to conventional therapy, and an effective one. The time may come when not offering this substantially more effective nutritional approach will be considered malpractice [emphasis added].*

Since this book was published, Americans overall have become sicker and healthcare spending has increased dramatically, as described in the next section. Thus, the time has come to embrace and leverage fasting as an efficacious, cost-effective treatment for a wide variety of diseases/illnesses.

BACKGROUND

According to the Centers for Medicare and Medicaid Services (CMS, 2025), National Health Expenditures (NHE) totaled a staggering $4.9 trillion in 2023 and accounted for 17.6% of US Gross Domestic Product (GDP). Medicare ($1.3 trillion) represented 21% of NHE, while Medicaid accounted for another 7.9% ($872 billion). The Center on Budget and Policy Priorities (2025) estimated that four national health insurance programs (Medicare, Medicaid, CHIP, and the ACA) represented 24%

of the entire federal budget. Annual health expenditures are predicted to continue increasing at rates above inflation and growth in GDP.

CMS figures for 2023 indicate that the private business sector accounted for 18% ($882 billion) of total national healthcare spending. A report from the Society for Human Resource Management (Mayer, 2024) estimated that average employer-sponsored healthcare costs per employee will increase from $14,823 in 2024 to $16,157 in 2025, a rise of 9%. These burgeoning healthcare costs are unsustainable and pose an immediate threat to the viability of many firms, especially smaller businesses that are unable to qualify for discounted pricing.

Households and individual consumers shouldered 27% ($1.323 trillion) of total healthcare expenditures in 2023 (CMS). In an article entitled, "Healthcare Insights: How Medical Debt is Crushing 100 Million Americans", John August (2024) from the Cornell ILR Scheinman Institute noted that 66.5% of personal bankruptcies in the US annually (an estimated 550,000 people) are primarily attributable to medical debt. Other adverse outcomes include delaying needed medical care, decreased credit scores leading to higher borrowing costs, and general declines in standard of living.

The shocking magnitude and seemingly uncontrollable inflation in US health-care spending have a crippling impact on our country, the business community, and individuals/families. Maintaining the status quo or making marginal changes are simply not acceptable. Bold action in the prevention and management of chronic disease and acute illness is needed, and needed now.

ANALYSIS

Purpose

The purpose of this chapter is to identify a unique approach to medical care very rarely used by practitioners, but it is as old as time. This chapter presents medically supervised fasting (MSF) as a safe, efficacious, cost-effective first-choice treatment for a variety of chronic diseases and minor illnesses. The rapidly expanding clinical research base (discussed below) justifies optimism about its potential as a treatment modality.

MSF is an opportunity for patients to assume greater responsibility and become more engaged and involved in the management of their own health and prevention (or mitigation) of disease. Healthcare professionals provide guidance and oversight of patients seeking to attain improved health outcomes. Additionally, medical oversight allows for greater benefits than general fasting alone due to the additional monitoring and ready response for needed healthcare intervention, if applicable.

The widespread utilization of MSF as a recognized medical treatment, would result in seismic changes in the US healthcare system (budgetary and patient care delivery). Thankfully, given the dawning "age of disruption" in federal, state, and local government, it is likely that this approach would be enthusiastically welcome by those focused on both the budget cutting impact of fasting and the promotion of the public's health. Leaders on both fronts might work to expand and promote its use.

Fasting Research

Focus on High Quality Journal Articles

Given the disturbing allegations and scathing conclusions in Dr. Casaba Szabo's newly published book (Unreliable: Bias, Fraud, and the Reproducibility Crisis in Biomedical Research, 2025), every effort was made to restrict citations in this chapter to articles from recognized, top-quality academic journals.

Definitions Within the empirical literature on fasting, researchers have tested a wide variety of schedules using different operational definitions for each one. In an effort to address these inconsistencies and the resultant confession that has arisen, Koppold, et al. (2024) conducted a Delphi methodology study with a multidisciplinary, multinational expert panel of 38 researchers and clinicians to formulate consensus definitions for 24 fasting-related terms. Two examples include the term "fasting", defined as "a voluntary abstinence from some or all foods or foods and beverages for preventive, therapeutic, religious, cultural, or other reasons" (p.1782), and the term "intermittent fasting", described as "repetitive fasting periods lasting up to 48 hours each including fasting regimens of 1 fasting day per week, 2 separate or consecutive fasting days per week, alternative-day fasting (ADF), and time-restricted eating (TRE)" (p. 1785). We applaud this effort and encourage consistent use of this nomenclature moving forward.

Literature Review Articles While much of the early research on fasting was done with animals, in the last 20 years there has been a proliferation of high quality experimental research with human subjects Cabo and Mattson (2019) reviewed the growing clinical literature on intermittent fasting in the New England Journal of Medicine and found solid evidence of its effectiveness in treating type 2 diabetes, obesity, cardiovascular disease, certain cancers, and neurologic disorders, such as Alzheimer's disease. Sun et al. [20 coauthors] published an impressive article in 2024 that consisted of an umbrella review of 23 meta-analyses evaluating the impact of intermittent fasting on 34 important health outcomes implicated in a wide variety of human disease processes. They confirmed that intermittent fasting had a beneficial impact on: (1) waist circumference, (2) fat mass, (3) low-density lipoprotein cholesterol, (4) high-density lipoprotein cholesterol, (5) total cholesterol,

(6) total triacyclglycerols, (7) fasting insulin, (8) systolic blood pressure, and (9) fat free mass. The authors concluded by calling her for more research addressing the precise mechanisms by which these health outcomes impact human functioning and well-being.

Sickness Associated Anorexia While medical fasting research has focused primarily on major diseases, like those cited earlier in the review by Cabo and Mattson (2019), intriguing research by Aviello, Cristiano, Luckman, and D'Agostino (2021), Van Niekerk, Loos, Nell, and Engelbrecht (2016), and Wilhelm, Surendar, and Karagiannis (2021) suggests that caloric restriction during infection- caused minor illness may also be beneficial. Van Niekerk et al. introduced and discussed the concept of sickness-associated anorexia (loss of appetite) or SAA. The authors noted that, in spite of the heavy metabolic cost of immune system activation, a "universal and cardinal manifestation" in both vertebrates and invertebrates is a pronounced decrease in appetite. They provide preliminary evidence suggesting that SAA is an evolution derived response, designed to enhance immune system functioning. An intriguing corollary proposition is also offended: Prior fasting may be a promising strategy to enhance vaccine effectiveness.

A comprehensive review by Wilhelm et al. (p. 1) concluded that: "The latest evidence suggests that dietary restriction may play an important regulatory role by influencing the activation and effector functions of immune cells." They also contend that the effectiveness of SAA may be contingent upon the nutritional reserves of the individual. For example, SAA would likely be harmful for someone who was severely malnourished. Aviello et al. noted that anorexia has "immediate beneficial outcomes for the host." However, they cite evidence suggesting that SAA appears to have a differential impact on bacterial as compared to viral infections.

The researchers in all three of these articles emphasize the compelling need for more, large scale clinical studies. Important unanswered questions include: the precise mechanisms by which SAA impacts the human immune system, the types of pathogens against which SAA is most effective, and the characteristics of patients that mediate the success of SAA in fighting infections.

A classic sleep study may provide a useful model for future research on SAA. Cohen, Doyle, Alper, Janicki-Deverts, and Turner (2009) recruited 153 healthy men and women, monitored their sleep habits for two weeks, then administered nasal spray containing a rhinovirus, quarantined the subjects for five days, and monitored them for signs of illness. Using this general format, a large sample of volunteers could be administered a similar pathogen, quarantined, and monitored for symptoms. For those who develop symptoms, three experimental groups could be created: (1) subjects who immediately begin fasting, (2) subjects who use common over-the-counter (OTC) medications, and (3) subjects who take no action. The experimental groups could then be compared on the duration and severity of experienced symptoms, the financial costs involved, and subject characteristics related to these outcomes. Similar large sample studies could be conducted with a variety of pathogens to determine the relative efficacy and cost savings of SAA in treating each of them.

Economic Impact Research Of particular relevance to this chapter is a recent article by Habka, Hsu, and Antoun (2025), entitled "Economic Evaluation of Fasting Mimicking Diet Versus Standard Care in Diabetic Patients on Dual or Triple Medications at Baseline in the United States: A Cost-Utility Model" in Value in Health. The authors developed and tested a model evaluating the impact of a periodic 5-day Fasting Mimicking Diet (FMD) followed for 3 years on health outcomes and cost-benefit figures over a 10-year timeframe.

Their results indicated that the FMD program resulted in: (1) 11.4% fewer diabetes complications, (2) 67.2% lower medication use, and (3) 45.0% fewer hypoglycemia events over a 10-year period. The net cost savings (primarily due to the decrease in medication use) was estimated to be $41,613 per patient.

For illustration purposes, if one assumes that 25% of the 34.1 million Americans with diabetes (CDC, 2020) are on dual or triple medications at baseline (.25 x 34.1 million = 8.5 million), the estimated cost savings over 10 years is $353.7 billion (8.5 million x $41, 613)!

Emerging New Research New applications of fasting as a potential treatment for a variety of health challenges continue to appear on a regular basis. Two noteable examples include the following. Caron, Kreher, Wu, and Przkora (2022) reported on promising results with intermittent fasting in the treatment of chronic pain. Lira-Junior, Arogáin, Crncalo, Ekberg, Chotirmall, Pettersson, Gustafsson, Biamar, and Bostanci (2024) conducted a small sample study indicating that intermittent fasting decreased periodontal inflammation.

Future Research Virtually every academic paper on the use of fasting in human subjects calls for more research to better understand the mechanisms that relate caloric restriction to health, to include longitudinal studies that address adverse events and longevity. When comparing fasting to traditional treatment options, large sample longitudinal randomized control trials are needed to accurately assess:

(1) clinical outcomes,
(2) cost,
(3) safety/side effects,
(4) patient satisfaction, and
(5) patient eligibility requirements.

It should be noted that fasting is not appropriate for everyone or for all medical conditions. According to Johns Hopkins Medicine (2025), fasting is contraindicated for the following populations: (1) children and teenagers younger than 18, (2) women who are pregnant or breast feeding, (3) people with type 1 diabetes, and (4) anyone with a history of eating disorders. This is but one example and presents a valid reason why discussions on fasting should occur in collaboration with medical care providers. However, many providers are unaware of the potential positive impact of fasting and may limit it as a viable option for patients.

SOLUTIONS AND RECOMMENDATIONS

A Call to Action—Federal Level

The President and/or Secretaries of HHS or VA could immediately direct the FDA (or an appointed independent medical board) to review the current clinical research literature on fasting to:

(1) determine if sufficient evidence presently exists to certify fasting as a first-choice treatment option for a particular disease (i.e., type 2 diabetes), based upon its documented efficacy and safety and
(2) identify and prioritize promising fasting applications that require additional research before certification is possible.

Once certified, the President or Department Secretaries could direct all federal healthcare programs and insurers to include fasting as a first-choice treatment for specific diseases, unless contraindicated for particular patients. Similar action would be expected in the private sector. These steps should result in decreased federal spending, lower deficits, and improved government credit ratings.

An integral component of this federally funded fasting research initiative should be the development of a national AI database, consisting of patient information (personal identifiers removed), treatment factors, and outcomes. Access to this information would yield critical insights concerning: (1) matching patients with optimal fasting regimens and (2) identifying those for whom fasting is contraindicated.

Working with Congress, the President and Department Secretaries can reallocate medical grant funding to support prioritized fasting research. Congress and the corporate sector could be solicited for additional and future funding, as needed.

The U.S. Department of Veterans Affairs (VA) of hospitals and clinics may offer an ideal environment in which to conduct rigorous fasting research. The federally funded agency provides a full range of in-patient and out-patient medical services to U.S. military veterans.

The VA has a longstanding commitment to conducting evidence-based research in-pursuit of innovations in healthcare, publishes an Annual State of Innovation

Report, and has delivered decades of impactful advances, including nuclear imaging technology, the cardiac peacemaker, new diabetes drugs, and the shingles vaccine. One major VA strategic priority for innovation is to increase veteran access to high-quality clinical trials.

It is also important to note that the VA takes a holistic approach to treating patients called Whole Health, which incorporates complementary and integrative healthcare in combination with conventional medical care. For example, the VA continues to conduct pioneering research on non-drug treatments for pain. Fasting as a potential treatment modality fits nicely within the VA's holistic model. Finally, given the present budget cutting across all federal agencies, the VA may be very interested in replicating the cost savings attributable to the use of the Fast Mimicking Diet to treat type 2 diabetes (Habka et al, 2025) discussed earlier.

A Call to Action—Healthcare Providers

To the extent that fasting is embraced by the public, increased patient demand will require significantly more healthcare providers with the requisite training in all aspects of fasting. This will involve continuing professional education for current providers and collegiate curriculum modifications for future providers.

Advanced Practice Registered Nurses (APRNs) provide a level of medical care supervision that may be in direct collaboration or consultation with a medical doctor and are foundationally prepared in a focus on holistic care modalities and non-pharmacological treatments for many chronic diseases (NONPF.com). Although similar in many ways, these care providers differ from their physician counterparts in their scope of practice and primary focus on patient-centered care. This holistic approach to supporting those with medical conditions, place APRNs in a unique position to champion alternative approaches to care delivery.

In fact, several articles have outlined the role APRNs can play in using fasting as a treatment modality. Nye, Cherrin, and Meirs (2024) acknowledge the health benefits of fasting and recommend the use medical supervision (regular physical evaluations, laboratory testing, dietary consult) along with cognitive behavioral modification support as a way to address lifestyle risk factors. Specifically, APRNs are pivotal in supporting the safety and effectiveness of MSF care management through patient education and counseling (e.g., types of fasting options and impact on body systems), development of patient appropriate medical fasting care plans, and engagement in interdisciplinary collaboration in support of holistic patient care.

As mentioned earlier, many healthcare providers (e.g., physicians and nurses) may not be fully aware of the potential positive health-related impact of fasting and simply view it as weight loss intervention. Therefore, the inclusion of continuing medical and nursing education is woefully needed for current practitioners. This can be provided through the delivery of a variety of available micro-credentials (e.g., Institute for Functional Medicine) and certifications in implementing health quality initiatives (which may include fasting protocols). Additionally, a review of the core preparatory health provider curriculum is needed to evaluate the current level of exposure health professions students have to alternative care delivery models (e.g., fasting).

A Call to Action—Health Insurance Companies

Firms that provide health insurance will play a pivotal role in the adaption of MSF as a treatment for a range of diseases/illnesses. Based upon the evidenced-based review and certification process discussed above by the FDA or other medical advisory board, fasting will be certified as a treatment for specific diseases or illnesses.

After certification has been obtained, health insurance organizations should: (1) formulate treatment and reimbursement protocols to incentivize patient use of MSF (unless contraindicated) and before prescription medications or surgery are authorized, (2) offer full-reimbursement for patient education on fasting to physicians and other healthcare professionals, and (3) provide full-reimbursement for medical supervision of fasting and any fasting-related laboratory testing. We also strongly recommend participation in the national AI database on fasting outcomes mentioned earlier.

A Call to Action—Businesses

The incessant increases in healthcare costs provide businesses with a powerful incentive to encourage and support the use of MSF as a frontline medical treatment. In order to facilitate these processes, several concrete steps can be taken. These include: (1) working with health insurance providers to encourage/require (unless contraindicated) fasting as an evidenced-based first step treatment for a specific list of conditions, (2) offering onsite fasting workshops to educate employees about the health benefits of fasting and perhaps a fasting "hotline" for questions, (3) incentivizing employees who try fasting, (4) establishing fasting support groups, and (5) when possible, providing funding for continuing research on fasting. Taken together, these actions should lead to substantially lower healthcare costs and an improved bottom line.

A Call to Action—Public Service Campaign

In order for a MSF initiative to be successful, a coordinated multi-pronged national public service campaign to educate consumers is clearly needed. The fundamental message is that fasting is an incredibly effective, generally very safe, and extremely cost-efficient way to treat a variety of chronic diseases and acute illnesses. It must be delivered via multiple media from reputable medical authorities and well-known celebrities. A convenient, free app may be a particularly impactful way to convey this information. The following basic issues must be addressed in clear and simple language:

What is fasting?
What are the different types of fasting?
How much does fasting cost?
How does fasting work?
What can I expect when fasting?
What processes control hunger during fasting?
Where can I find additional information about fasting?
Where can I find medical professionals with expertise in fasting?
How do I know if I am able to fast?
How to talk with my health provider about my eligibility for a medically supervised fast?

Time Magazine (Haupt, May 12, 2025) provided an excellent set of five questions that patients, as self-advocates, should ask at doctor's appointments. To this list, we would add the following five questions related to fasting.

1. Given my diagnosis, is fasting a possible treatment option?
2. Is fasting contraindicated for me? If so, why?
3. Can you explain how fasting might work for me and what I can expect?
4. Can you recommend an app to help guide my fasting?
5. Can you, or someone you refer me to, medically supervise my fast?

For anyone interested in a comprehensive, informative history of fasting, the book, *The Oldest Cure in the World: Adventures in the Art and Science of Fasting*, by Steven Hendricks (2022) is highly recommended.

FUTURE DIRECTIONS

Overcoming Opposition

The widespread introduction and use of fasting as a medical treatment would likely result in considerable disruption in the US healthcare industry. Thus, one could reasonably anticipate determined, organized, and well-funded opposition. Likely sources would include: (1) the pharmaceutical industry, (2) OTC medication manufacturers, (3) the hospital industry, (4) the medical profession, and (5) the public.

Pharmaceutical Industry Chacko (2025) from Statifacts calculated that the total size of the US pharmaceutical market in 2024 was $634.34 billion, and predicted to rise to $670.69 billion in 2025 and $1.11 trillion by 2034. Manufacturing and selling prescription drugs has been extremely profitable for several large US and international companies.

Widespread adoption of MSF as a treatment for chronic disease and acute illness can be expected to dramatically decrease the size of pharmaceutical market, seriously threatening the profitability and viability of domestic drug firms. Consequently, determined opposition from Big Pharma can be anticipated and should not be under-estimated.

This opposition could take several forms, from political lobbying/campaign contributions at the federal and state levels, to a variety of influence strategies with health insurance providers, hospitals, and medical prescribers. Writing in the AMA Journal of Ethics, From the Editor, Medicine and the Market, Kushnick (2015) asserted that: "Pharmaceutical companies affect not only physicans' prescribing practices, but also which drugs are developed, how much they cost, and their availability in ways influenced by financial motives."

OTC Manufacturers Similar to the pharmaceutical industry, makers of OTC remedies can expect to see pronounced declines in their sales if fasting is widely utilized. Statistica (2025) estimated that the size of the US OTC market in 2025 to be $42.76 billion, with the largest portion being cold & cough remedies, totaling $11.71 billion (27.4%). The per capita cost was $124.44 or nearly $500.00 ($497.76) for a family of four. Opposition strategies will likely paralled those employed by the pharmaceutical industry discussed above.

Hospital Industry According to the American Hospital Association's Fast Facts on US Hospitals, 2025, there are 6,093 hospitals with 913,136 staffed beds. Grandview Research (2024) estimated the total US hospital services market in 2024 was $1.6 trillion, almost one-third of overall national healthcare spending.

Broad utilization of MSF as a first-choice treatment for many diseases/illnesses can be expected to result in a dramatic decrease in the demand for hospital beds, many surgical procedures, and a broad spectrum of diagnostic testing. These disruptions will pose compelling existential threats to many institutions, particularly smaller hospitals and those in rural areas. Oppositional strategies are likely to be similar to those discussed above pertinent to the pharmaceutical and OTC industries.

Medical Profession The proliferation of MSF in the US provides a significant opportunity to change the very foundation of the health care delivery system by both reducing *and* modifying health care services to treat a wide range of chronic diseases and illnesses. Medical specialties involved in treating the conditions found by Cabo and Mattson (2019) to be effectively impacted by intermittent fasting ("type 2 diabetes, obesity, cardiovascular disease, certain cancers, and neurologic disorders, such as Alzheimer's disease") would be particularly hard hit. Medical providers in these areas could experience huge declines in their income/patient load and the potential need for retraining in another specialty, possibility involving a more holistic/preventive approach to healthcare utilizing therapeutic fasting. Anyone facing serious threats to their likelihood can be expected to fight back and oppose the casual nexus.

A significant factor influencing this opposition is the lack of medical education preparation and acceptance of fasting as a viable treatment option. Traditional medical education (especially in westernized countries) rarely includes fasting in the core curriculum for healthcare providers (physicians and nurses) and if mentioned, it may only be relegated to concepts covered by integrative medicine curricula. In fact, even subjects such as nutrition remain largely limited in most educational settings (Eldin, et al., 2024). The promotion of MSF as an approved treatment option also places greater emphasis on nutrition education and improved patient outcomes.

Public Knowledge and Misperceptions Two of the most challenging obstacles to the acceptance and utilization of fasting as a legitimate medical treatment may be the public's current lack of knowledge and existing misperceptions. Our sense as educators is that the US public is generally unaware of what fasting is and how it can be used to treat a range of diseases/illnesses. While there are popular fads focusing on various intermittent fasting regimens for weight loss, fundamental knowledge about fasting is generally lacking. Common misperceptions can also be problematic. For example, Runge (2025, p. 194) noted a widespread belief among Americans that there is "a pill for everything, even though there isn't". Natural remedies like fasting are often not considered as possible treatments.

Also, given the societal focus on instant gratification, the ready availability of a wide variety of high-calorie, high-fat food and drink options, and the surging incidence of adulty obesity, the thought of possibly enduring intense hunger while fasting is anathema to many people. In fact, counter arguments concerning the role of hunger in fasting include: (1) with sickness associate anorexia, hunger is not present during illness, (2) many intermittent fasting options involve restricted eating only during specific times over a 24-hour period, and (3) as originally noted by Fuhrman (1995) and confirmed by Grundler, Mesnage, Ruppert, Kouretas, and Toledo (2024), even in long-term, water-only fasting, hunger typically vanishes by the second or third day of the fast.

While public opposition to fasting is certain to occur, with appropriate national educational programs (especially addressing the role of hunger and impulse control while fasting) and insurance incentives, we believe that public opinion can be slowly swayed in favor of fasting. Using the pragmatism of William James, we encourage those who are medically able to fast to "try it and see if it works". Our experience suggests that most people are pleasantly surprised at how relatively easy fasting is and how good they feel.

CONCLUSIONS

Medical research has documented that fasting represents an efficacious, safe, and cost-effective treatment for an expansive range of human diseases/illnesses. The widespread adoption of fasting holds the promise of positioning the US on the cusp of a historic inflection point in national healthcare costs. Instead of never ending annual increases, fasting offers an opportunity to dramatically reverse the trend and begin an era of continuous decline.

REFERENCES

American Hospital Association. (2025) Fast facts on U.S. hospitals, 2025, https://www.aha.org/statistics/fast-facts-us-hospitals. Retrieved May 30, 2025.

August, J. (2024) Healthcare insights: How medical debt is crushing 100 million Americans. Cornell ILR Scheinman Institute, Oct. 21, 2024. https://www.ilr.cornell.edu/scheinman-institute/blog/john-august-healthcare/healthcare-insights-how-medical-debt-crushing-100-million-americans

Aviello, G., Cristiano, C., Luckman, S. M., & D'Agostino, G. (2021). Brain control of appetite during sickness. *British Journal of Pharmacology*, *178*(10), 2096–2110. DOI: 10.1111/bph.15189 PMID: 32627171

Cabo, R., & Mattson, M. P. (2019). Effects of intermittent fasting on health, aging, and disease. *The New England Journal of Medicine*, *381*(26), 2541–2551. DOI: 10.1056/NEJMra1905136 PMID: 31881139

Caron, J. P., Kreher, M. A., Mickle, A. M., Wu, S., Przkora, R., Estores, I. M., & Sibille, K. T. (2022). Intermittent fasting: Potential utility in the treatment of chronic pain across the clinical spectrum. *Nutrients*, *14*(12), 2536. DOI: 10.3390/nu14122536 PMID: 35745266

Center on Budget and Policy Priorities. (2025) Policy basics: Where do our federal tax dollars go? https://www.chpp.org/research/federal-budget/where-do-our-federal-tax-dollars-go. Retrieved February 22, 2025.

Centers for Medicare and Medicaid Service – CMS. (2025) National health expenditures (NHE) fact sheet. https://www.cms.gov/data-research/statistics-trents-and-reports/national-health-expenditures-data/nhe-fact-sheet. Retrieved January 20, 2025.

Cohen, S., Doyle, W.J., Alper, C.M., Janicki-Deverts, D. & Turner, R.B. (2009). Sleep habits and susceptibility to the common cold. Archives of Internal Medicine, Jan, 169 (1), 62-67. DOI: 10.1001/archinternmed.2008.505

Eldin, M. M., Huynh, C., Eldin, R. A., Khan, S., Nguyen, B., & Kim, G. (2024). 8 The current state of nutrition education in medical schools in the United States: An analysis of curriculum, faculty perspectives, and resources. *BMJ Nutrition, Prevention & Health*, *7*, A4.1–A4. Advance online publication. DOI: 10.1136/bmjnph-2024-nnedprosummit2023.8

Fuhrman, J. (1995). *Fasting and eating for health: A Medical doctor's program for conquering disease*. St. Martin's Griffin.

Grandview Research. (2024) U.S. hospital services market size and outlooks, https://www.grandviewresearch.com/horizon/outlook/hosptial-servicesmarket. Retrieved May 30, 2025.

Grundler, F., Mesnage, R., Ruppert, P. M. M., Kouretas, D., & Toledo, F. W. (2024). Long-term fasting-induced ketosis in 1610 subjects: Metabolic regulation and safety. *Nutrients*, *16*(12), 1849. DOI: 10.3390/nu16121849 PMID: 38931204

Habka, D., Hsu, W. C., & Antoun, J. (2025). Economic evaluation of fasting mimicking diet versus standard care in diabetic patients on dual or triple medications at baseline in the United States: A cost-utility analysis. *Value in Health*, *28*(1), 51–59. DOI: 10.1016/j.jval.2024.08.003 PMID: 39343090

Haupt, A. (2025, May 12). 5 questions you should always ask at doctor's appointments. *Time*, •••, 8.

Hendricks, S. (2022) The oldest cure in the world: Adventures in the art and science of fasting. New York: Abrams Press Johns Hopkins Medicine (2025) Intermittent fasting: What is it, and how does it work? https://www.hopkinsmedicine.org/health/wellness-and-prevention/intermittent-fasting-what-is-it-and-how-does-it-work. Retrieved January 20, 2025.

Koppold, D. A., Breinlinger, C., Hanslian, E., Kessler, C., Cramer, H., Rajput Khokhar, A., Peterson, C. M., Tinsley, G., Vernieri, C., Bloomer, R., Boschmann, M., Bragazzi, N., Brandhorst, S., Gabel, K., Goldhamer, A. C., Grajower, M., Harvie, M., Heilbronn, L., Home, B., & Michalsen, A. (2024). International consensus on fasting terminology. *Cell Metabolism*, *36*(8), 1779–1794. DOI: 10.1016/j.cmet.2024.06.013 PMID: 39059384

Kushnick, H. L. (2015) Medicine and the market AMA Journal of Ethics, From the Editor, August 2015, https://journalofethics.ama-assn.org/article/medicine-and-market/2015-08

Lira-Junior, R., Aogain, M. M., Crncalo, E., Ekberg, N. R., Chotirmall, S. H., Pettersson, S., Gustafsson, A., Brismar, K., & Bostanci, N. (2024). Effects of intermittent fasting on periodontal inflammation and subgingival microbiota. *Journal of Periodontology*, *95*(7), 640–649. DOI: 10.1002/JPER.23-0676 PMID: 38655661

Luengo-Fernandez, R., Walli-Attaei, M., Gray, A., Torbica, A., Maggioni, A. P., Huculeci, R., Bairami, F., Aboyans, V., Timmis, A. D., Vardas, P., & Leal, J. (2023). Economic burden of cardiovascular diseases in the European Union: A population-based cost study. *European Heart Journal*, *44*(45), 4752–4767. DOI: 10.1093/eurheartj/ehad583 PMID: 37632363

Mayer, K. (2024) Employers project 8% - 9% rise in health care costs for 2025. Society for Human Resource Management, https://www.shrm.org/topics-tool/news/benefits-compensation/employers-project-8-9-rise-in-health-care-costs-for-2025. Retrieved May 26, 2025.

Niekerk, G., Loos, B., Nell, T., & Engelbrecht, A.M. Autophagy-A free meal in sickness-associated anorexia, Autophagy, 12 (4), 727-734, .DOI: 10.1080/15548627.2016.1147672

Nye, K., Cherrin, C., & Meires, J. (2024). Intermittent fasting: Exploring approaches, benefits, and implications for health and weight management. *The Journal for Nurse Practitioners, 20*(3), 104893. DOI: 10.1016/j.nurpra.2023.104893

Runge, M. (2025). *The great healthcare disruption: big tech, bold policy, and the future of american medicine*. Forbes Books.

Statifacts (2025) U.S. pharmaceutical market – Industry report. https://www.statifacts.com/outlook/us-pharmaceutical-market. Retrieved May 29, 2025.

Statista (2025) OTC pharmaceuticals – United States – market forecast. https://www.statista.com/outlook/hmo/otc-pharmaceuticals/united-states. Retrieved May 29, 2025.

Sun, M. L., Yao, W., Wang, X. Y., Gao, S., Varady, K. A., Forslund, S. K., Zhang, M. Z. Y., Cao, F., Zou, B. J., Sun, M. H., Liu, K. X., Bao, Q., Xu, J., Qin, X., Xiao, Q., Wu, L., Zhao, Y. H., Zhang, D. Y., Wu, Q. J., & Gong, T. T. (2024, April). Intermittent fasting and health outcomes: An umbrella review of systematic reviews and meta-analyses of randomized controlled trials. *EClinicalMedicine, 70*, 102519. DOI: 10.1016/j.eclinm.2024.102519 PMID: 38500840

Szabo, C. (2025). *Unreliable: Bias, fraud, and the reproducibility crisis in biomedical research*. Columbia University Press. DOI: 10.7312/szab21623

Wilhelm, C., Surendar, J., & Karagiannis, F. (2021) Enemy or ally? Fasting as an essential regulator of immune responses. Trends in Immunology, May, 42 (5), 389-400. .DOI: 10.1016/j.it.2021.03.007

ADDITIONAL READING

Goldhamer, A. (2025). *The science and power of therapeutic fasting*. Van Edward Publishing. ISBN: 9798263684501amazon

Kalam, F., James, D. L., Li, Y. R., Coleman, M. F., Kiesel, V. A., Cespedes Feliciano, E. M., . . . Kleckner, A. S. (2023). Intermittent fasting interventions to leverage metabolic and circadian mechanisms for cancer treatment and supportive care outcomes. *JNCI Monographs, 2023*(61), 84–103. https://escholarship.org/uc/item/49c622d6#author

Koppold, D. A., Michalsen, A., & Hanslian, E. (2024). Effectiveness of prolonged fasting in treating human chronic diseases: Clinical evidence and empirical insights from a specialized university medical center. In *Intermittent and periodic fasting, aging and disease* (pp. 243–267). Springer., https://link.springer.com/chapter/10.1007/978-3-031-49622-6_10 DOI: 10.1007/978-3-031-49622-6_10

Msane, S., Khathi, A., & Sosibo, A. (2024). Therapeutic potential of various intermittent fasting regimens in alleviating type 2 diabetes mellitus and prediabetes: A narrative review. *Nutrients, 16*(16), 2692. https://pubmed.ncbi.nlm.nih.gov/39203828/. DOI: 10.3390/nu16162692 PMID: 39203828

National Institute on Aging. (2020). *Research on intermittent fasting shows health benefits*. Retrieved from https://www.nia.nih.gov/news/research-intermittent-fasting-shows-health-benefits

Patikorn, C., Roubal, K., Veettil, S. K., Chandran, V., Pham, T., Lee, Y. Y., Giovannucci, E. L., Varady, K. A., & Chaiyakunapruk, N. (2021). Intermittent fasting and obesity-related health outcomes: An umbrella review of meta-analyses of randomized clinical trials. *JAMA Network Open, 4*(12), e2139558. https://jamanetwork.com/journals/jamanetworkopen/fullarticle/2787246. DOI: 10.1001/jamanetworkopen.2021.39558 PMID: 34919135

Semnani-Azad, Z., Khan, T. A., Chiavaroli, L., Chen, V., Bhatt, H. A., Chen, A., Chiang, N., Oguntala, J., Kabisch, S., Lau, D. C. W., Wharton, S., Sharma, A. M., Harris, L., Leiter, L. A., Hill, J. O., Hu, F. B., Lean, M. E. J., Kahleová, H., Rahelic, D., & Sievenpiper, J. L. (2025). Intermittent fasting strategies and their effects on body weight and other cardiometabolic risk factors: Systematic review and network meta-analysis of randomized clinical trials. *BMJ (Clinical Research Ed.), 389*, e082007. https://pubmed.ncbi.nlm.nih.gov/40533200/. DOI: 10.1136/bmj-2024-082007 PMID: 40533200

KEY TERMS AND DEFINITIONS

Big Pharma: The collection of large, international companies that produce pharmaceutical drugs for use in treating illness and disease.

Medically Supervised Fast (MSF): A planned reduction in individual caloric intake that is formulated and overseen by a healthcare professional with education and experience in supervising fasts.

National Health Expenditures (NHE): The total annual dollar amount spent in the United States on health-related products and services.

Time Restricted Eating (TRE): A type of intermittent fasting that continues caloric intake to specific periods of time during a 24-hour day.

Chapter 8
Opportunities in Mental Healthcare Reform

Mahendra Ramachandran
http://orcid.org/0009-0001-1692-6065
Independent Researcher, USA

Sarah Prabhu
http://orcid.org/0009-0001-1692-6065
National Alliance on Mental Illness (NAMI) - Santa Clara County, USA

ABSTRACT

This chapter reviews mental healthcare reform in the US, highlighting transinstitutionalization due to inadequate community support post-deinstitutionalization. It details legislative efforts, persistent access barriers (financial, attitudinal, structural, stigma), and the societal costs of delayed treatment. Proposed reforms include prioritizing affordability, combating stigma, strengthening primary care, and investing in early intervention. The text also explores nutritional psychiatry, the gut-brain axis, and the transformative potential of precision psychiatry via biomarkers and AI. Despite implementation hurdles, it advocates for collaborative efforts to achieve personalized mental healthcare and treat mental illnesses as brain diseases, not personal failings.

INTRODUCTION

The landscape of healthcare reform has seen remarkable progress in addressing physical health conditions, yet mental health remains an overlooked and underfunded area. While policies and laws promoting mental health parity exist, they lack enforcement mechanisms, leading to a continued disparity between psychological

DOI: 10.4018/979-8-3373-2577-4.ch008

and physical health care. Mental illnesses affect millions globally, with depression alone costing the economy over $1 trillion annually in lost productivity. However, solutions remain fragmented, and opportunities for meaningful reform remain under-explored.

In this chapter, we will examine the historical account of mental health laws in the United States and delve into current challenges within the mental health care system and propose strategic reforms. We will explore how early intervention, investment in diagnostic tools, and systemic policy changes can transform mental health care into a proactive rather than reactive system.

BACKGROUND: HISTORICAL OVERVIEW OF MENTAL HEALTH LAW IN THE UNITED STATES

Over the last hundred years, mental health law in the United States has undergone extensive and cyclical transformation, moving from a punitive, institutional model toward a vision of community-based care. This evolution towards community-based care has been driven by persistent advocacy from a variety of stakeholders, including family members, clinicians, and disability advocates. A paper published by George, P., Jones, N., Goldman, H., and Rosenblatt, A., 2023, highlights the federal and state legislative milestones that marked these healthcare reforms. However, a central, unintended consequence of these reforms has been the phenomenon of "transinstitutionalization," where the reduction in psychiatric hospital populations, mainly due to inadequate community infrastructure and funding, resulted in a significant increase in individuals with mental illness within the criminal justice system. Despite progress in recognizing patient rights and striving for insurance parity, achieving comprehensive and equitable mental health services remains an ongoing challenge, highlighting the dynamic nature of this public healthcare need.

From Punishment to Public Health: Early 20th Century Foundations

Before the 20th century, the societal response to mental illness was predominantly punitive and custodial. Individuals with mental health conditions were often confined in jails and almshouses alongside criminals and the impoverished. A shift began in the mid-19th century with the "moral treatment" movement, championed by reformers like Dorothea Dix, who advocated for the creation of dedicated psychiatric asylums to provide more humane environments. However, these institutions often fell into neglect and overcrowding by the end of the century.

The early 20th century saw the rise of the "Mental Hygiene movement," which introduced psychiatric hospitals and clinics as part of a public health initiative. Influential figures like Clifford Beers, whose autobiography "A Mind That Found Itself" exposed the harsh realities of mental institutions, spurred advocacy for the prevention of mental illness. As shown in Figure 1, this history though appears to be a simple linear progression, however, has a series of cyclical reforms, often initiated in response to the failures of previous eras and sustained by advocacy. This pattern underscores a continuous societal effort to balance humane care and individual rights with the practicalities of funding and public safety.

Figure 1. shows the key mental health laws that were passed in the US.

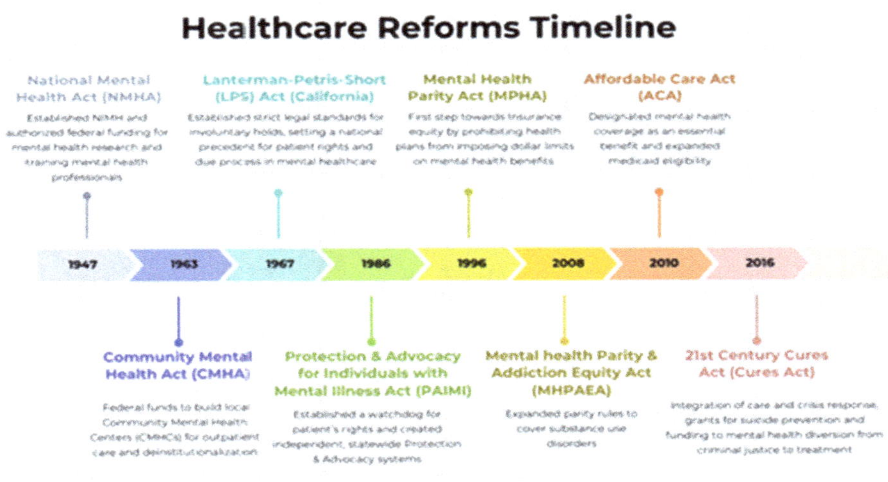

The Dawn of Federal Involvement: Post-World War II Shifts (1940s-1950s)

The alarming rates of mental health issues observed among draftees and veterans during World War II underscored a national mental health crisis that transcended state boundaries, necessitating federal intervention. On July 3, 1946, President Harry S. Truman signed the National Mental Health Act (NMHA) of 1946 into law. The NMHA law established the National Institute of Mental Health (NIMH). It allocated federal funds for crucial areas: research into psychiatric disorders, professional training for mental health clinicians, and preventive services. The overarching aim was to facilitate the development of more effective methods for the prevention, diagnosis, and treatment of mental illness.

The Act's focus on scientific inquiry and professionalization represented a significant departure from earlier custodial or moral treatment models, laying the groundwork for a more biomedical and evidence-based approach to mental illness. This federal leadership in research funding subsequently contributed to the development of several new psychiatric drugs. *Figure 2* shows the timeline of the development of antipsychotic drugs since 1940.

Figure 2. Saloni Dattani (2024). - "Antipsychotic medications: a timeline of innovations and remaining challenges" Published online at OurWorldinData.org.

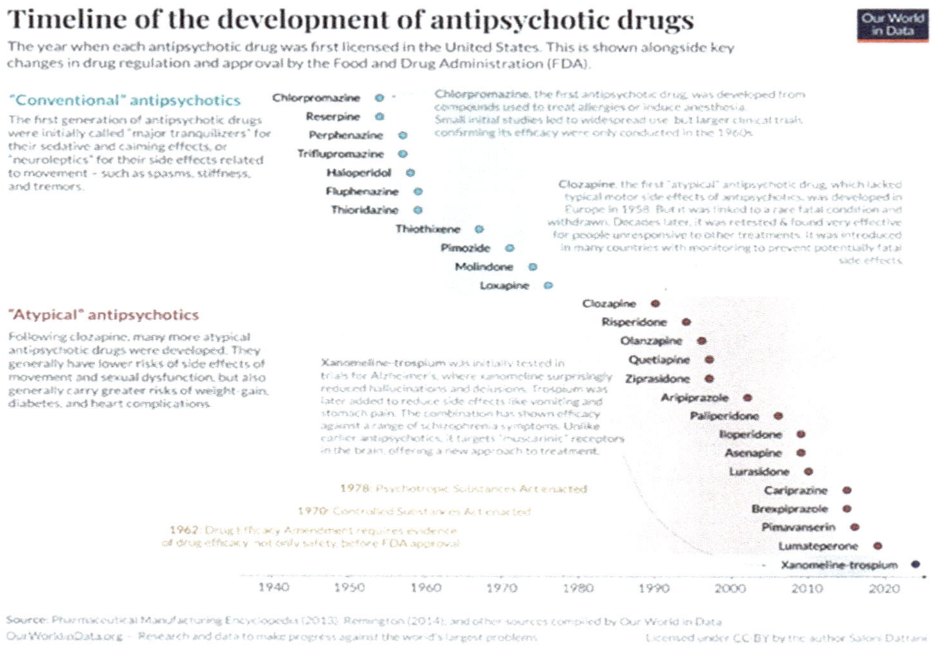

Retrieved from: 'https://ourworldindata.org/antipsychotic-medications-timeline'

Despite this federal action, the mid-20th century marked the peak of institutionalization, with over 500,000 individuals in psychiatric institutions in 1955, equivalent to 339 beds per 100,000 people.

As psychiatric institutions were seeing a rise in the number of admissions, some states like Texas, initiated reforms that formed the foundational ideas to shift from custodial care to treatment with a focus on basic human rights. The Texas Mental Health Code of 1957 defined the state's responsibility for mental health services and established patient rights, including visitation, religious freedom, and confidentiality.

The code also formalized voluntary admission processes and replaced stigmatizing terms like "lunacy" with "mental illness" to improve the undesirable conditions in overcrowded state hospitals.

The Deinstitutionalization Era and Its Paradox (1960s-1970s)

A monumental shift occurred with the Community Mental Health Act (CMHA) of 1963, signed by President John F. Kennedy. Its primary goal was to shift mental health treatment from large state hospitals to smaller, community-based settings, fostering individualized care and social freedom. The Act authorized federal funding for the construction of Community Mental Health Centers (CMHCs) nationwide.

As reported by Lamb, H. R. and Bachrach, L. L., 2001, the CMHA's vision was severely undermined by insufficient funding and policy gaps, creating a "deinstitutionalization paradox". CMHA's ambitious plan for 1,500 Community Mental Health Centers was never realized; only about half were built, partly due to budget constraints from the Vietnam War. This gap between legislative intent and practical execution led to unprecedented levels of homelessness and forced the criminal justice system into the role of a de facto mental healthcare provider.

The 1965 passage of the Institutions for Mental Diseases (IMD) exclusion for Medicaid further accelerated deinstitutionalization. This provision prohibited federal reimbursement for care in IMDs for adults aged 21-64, creating a financial disincentive for states to maintain large psychiatric hospitals and encouraging the transfer of patients to other facilities.

State-level legislation also played a crucial role. California's Lanterman-Petris-Short (LPS) Act of 1967 set a new standard for civil commitment, aiming to end inappropriate and indefinite involuntary commitments. The LPS Act established strict criteria, limiting involuntary detention to individuals who were a "danger to themselves, a danger to others, or gravely disabled" due to a mental illness. While protecting civil liberties and promoting treatment in the "least restrictive setting," the Act made involuntary commitment more difficult, contributing to the deinstitutionalization trend. Recent amendments, like California's Senate Bill 43, have expanded these terms to include individuals with severe substance use disorders or those who cannot ensure their own personal safety.

Transinstitutionalization: The Criminalization of Mental Illness

The era of deinstitutionalization saw a dramatic fall in the number of state psychiatric hospital beds, from a peak of 339 per 100,000 population in 1955 to fewer than 12 per 100,000 by 2016. By early 2023, the number stood at 10.8 beds per

100,000, a decrease of nearly 94% from its peak, while experts estimate a minimum need of 30 to 60 beds per 100,000.

This reduction coincided with a sharp increase in the number of individuals with mental illness in jails and prisons. As stated in Toynbee (2015), this inverse relationship aligns with the Penrose Hypothesis, proposed in 1939, which posits that as psychiatric bed availability decreases, the prisoner population increases. This phenomenon, known as "transinstitutionalization" or the "criminalization of mental illness," describes the process by which individuals discharged from hospitals or denied admission due to a lack of resources end up in the criminal justice system. By 2012, there were nearly ten times more individuals with mental illness in prisons than in psychiatric hospitals, a stark indicator of systemic failure. Figure 3 shows the data on the inverse relationship between decrease in number of psychiatric beds to increase in prisoner population in US for the past six decades.

Figure 3. The Penrose hypothesis predicts a negative (inverse) correlation between the number of psychiatric hospital beds and the number of people incarcerated in prisons. This historical data for the US strongly reflects this trend, driven by deinstitutionalization policy. The data point for the incarcerated population in 2020 reflects a notable drop, primarily due to accelerated releases and reduced admissions during the initial COVID-19 pandemic response.

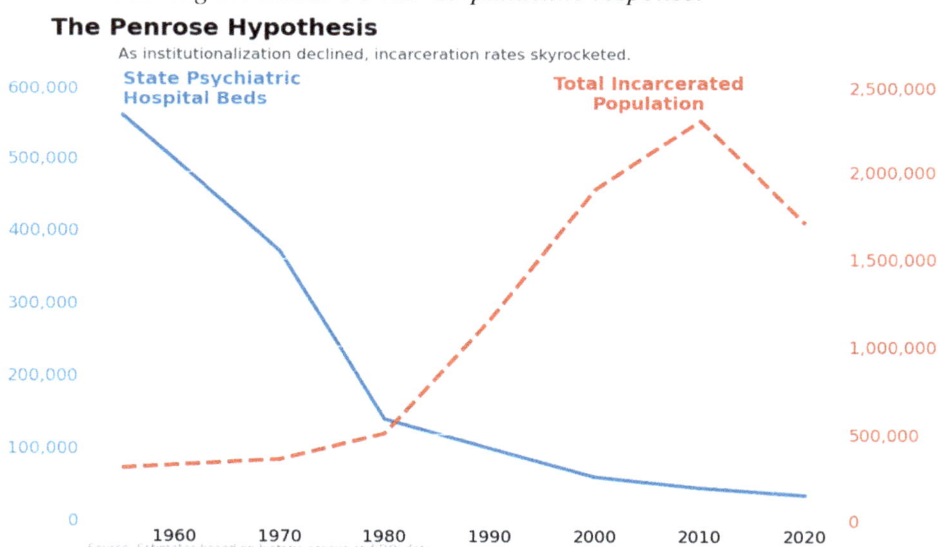

Data taken from: [1] US Department of Justice, Bureau of Justice Statistics. (2021, December). Prisoners in 2020 – Statistical Tables. Retrieved from https://bjs.ojp.gov/content/pub/pdf/p20st.pdf [2] US Department of Health and Human Services, Substance Abuse and Mental Health Services Administration, National Association of State Mental Health Program Directors Research Institute, Inc. (NRI). (2025). Use of State Psychiatric Hospitals, 2025. Retrieved from https://nri-inc.org/media/4bofjpqy/smha-use-of-state-psychiatric-hospitals-july-2025-final.pdf.

In her book Insane: America's Criminal Treatment of Mental Illness, Roth, A. (2018) investigates the widespread incarceration of the mentally ill in the US since transinstitutionalization and what she sees as impossible burdens placed on correctional officers to act as mental health providers when they are not adequately trained. The increase in the number of prison inmates with mental illness is due to the poor execution of deinstitutionalization, done without adequate development of supportive housing, social services, or community mental health infrastructure.

As reported in Schildbach S, Schildbach C. (2018) and Prins, S.J. (2011), this vulnerability was amplified by the "War on Drugs," which criminalized addiction, a condition often co-occurring with mental illness. The result is a regression to earlier, punitive approaches, with correctional facilities ill-equipped to provide care. Approximately 37% of state and federal prisoners and 44% of local jail inmates have a mental illness, about twice the rate of the general adult population. A staggering 63% of incarcerated individuals with a history of mental illness receive no treatment while in state and federal prisons. This lack of care can worsen symptoms and lead to higher rates of reincarceration, creating a costly "revolving door" that shifts the burden from healthcare to corrections with worse outcomes.

Reforming the System: Rights, Advocacy, and Parity (1980s-2000s)

The Mental Health Systems Act (MHSA) of 1980, signed by President Jimmy Carter, aimed to reform the system by providing federal grants for comprehensive, community-based care, with a focus on chronically ill individuals, children, and older adults. It also included a patient Bill of Rights. However, the Act was short-lived; most of its provisions were repealed in 1981 by President Ronald Reagan, reflecting a shift in political ideology toward smaller government and reduced federal spending. This "stop-start" pattern of federal policy created instability for long-term planning required to provide mental health services.

In response to reports of abuse and neglect, Congress passed the Protection and Advocacy for Mentally Ill Individuals Act of 1986 (PAIMI Act). This Act established independent, state-level protection and advocacy (P&A) systems to safeguard the rights of individuals with mental illness by investigating abuse and civil rights violations. In 2000, its authority was expanded to cover individuals living in the community. The PAIMI Act institutionalized mental health advocacy by establishing a legal framework for patient rights and oversight.

The Mental Health Amendments of 1990 re-established a federal framework for services, with a focus back on individuals with "serious mental illnesses" and "seriously emotionally disturbed children". It mandated state-level planning councils and authorized funding for research and training, particularly for underserved populations.

The push for equitable insurance coverage began with the Mental Health Parity Act (MHPA) of 1996. This first federal parity law prohibited large group health plans from imposing stricter annual or lifetime dollar limits on mental health benefits compared to medical benefits. While its impact was limited, it was a crucial first step.

A more comprehensive law, the Mental Health Parity and Addiction Equity Act (MHPAEA) of 2008, significantly expanded these requirements. It extended parity to substance use disorders (SUDs). It prohibited more restrictive financial requirements (like copays) and treatment limitations (like visit limits) for mental health and SUD benefits compared to medical/surgical benefits. These parity laws have improved financial protection and increased the use of mental health services. However, enforcement remains a challenge, with many insurers failing to fully comply with the law, highlighting a gap between legislative intent and practical access to care.

Judicial decisions have also profoundly shaped mental health laws. Landmark cases like Rouse v. Cameron (1966) established a right to treatment for committed patients, and Wyatt v. Stickney (1972) affirmed a constitutional right to individual treatment. O'Connor v. Donaldson (1975) held that states cannot confine a non-dangerous individual capable of surviving safely in freedom, tying involuntary commitment to dangerousness. Addington v. Texas (1979) established that commitment requires "clear and convincing evidence" of mental illness and dangerousness. These cases compelled states to reform their laws and improve conditions, serving as a vital catalyst for change.

Modern Landscape and Future Directions (2010s-Present)

The Affordable Care Act (ACA) of 2010 significantly advanced mental health coverage by designating mental health and SUD services as one of ten essential health benefits (EHBs) for most health plans, ensuring coverage for pre-existing conditions and prohibiting annual or lifetime dollar limits on these benefits. The ACA has improved access to care for millions, as insured adults are far more likely to receive mental health treatment. Nevertheless, challenges persist, including high out-of-pocket costs for privately insured individuals and potential cuts to programs like Medicaid, which covers nearly a third of adults with mental health disorders.

The 21st Century Cures Act of 2016 was another milestone, with its "Helping Families in Mental Health Crisis" division addressing prevention, treatment, and interactions with the criminal justice system. The Act strengthened mental health parity regulations, provided grants for community resources and suicide prevention, and funded de-escalation training for law enforcement. It also included provisions to divert individuals with mental illness from incarceration to treatment, aiming for a more patient-centered system.

The Federal Communications Commission (FCC) proposed a 3-digit, easy-to-remember number for suicide prevention in a report to Congress in August 2019, which was later enacted by President Trump on October 17, 2020, as the National Suicide Hotline Designation Act of 2020. The 9-8-8 number became available nationwide as the suicide prevention lifeline and the Veterans' crisis line.

Despite these legislative efforts, the problem of transinstitutionalization persists. The enforcement gap in parity laws continues to create barriers to care, and funding cuts threaten to worsen the situation. There is a broad consensus that simply increasing the number of psychiatric hospital beds will not solve the overrepresentation of individuals with serious mental illness in jails. Instead, a nuanced approach is needed that focuses on diverting individuals from the criminal justice system to community-based treatment. Community-based treatment requires a substantial investment in the behavioral health workforce and infrastructure, with an emphasis on integrating care for mental health and substance use. Reversing the Penrose Effect requires a sustained, comprehensive investment in community services to ensure individuals receive the proper care in the right setting.

ANALYSIS

Having understood the historical perspective of mental health laws and their impact on US society, this chapter focuses on the importance of early detection and intervention in mental healthcare, the barriers to access treatment, and their consequences. We will summarize the recommendations from our analysis and highlight the upcoming advances in diagnostics and treatment for mental healthcare.

Delayed Care

According to the National Institute of Mental Health (NIMH), approximately 59.3 million adults (1 in 5) in the US live with a mental health diagnosis. While 80% of people who live with a mental health disorder eventually seek professional help, studies show that there is an average delay of 11 years before they make their first contact with a clinician since they started experiencing the mental health symptoms.

Tom Insel, the former director of NIMH, states, "Early detection and intervention are the foundations for better outcomes" in addressing these disorders (Insel, 2014). Early intervention programs for psychosis have shown "better outcomes than routine management" (Buoli et al., 2013).

The biggest obstacle to treatment at this stage of illness is the patient's unwillingness to comply with treatment due to stigma or lack of insight combined with the patient's rights that hinder assistance from family members. Most mental health diagnoses are made after an acute episode that results in hospitalization or incarceration. Behavioral symptoms are often late manifestations of underlying neurodevelopmental processes, meaning that a focus solely on symptom-based diagnosis misses critical opportunities for early detection and intervention. The delay in accessing mental health services, often spanning years, contributes to poorer treatment outcomes, particularly in severe conditions like psychosis.

Multiple studies have documented a substantial delay between the onset of mental illness symptoms and the initiation of treatment.

· 50% of all lifetime mental illness begins by age 14, and 75% by age 24. However, the average delay between the onset of mental illness symptoms and treatment is 11 years (SAMHSA, 2021).
· The median number of years between the onset of the first mental disorder and the first treatment contact is 11 years (Wang et al., 2004).
· For psychosis, "the duration of untreated psychosis exceeds 100 weeks" (Insel, 2014), which is more than 1.9 years.
· Buoli et al. (2013) found a mean duration of untreated illness of 2.37 years for schizophrenia, with significant country-specific differences (Italy: 4.14 years; Russia: 1.16 years).

In essence, the delay in diagnosis is mainly due to the fragmented structure of the healthcare system that does not have a holistic, integrated primary health and behavioral health services for youth.

However, identifying individuals at high risk, especially adolescents, presents both scientific and ethical dilemmas due to the unpredictability of developmental trajectories and concerns about mislabeling. The Bipartisan Policy Center's Youth Mental Health and Substance Use Task Force, in its January 7, 2025 report "*Redesigning the Health Care Delivery System to Better Meet the Needs of Youth*," concluded that the current health care system needs significant structural reforms to better serve young people.

Barriers to Mental Health Care Access

In this section, we will explore the barriers to mental healthcare access, the impact of treatment delays, and the broader societal consequences of neglecting mental health.

Access to healthcare is complex and involves multiple dimensions: approachability, availability, affordability, acceptability, and appropriateness (Coombs et al., 2021). Figure 4 shows the ranking of mental health care access across US states.

Figure 4. The Access Ranking indicates how much access to mental health care exists within a state. The access measures include access to insurance, access to treatment, the quality and cost of insurance, access to special education, and the availability of the mental health workforce. A high Access Ranking (1-13) indicates that a state provides relatively more access to insurance and mental health care than those ranked 39-51. 2024.State of Mental Health in America. Mental Health America.

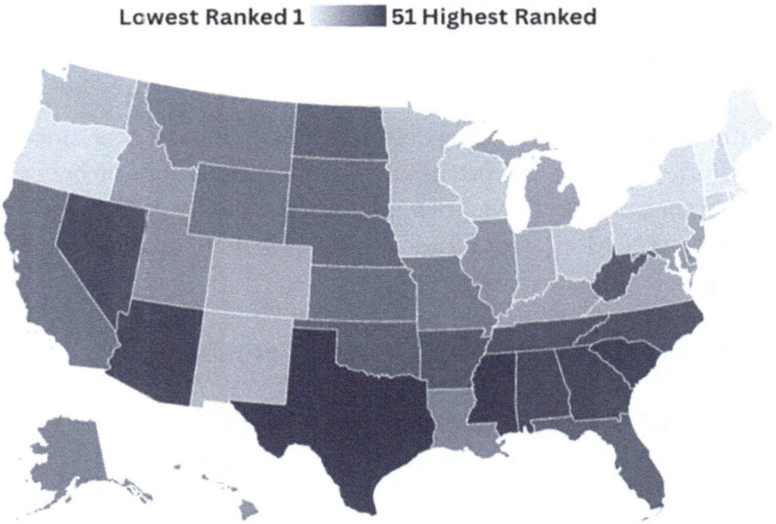

[https://mhanational.org/issues/state-mental-health-america]

Financial, attitudinal, and structural barriers remain prominent and disproportionately affect vulnerable populations. The lack of routine screening, particularly for maternal depression, has profound, intergenerational negative impacts on child health and development, violating the fundamental rights of these children. Early intervention, though challenging to implement effectively, is crucial for improving long-term outcomes.

Affordability

Financial concerns remain a leading obstacle, even after healthcare reforms.

· Post-ACA reforms, approximately one-fifth of US adults with mental health conditions still lack a usual source of care, and more than half report affordability-related barriers to accessing healthcare. (Sherrill and Gonzales, 2017 & Coombs et al. 2021)

· Mojtabai (2021) states that "Not being able to afford the cost of mental health care was the most commonly reported barrier… with no significant change over time."

Attitudinal and Structural Barriers

According to Mojtabai (2021), despite some improvements in insurance coverage, non-financial barriers are also on the rise for low-income adults. Here are some of the key observations:

· Attitudinal and structural barriers increased following ACA implementation.
· Specific increases in attitudinal barriers include fear of being committed against their will and belief that treatment would not be helpful.
· Structural barriers, such as not knowing where to receive treatment and not having time, also increased.

Disparities among certain demographic groups

· Males in the Hispanic community who worry about affording emergent or routine healthcare were associated with "no usual source of care" (Coombs et al., 2021).
· The US has a wider gap in healthcare access barriers between persons with and without mental health conditions than several other countries (Corscadden et al., 2018, cited in Coombs et al., 2021).
· Rural Americans face unique barriers, including longer travel distances to hospitals and limited broadband access for telehealth.

Stigma: Barrier to treatment

Stigma associated with mental health challenges significantly impacts access and engagement with services. Stigma can come from various sources – self-stigma, stigma from society, or stigma from discriminatory policies, laws, and systems.

Prejudices, media portrayal of mental illness, cultural beliefs are some of the reasons for self-stigma that prevents people from seeking help when they start experiencing symptoms of mental illness. Even when individuals actively seek help, societal stigma may limit family support, or their needs may be overlooked by primary care physicians focused primarily on physical illness.

Self-stigma occurs when individuals internalize stereotypes, leading to what Corrigan et al. (2009) call the "Why Try" effect—a cycle in which diminished self-esteem leads people to opt out of life opportunities such as employment or independent living. Mojtabai (2021) notes that negative news coverage of mental illness may have contributed to negative attitudes toward seeking mental health treatment.

Public misconceptions and the desire for social distancing drive social stigma. Pescosolido (2013) identify persistent prejudice that remains even as medical knowledge improves, fostering "benevolent" but coercive attitudes.

Finally, structural stigma refers to the "societal-level conditions, cultural norms, and institutional policies" that restrict opportunities (Hatzenbuehler & Link, 2014); recent work by the Lancet Commission (Thornicroft et al., 2022) highlights how this manifests globally in discriminatory laws and funding disparities that systematically bar individuals from full societal participation.

Stigma exacerbates mental health conditions and acts as a significant barrier to healthcare access compounding the suffering of those seeking help. (Coombs et al., 2021).

Role of Primary Care:

While contact with primary care can reduce negative pathways to specialized care, it can also lead to delays in appropriate referrals for severe conditions like psychosis. Patients who were in contact with primary care had a reduced likelihood of negative pathways to care but also had longer referral delays to early intervention services for first-episode psychosis (Anderson et al., 2013). The longer delays in referral to psychiatry by primary care physicians suggest that primary care providers need additional training in the recognition of early psychosis and protocols for referral.

Type of Delay	Description	Primary Driver
Identification Delay	Patients have symptoms, but PCP focuses on somatic (physical) causes first.	Diagnostic Overshadowing
Treatment Delay	Diagnosis is made, but medication dosage is too low or not changed when ineffective.	Clinical Inertia
Prioritization Delay	Mental health is deprioritized during a visit to focus on diabetes/heart issues.	Competing Demands

Economic & Systemic Hurdles

During a recent Precision Mental Health symposium at Stanford (2025) on the title of "Bridging Psychiatry, Neuroscience and AI" (https://medstanford.edu/pmhw), Dr. Tom Insel highlighted that the mental healthcare landscape faces a series of fundamental challenges that impede progress, despite the availability of effective treatments.

Drawing from his extensive experience, in mental health research, policy, and technology, he classified the mental health system landscape into four key domains—Diagnosis, Treatment, Setting, and Payment as shown in Figure 5. He highlighted the need for reform in the 4th domain – Payment.

Figure 5. The Landscape of the mental health system comprises four key domains. Abbreviations: SDOH- Social determinants of health, ER-Emergency room, IOP-Intensive outpatient program, PHP-Partial hospitalization program, AI- Artificial intelligence.

DIAGNOSIS	**TREATMENT**	**SETTING**	**PAYMENT**
Symptoms	Medical	Online/App	Free (e.g., AI)
Signs	Psychological	Offline Outpatient	Out of Pocket
Labs	Neurotech	Crisis/ER	Public Insurance
Social Determinants of Health	Rehabilitative	Intensive Outpatient Program/ Partial Hospitalization	Private Insurance
Function	Combined	Inpatient	Uninsured

Retrieved from: https://medstanford.edu/pmhw

When, how and who is able to pay will determine the adoption of important advances in early diagnosis and treatment of mental health conditions. While there has been significant progress in diagnosis and treatment, the adoption of these innovations and their accessibility have been hindered due to economic realities of the payment system across various settings.

Impact of Untreated Mental Illness

A delay in treating mental illness leads to a decrease in the quality of life for the individual and increase the economic burden to the society. Suppose we compare this to someone who shows early symptoms of cancer and does not seek treatment until the symptoms progress to an advanced stage of cancer. At this point, even the treatment that could have helped earlier in the diagnosis may no longer be effective. Similarly, the delays in seeking treatment can worsen the individual's social functioning and quality of life.

According to several studies (Reichert, A. & Jacobs, R., 2018; Penttilä et al., 2014; and Buoli et al., 2013), prolonged waiting periods for treatment are associated with worse patient outcomes. Individuals whose mental disorders begin in childhood or adolescence tend to experience longer treatment delays. According to Wang et. Al. (2014), patients with early-onset disorders typically do not make their first treatment contacts until early adulthood. As minors rely on adults for access to care, the delay in starting treatment from the onset of the symptoms depends on their guardians' ability and receptiveness to advocate for care for their loved ones.

Several studies examining the impact of waiting times for treatment have shown that prolonged delays in starting treatment led to increased symptom severity, a poorer response to delayed treatment, and worsening social functioning.

Economic and Social Burden

Mental illness imposes high costs on individuals, families, and global economies. According to the WHO fact sheet, 15% of working-age adults were estimated to have a mental disorder in 2019. It is estimated that globally, 12 billion working days are lost every year to depression and anxiety, for $1 trillion per year in lost productivity. This does figure from WHO does not take into account the loss of productivity arising from the emotional and economic toll on caregivers of people living with serious mental health conditions.

Abramson, B. Boerma, J., & Tsyvinski, A. (2024) made the following observations in their recent paper "Macroeconomics of Mental Health".

· Mental illness is widespread and costly in the United States, affecting over 20% of adults, with approximately 5.5% experiencing serious mental illness.
· Depression and anxiety globally account for 8% of all years lived with disability.
· The aggregate cost of mental illness is estimated at 1.7% of consumption annually, or $189 billion.
· The average consumption equivalent cost is 15.6% for individuals with serious mental illness and 10.3% for those with mild disease.
· Welfare costs are higher for younger individuals (below age 55), averaging 2.4%, compared to 1.0% for older individuals (above age 55).
· Among younger individuals, the middle class (wealth between $25,000 and $100,000) incurs the most significant welfare cost at 3.4%.
· The total societal burden, including healthcare and suicide-related costs, is estimated at $282 billion annually, which is 30% larger than previous epidemiological estimates. This higher estimate is attributed to the model's ability

to account for the dynamic effects of mental illness on consumption, labor, savings, and asset allocation decisions.

There are approximately 8.4 million Americans providing care specifically to an adult with mental or emotional health issue and the estimated economic value of unpaid caregiving in the US is roughly $600 billion annually (which includes caring for someone with mental illness). (Reinhard, S. C. et.al., 2023 and Report on Pins and Needles: Caregivers of adult with mental illness, 2020)

Maternal Depression's Far-Reaching Consequences

Neglecting maternal depression has severe, long-term impacts on children and constitutes a violation of their rights. Here are several observations by Mokwena (2021) in her work:

· Neglecting to diagnose and treat maternal depression compromises current and future health, developmental, and social outcomes of the affected children, and therefore violates their constitutional rights.
· Maternal depression is linked to low birth weight, intrauterine growth restriction, premature delivery, and poor breastfeeding outcomes.
· It leads to "malnutrition," which is a "primary cause of child morbidity and mortality".
· Long-term impacts include compromised cognitive development and language acquisition in children, deviant behaviors, and economic disadvantages in later life.
· Maternal depression has also been linked to a significant risk of suicide or infanticide.

RECOMMENDATION

The collective evidence strongly underscores the critical need for a multifaceted approach to improve mental healthcare access and outcomes. Addressing the persistent delays in treatment and the multifaceted barriers is of paramount importance.

· Targeted public education campaigns are essential to reduce and ultimately eradicate stigma, while increasing awareness, normalizing help-seeking behaviors, and supporting early identification and treatment.

· Prioritize Affordability and Accessibility: Policymakers must focus on reducing financial barriers, which remain a significant hurdle, and ensure physical and timely access to services, especially in underserved areas.

· Implement a multi-pronged approach to tackle economic, attitudinal, and structural barriers. We recommend the following approaches:

- o Expand the use of new technologies, such as telehealth and mobile interventions.
- o Promote patient-centered approaches to improve engagement, such as reducing waiting times for specialized services.
- o Integrating mental health screening to detect early onset mental illness.
- o Strengthen mental health coverage provisions in insurance plans.

· Combat Stigma and Enhance Awareness: Public education campaigns and training for healthcare professionals are essential to reduce stigma and improve the identification and referral of individuals with mental health challenges to speciality care (psychiatrists) just as would be done for other physical health conditions.

· Strengthen Primary Care's Role: Primary care providers should receive enhanced training to recognize early signs of mental illness, particularly severe conditions such as psychosis, with clear referral pathways to specialized services.

· Invest in Early Intervention: Given the long-term benefits, it is crucial to allocate resources to research and implement effective early detection and intervention strategies, particularly for young individuals and high-risk populations with robust oversight.

· The investment in early intervention includes exploring novel, less intrusive interventions and diagnostic tools that can benefit even those incorrectly identified as at-risk.

· Enforce Early and Periodic Screening, Diagnostic and Treatment (EPSDT) compliance to shift our current system from a "crisis-oriented" model to one focused on prevention and early intervention.

· Enable pediatric providers to bill for behavioral health services before a formal diagnosis is made. This "early action" approach will prevent families from waiting until a child is severely ill to get insurance coverage to help facilitate early intervention.

· Integrate Maternal Mental Health into Routine Care: Mandatory and routine screening for maternal depression in public health services is critical to improve child health and development outcomes, uphold children's rights, and prevent intergenerational cycles of disadvantage.

· Monitor and Evaluate Policies: Continuous monitoring of healthcare reforms and policies is essential to ensure they effectively address the diverse barriers to mental health care and achieve the desired improvements in service utilization and patient outcomes.

· Rethinking Recovery: Focus on developing diagnostic tools that are not focused on symptoms but on biomarkers that promote timely access to treatment. Investing in training medical providers in ways to engage patients in treatment using peer support, and establishing a payment system that values quality and outcomes of care provided.

FUTURE DIRECTIONS: TECHNOLOGICAL DEVELOPMENTS IN MENTAL HEALTH

In this section, we will examine emerging new technologies and treatments for mental health conditions. We will examine the influence of nutrition and the gut microbiome on brain health and explore emerging digital mental health (DMH) tools in early detection of mental illness. Furthermore, we will examine the potential and challenges of leveraging machine learning and DMH technologies for precision psychiatry, including concerns around data privacy and the diagnostic process.

Nutritional Psychiatry and the Impact of Diet

A balanced diet is crucial for overall well-being, affecting both physical and mental health. Nutrition is considered an essential factor in brain development and the prevention of mental disorders. Nutritional psychiatry aims to understand how diet modulates neurobiological pathways, how nutraceuticals can correct deficiencies, and how nutrient quality affects mental health.

Dal and Bilici (2024) conducted a comprehensive examination of literature to review the potential role of nutrition on mental health conditions and evaluate the effectiveness of dietary interventions. In their review paper, they cite several studies that use dietary interventions for mental illness. We have listed some key studies below:

· Studies by Parletta et al. (2017) show that a Mediterranean diet, particularly when supplemented with fish oil, can improve depression and mental health scores. Their study found scores to be "1.68 and 1.52 times, respectively, compared to the control group."

· A dietary intervention based on 11 food groups called ModiMedDiet, reported by Jacka F.N. et al (2017), aligned with depression prevention recommendations, showed "a significantly... greater improvement in depression scores" compared to a control group.

· According to Ardekani A.M. et al. (2023), the Mediterranean-DASH (Dietary Approaches to Stop Hypertension) Intervention for Neurodegenerative Delay (MIND) diet may have a beneficial impact on mental health due to its antioxidant and anti-inflammatory properties, as well as reduced consumption of red meat and sweets. Adherence to the MIND diet has been "inversely associated with the probability of depression and psychological distress" as reported by Salari-Moghaddam et al (2019).

· Diets rich in refined sugars and saturated fats are linked to altered microbiota, reduced gut barrier function, altered neurotransmitter metabolism, and increased mental health risks. In their research, Shoubridge, A.P., Choo, J.M., Martin, A.M., et al. (2022) cite that nitrated cured meats have been associated with a "markedly increased rate of hospitalisation for acute mania".

Ongoing research across various aspects of nutritional psychiatry holds significant potential to improve brain function and mental health.

The Gut-Brain Axis and Microbiome's Role in Mental Health

The gut microbiome refers to the community of trillions of microorganisms that live in our digestive system. These microbes play an important role in both our physical and mental health. The gut is often called the "second brain" because it has its own complex nervous system, known as the enteric nervous system (ENS), which operates independently of the brain. This system contains millions of neurons and controls digestion, gut movement, and enzyme release without needing direct input from the brain. The gut also produces many of the same neurotransmitters as the brain, including large portions of the body's serotonin, which influences mood and emotional regulation. Through constant two-way communication with the brain via nerves, hormones, and the immune system, the gut can affect emotions, stress response, and mental health. When the gut microbiome is imbalanced, it can affect mood, thinking and behavior and has been found to be linked to mental health conditions such as anxiety and depression.

In a recent review of the gut microbiome's central role in influencing mental well-being, Gupt, A., Naudiyal, S., Rani, A. et al. (2024) define the "gut-brain axis" as the crucial bidirectional communication between the gastrointestinal tract and the brain and suggest notable pathways of Influence:

· Neuroendocrine System (HPA axis): Gut microbiota alters nutrient availability, thereby influencing the release of peptides from enteroendocrine cells, which, in turn, affect the gut-brain axis. The HPA axis regulates digestion, mood, emotions, energy expenditure, and stress response.

· Short-Chain Fatty Acids (SCFAs): Metabolites such as Acetate, Butyrate, and Propionate (produced by fermentable fibers) are absorbed in the small intestine and influence the microbial profile. Butyrate has anti-inflammatory and immuno-modulatory properties and can affect the central nervous system.
· Secondary Bile Acids (SBAs): Act as a link between the gut microbiota and the brain and are essential for nutrient absorption, digestion, and the elimination of toxic metabolites.
· Vagus Nerve: Recognized as a significant mediator of microbiome-brain interactions.
· Endocannabinoid System: The gut microbiome can regulate genes in the endocannabinoid system, influencing the central nervous system's responses to stressors and maintaining the balance between excitatory and inhibitory signals in the brain.
· Dysbiosis: An imbalance in gut microbiota ("dysbiosis") is linked to digestive issues (e.g., irritable bowel syndrome), chronic fatigue, food intolerances, and mental health symptoms like anxiety, depression, and brain fog.
· Dietary Influence on Microbiota: Diet significantly affects gut microbiota composition, influencing digestion, absorption, metabolism, and the extraction of beneficial molecules.

Ongoing research in the gut-brain axis has the potential to shed further light on the role of gut bacterial species and their impact on our mental health.

Pillars of Precision Psychiatry: New Avenues for Biomarker Discovery

Psychiatry is often considered more challenging than many other branches of medicine because it deals with the brain and mind, which is extremely complex and not yet fully understood. Unlike conditions such as diabetes or cancer, most psychiatric disorders do not have clear biological markers that can be measured with a single lab test or scan. Diagnosis relies heavily on patient-reported symptoms, behavior, and clinical judgment, all of which can be influenced by culture, language, and social context.

Precision psychiatry is an emerging approach to mental health care that aims to tailor prevention, diagnosis, and treatment to the individual rather than relying on a one-size-fits-all model. It draws on information from genetics, brain imaging, psychology, life experiences, and environmental factors to better understand why people experience mental illness differently and why the same treatment may work well for one person but not another. By integrating these diverse data sources, precision psychiatry seeks to improve early identification of mental health conditions, select treatments with a higher likelihood of success, and reduce trial-and-error prescribing.

Here are some key advancements in this area emerging from:

1. **Genetics and Epigenetics**: The influence of a person's genes on their health is a well-known fact. The emerging field of epigenetics explains why some people do not develop an illness even if they have the gene for the illness. This is because the gene expression – the turning on and off of the genes – is influenced by the environment such as stress and trauma. The influence of gene expression without involving a change in DNA sequence is called epigenetics. Genome-wide association studies (GWASs) reveal such genetic influences, identifying over 100 risk loci for major depressive disorders (MDD). Polygenic Risk Scores (PRSs) aggregate these minor genetic effects to estimate individual predispositions. These studies show promise for understanding and developing treatments for conditions like bipolar disorder.
2. **Pharmacogenomic Testing** analyzes an individual's DNA to predict how they will respond to a particular medication. This test is particularly useful in treating cancer, chronic pain, and psychiatric illnesses. It helps the doctors determine which medication will be most effective, the right dose, and potential side-effects it may cause. Psychiatric treatment often involves trial and error methods of treatment where the first anti-depressant prescribed may not work and produce undesirable side effects. Many patients give up hope and discontinue treatment due to this. Pharmacogenetic testing helps improve patient engagement by providing individualized precision treatment that is effective, with minimal side-effects. (Haga, S. B. & LaPointe, N. M. 2013). In psychiatry, this test involves testing for cytochrome P450 (CYP) genes with a simple cheek swab. Cytochrome P450 genes are a large family of liver enzymes that play a crucial role in the metabolism of drugs in the body. These genes have variations in their DNA which account for the reason why different people have different side effects to the same medication. Cytochrome P450 genes (e.g., CYP2D6, CYP2C19, CYP3A4/5), are the most established genetic tool, optimizing psychotropic drug metabolism and influencing treatment response and side effects. The US Food and Drug Administration (FDA) has already incorporated pharmacogenetic information into drug labels for many psychotropics.
   - According to van Westrhenen, R., Young, A. H., Heilbronner, U., et al. (2025), a new intervention for implementing pharmacogenetics in psychiatry, called PSY-PGx, is currently being evaluated in real-world utility.
   - In a recent study by Chen, Y., Wang, P., and Li, Z. (2025), epigenetic factors, such as DNA methylation, are explored for predicting or

monitoring treatment response, including cognitive-behavioral therapy (CBT).

3. **Advanced Neuroimaging:** Neuroimaging provides objective insights into brain function, serving as a direct measure of brain activity. Neuroimaging also helps identify brain circuit biotypes for more effective treatment selection.
    - o At Stanford Precision Psychiatry Center, their study analyzed functional MRI scans from 801 unmedicated patients to identify six distinct "biotypes" of depression and anxiety defined by specific patterns of brain circuit dysfunction. Unlike traditional diagnostic labels, these biotypes were distinguished by unique symptom profiles, performance on cognitive tests, and varied responses to different medications and behavioral therapies. These findings suggest a new, precision-medicine approach for psychiatry that moves to biologically grounded classifications that help guide personalized treatment. (Tozzi, L., Zhang, X., Pines A., et.al, 2024)
    - o According to Miranda, L., Paul, R., Pütz, B., & Koutsouleris, N. (2021), Functional Magnetic Resonance Imaging (fMRI) detects subtle changes in brain networks, aiding disease subtyping and symptom validation.
    - o Neuner, I., Veselinović, T., Ramkiran, S. et al. (2022) reported that the use of Ultra-High Field MRI (7T-UHF-MRI) offers superior resolution for individual-level, prognosis-relevant changes, capturing detailed structural, neurochemical, and metabolic information.
    - o Electroencephalography (EEG) is a cost-effective, high-temporal resolution tool for identifying MDD biomarkers. AI-driven EEG analysis, using deep learning (CNNs, CNN-LSTMs), shows high accuracy in predicting depression and treatment outcomes, with potential for portable diagnostic tools. Kaur, G., Aggarwal, H., Goel, N. (2025).
4. **Immunopsychiatry**: Research by Miller et al. (2025), showed that 30% of individuals with depression have a higher level of inflammation. They found that there is a link between immune system and the brain. When the body is inflamed, it can change how the brain works, including the way brain cells communicate. Validated biomarkers, like C-reactive protein (CRP), are already used in studies to measure inflammation. This means they could open new ways to treat mental health conditions.
5. **Wearable Technologies**: Digital phenotyping is a method of measuring and understanding human behavior and mental health using data collected from digital devices, like smartphones and wearable technologies. It involves analyzing patterns such as movement, sleep, phone usage, typing speed, voice features, and social interaction (for example, calls or texts), often collected passively and continuously during everyday life. This passive sensing enables continuous

patient monitoring, providing timely insights to clinicians, and supporting the development of cost-effective diagnostic and monitoring tools. Smith, et al. al. (2023), Koch, et. al. (2024), Castro Martínez, J. C. (2023).

The Transformative Role of Artificial Intelligence

Machine Learning (ML) and Artificial Intelligence (AI) are central to integrating these diverse data streams for precision psychiatry. AI models can analyze complex patterns to achieve more precise diagnoses, personalized treatment recommendations, and predictive algorithms. Deep learning methods excel at extracting subtle features from neuroimaging data, often outperforming traditional ML approaches in terms of accuracy. These computational tools are vital for managing high data variability and interpreting large datasets, helping to identify individualized "neurobiological fingerprints." AI may also improve efficiency and access to mental care and reduce costs. Machine learning has been applied to analyze multi-modal data, including text, audio, and video, for objective assessment of psychiatric symptoms.

Challenges to Implementation and the Path Forward

Despite its promise, precision psychiatry faces significant hurdles for widespread clinical adoption, particularly in the US.

· Data Issues: A lack of standardized acquisition protocols and evaluation methods (especially EEG and fMRI) hampers direct comparisons and replication. Large, publicly available, multi-site datasets are critically needed for robust AI model training and to overcome limitations from small, heterogeneous datasets.
· Generalizability and Bias: Studies often use small, heterogeneous samples, limiting real-world applicability. Geographic data concentration can also introduce biases, affecting generalizability to diverse US populations.
· Clinical Integration and Interpretability: Integrating AI tools into existing clinical workflows is complex. Clinicians require explainable AI (XAI) models that are transparent and interpretable to build trust and facilitate adoption, moving beyond mere accuracy.
· Regulatory Hurdles: Strict regulatory guidelines, including FDA mandates for thorough validation via multi-center trials, are necessary before AI tools can be widely deployed. The current literature often lacks rigorous external validation.

To truly realize the potential of precision psychiatry in the United States and globally, a collaborative approach involving academia, industry, funding agencies, patients, payors, and policymakers is essential. Future research must prioritize harmonized methodologies, large-scale clinical trials with diverse populations, and prospective validations in real-world settings.

Longitudinal studies are also desperately needed to capture the chronic, episodic, and progressive nature of mental illnesses. By addressing these areas, precision psychiatry can transform mental healthcare, improve patient outcomes, and alleviate the immense burden on individuals and the healthcare system.

The journey towards truly personalized mental healthcare is complex, but emerging insights and tools offer a clear, hopeful roadmap.

CONCLUSION

Mental health care is at a critical crossroads. While challenges remain, the opportunities for transformation are immense. By focusing on education to reduce stigma, early intervention, investment in research for biomarker-based diagnostic tools, and improving accessibility to treatment through value-based payment options, we can redefine mental health care for future generations.

Mental health must be treated with the same urgency, scientific rigor, and policy support as physical health. Only when mental health is integrated into care pathways with the same seriousness as physical health, will we have a truly reformed and responsive healthcare system. The time is ripe for policymakers, healthcare leaders, and communities to act - invest in evidence-based treatment, expand access, and champion the cultural change needed to ensure that every person receives compassionate, science-informed mental healthcare. When mental illnesses are diagnosed and treated as brain diseases rather than personal failings, care will become more equitable, and society will move toward a stronger future where every individual can thrive.

REFERENCES

Abramson, B., Boerma, J., & Tsyvinski, A. (2024). Macroeconomics of Mental Health, NBER Working Paper 32354, DOI: 10.3386/w32354

Anderson, K. K., Fuhrer, R., Schmitz, N., & Malla, A. K. (2013). Determinants of negative pathways to care and their impact on service disengagement in first-episode psychosis. *Social Psychiatry and Psychiatric Epidemiology*, *48*(1), 125–136. DOI: 10.1007/s00127-012-0571-0 PMID: 22976337

Ardekani, A. M., Vahdat, S., Hojati, A., Moradi, H., Tousi, A. Z., Ebrahimzadeh, F., & Farhangi, M. A. (2023). Evaluating the association between the Mediterranean-DASH Intervention for Neurodegenerative Delay (MIND) diet, mental health, and cardio-metabolic risk factors among individuals with obesity. *BMC Endocrine Disorders*, *23*(1), 29. DOI: 10.1186/s12902-023-01284-8 PMID: 36726099

Buoli, M., Dell'osso, B., Zaytseva, Y., Gurovich, I. Y., Movina, L., Dorodnova, A., Shmuckler, A., & Altamura, A. C. (2013). Duration of untreated illness (DUI) and schizophrenia sub-types: A collaborative study between the universities of Milan and Moscow. *The International Journal of Social Psychiatry*, *59*(8), 765–770. DOI: 10.1177/0020764012456807 PMID: 23034286

Castro Martínez, J. C., & Santamaría-García, H. (2023). Understanding mental health through computers: An introduction to computational psychiatry. *Frontiers in Psychiatry*, *14*, 1092471. DOI: 10.3389/fpsyt.2023.1092471 PMID: 36824671

Chen, Y., Wang, P., & Li, Z. (2025). Exploring genetic and epigenetic markers for predicting or monitoring response to cognitive-behavioral therapy in obsessive-compulsive disorder: A systematic review. *Neuroscience and Biobehavioral Reviews*, *174*, 106192. DOI: 10.1016/j.neubiorev.2025.106192 PMID: 40324706

Coombs, N. C., Meriwether, W. E., Caringi, J., & Newcomer, S. R. (2021). Barriers to healthcare access among US adults with mental health challenges: A population-based study. *SSM - Population Health*, *15*, 100847. DOI: 10.1016/j.ssmph.2021.100847 PMID: 34179332

Corrigan, P. W., Larson, J. E., & Rüsch, N. (2009). Self-stigma and the "why try" effect: Impact on life goals and evidence-based practices. *World Psychiatry; Official Journal of the World Psychiatric Association (WPA)*, *8*(2), 75–81. DOI: 10.1002/j.2051-5545.2009.tb00218.x PMID: 19516923

Dal, N., & Bilici, S. (2024). An Overview of the Potential Role of Nutrition in Mental Disorders in the Light of Advances in Nutripsychiatry. *Current Nutrition Reports*, *13*(2), 69–81. DOI: 10.1007/s13668-024-00520-4 PMID: 38329691

George, P., Jones, N., Goldman, H., & Rosenblatt, A. (2023). Cycles of reform in the history of psychosis treatment in the United States. *SSM. Mental Health*, *3*, 100205. DOI: 10.1016/j.ssmmh.2023.100205 PMID: 37388405

Gupt, A., Naudiyal, S., Rani, A., & Kumar, S. (2024). Mental Health and the Microbiome: A Review of Psychological Impacts of Gut Microflora. *Current Pharmacology Reports*, *10*(4), 223–236. DOI: 10.1007/s40495-024-00357-z

Haga, S. B., & LaPointe, N. M. (2013). The potential impact of pharmacogenetic testing on medication adherence. *The Pharmacogenomics Journal*, *13*(6), 481–483. DOI: 10.1038/tpj.2013.33 PMID: 23999596

Hatzenbuehler, M. L., & Link, B. G. (2014). Introduction to the special issue on structural stigma and health. *Social Science & Medicine*, *103*, 1–6. DOI: 10.1016/j.socscimed.2013.12.017 PMID: 24445152

Insel, T. R. (2014). Mental disorders in childhood: Shifting the focus from behavioral symptoms to neurodevelopmental trajectories. *Journal of the American Medical Association*, *311*(17), 1727–1728. DOI: 10.1001/jama.2014.1193 PMID: 24794359

Jacka, F. N., O'Neil, A., Opie, R., Itsiopoulos, C., Cotton, S., Mohebbi, M., Castle, D., Dash, S., Mihalopoulos, C., Chatterton, M. L., Brazionis, L., Dean, O. M., Hodge, A. M., & Berk, M. (2017). A randomised controlled trial of dietary improvement for adults with major depression (the 'SMILES' trial). *BMC Medicine*, *15*(1), 23. DOI: 10.1186/s12916-017-0791-y PMID: 28137247

Kaur, G., Aggarwal, H., & Goel, N. (2025). Artificial intelligence driven neuropsychiatry: A systematic review of electroencephalography-based computational techniques for major depressive disorder prediction. *Neuroscience*, *581*, 179–207. DOI: 10.1016/j.neuroscience.2025.07.010 PMID: 40639536

Koch, E., Pardiñas, A. F., O'Connell, K. S., Selvaggi, P., Collados, J. C., Babic, A., Marshall, S. E., Eycken, E. V., Angulo, C., Lu, Y., Sullivan, P. F., Dale, A. M., Molden, E., Posthuma, D., White, N., Schubert, A., Djurovic, S., Heimer, H., Stefánsson, H., & Andreassen, O. A. (2024). How Real-World Data Can Facilitate the Development of Precision Medicine Treatment in Psychiatry. *Biological Psychiatry*, *96*(7), 543–551. DOI: 10.1016/j.biopsych.2024.01.001 PMID: 38185234

Lamb, H. R., & Bachrach, L. L. (2001). Some Perspectives on Deinstitutionalization. *Psychiatric Services (Washington, D.C.)*, *52*(8), 999–1118. DOI: 10.1176/appi.ps.52.8.1039 PMID: 11474048

Miller, A. H., Berk, M., Bloch, G., Briquet-Laugier, V., Brouillon, C., Cuthbert, B. N., Dantzer, R., Davis, M. C., De Picker, L. J., Drevets, W. C., Eyre, H. A., Hack, L. M., Harrison, N. A., Krystal, A. D., Lombardo, G., Mondelli, V., Pariante, C. M., Pulvirenti, L., Salvadore, G., & Leboyer, M. (2025). Advancing precision psychiatry and targeted treatments: Insights from immunopsychiatry. *Brain, Behavior, and Immunity, 125*, 319–329. DOI: 10.1016/j.bbi.2025.01.002 PMID: 39828008

Miranda, L., Paul, R., Pütz, B., Koutsouleris, N., & Müller-Myhsok, B. (2021). Systematic Review of Functional MRI Applications for Psychiatric Disease Subtyping. *Frontiers in Psychiatry, 12*, 665536. DOI: 10.3389/fpsyt.2021.665536 PMID: 34744805

Mojtabai, R. (2021). US. Health Care Reform and Enduring Barriers to Mental Health Care Among Low-Income Adults With Psychological Distress. *Psychiatric Services (Washington, D.C.), 72*(3), 338–342. DOI: 10.1176/appi.ps.202000194 PMID: 33467868

Mokwena, K. E. (2021). Neglecting Maternal Depression Compromises Child Health and Development Outcomes, and Violates Children's Rights in South Africa. *Children (Basel, Switzerland), 8*(7), 609. DOI: 10.3390/children8070609 PMID: 34356588

Neuner, I., Veselinović, T., Ramkiran, S., Rajkumar, R., Schnellbaecher, G. J., & Shah, N. J. (2022). 7T ultra-high-field neuroimaging for mental health: An emerging tool for precision psychiatry? *Translational Psychiatry, 12*(1), 36. DOI: 10.1038/s41398-022-01787-3 PMID: 35082273

Parletta, N., Zarnowiecki, D., Cho, J., Wilson, A., Bogomolova, S., Villani, A., Itsiopoulos, C., Niyonsenga, T., Blunden, S., Meyer, B., Segal, L., Baune, B. T., & O'Dea, K. (2017). A Mediterranean-style dietary intervention supplemented with fish oil improves diet quality and mental health in people with depression: A randomized controlled trial (HELFIMED). *Nutritional Neuroscience, 22*(7), 474–487. DOI: 10.1080/1028415X.2017.1411320 PMID: 29215971

Pescosolido, B. A. (2013). The public stigma of mental illness: What do we think; what do we know; what can we prove? *Journal of Health and Social Behavior, 54*(1), 1–21. DOI: 10.1177/0022146512471197 PMID: 23325423

Prins, S. J. (2011). Does Transinstitutionalization Explain the Overrepresentation of People with Serious Mental Illnesses in the Criminal Justice System? *Community Mental Health Journal, 47*(6), 716–722. DOI: 10.1007/s10597-011-9420-y PMID: 21655941

Reichert, A., & Jacobs, R. (2018). The impact of waiting time on patient outcomes: Evidence from early intervention in psychosis services in England. *Health Economics*, *27*(11), 1772–1787. DOI: 10.1002/hec.3800 PMID: 30014544

Reinhard, S. C., Caldera, S., Houser, A., & Choula, R. B. (2023). Valuing the Invaluable 2023 Update: Strengthening Supports for Family Caregivers. Washington, DC: AARP Public Policy Institute. March 8, 2023. DOI: 10.26419/ppi.00082.006

Roth A. (2018). Insane: America's Criminal Treatment of Mental Illness

Salari-Moghaddam, A., Keshteli, A. H., Mousavi, S. M., Afshar, H., Esmaillzadeh, A., & Adibi, P. (2019). Adherence to the MIND diet and prevalence of psychological disorders in adults. *Journal of Affective Disorders*, *256*, 96–102. DOI: 10.1016/j.jad.2019.05.056 PMID: 31170621

Schildbach, S., & Schildbach, C. (2018). Criminalization Through Transinstitutionalization: A Critical Review of the Penrose Hypothesis in the Context of Compensation Imprisonment. *Frontiers in Psychiatry*, *9*, 534. DOI: 10.3389/fpsyt.2018.00534 PMID: 30410452

Shoubridge, A. P., Choo, J. M., Martin, A. M., Keating, D. J., Wong, M.-L., Licinio, J., & Rogers, G. B. (2022). The gut microbiome and mental health: Advances in research and emerging priorities. *Molecular Psychiatry*, *27*(4), 1908–1919. DOI: 10.1038/s41380-022-01479-w PMID: 35236957

Smith, K. A., Blease, C., Faurholt-Jepsen, M., Firth, J., Van Daele, T., Moreno, C., Carlbring, P., Ebner-Priemer, U. W., Koutsouleris, N., Riper, H., Mouchabac, S., Torous, J., & Cipriani, A. (2023). Digital mental health: Challenges and next steps. *BMJ Mental Health*, *26*(1), e300670. DOI: 10.1136/bmjment-2023-300670 PMID: 37197797

Substance Abuse and Mental Health Services Administration. (2021). Key substance use and mental health indicators in the United States: Results from the 2020 National Survey on Drug Use and Health (HHS Publication No.PEP21-07-01-003, NSDUH Series H-56). Rockville, MD: Center for Behavioral Health Statistics and Quality, Substance Abuse and Mental Health Services Administration. Retrieved from https://www.samhsa.gov/data/

Thornicroft, G., Sunkel, C., Alikhon Aliev, A., Baker, S., Brohan, E., El Chammay, R., Davies, K., Demissie, M., Duncan, J., Fekadu, W., Gronholm, P. C., Guerrero, Z., Gurung, D., Habtamu, K., Hanlon, C., Heim, E., Henderson, C., Hijazi, Z., Hoffman, C., & Winkler, P. (2022). The Lancet Commission on ending stigma and discrimination in mental health. *Lancet*, *400*(10361), 1438–1480. DOI: 10.1016/S0140-6736(22)01470-2 PMID: 36223799

Toynbee, M. (2015). The Penrose hypothesis in the 21st century: Revisiting the asylum. *Evidence-Based Mental Health, 18*(3), 76. DOI: 10.1136/eb-2015-102115 PMID: 26116302

Tozzi, L., Zhang, X., Pines, A., Olmsted, A. M., Zhai, E. S., Anene, E. T., Chesnut, M., Holt-Gosselin, B., Chang, S., Stetz, P. C., Ramirez, C. A., Hack, L. M., Korgaonkar, M. S., Wintermark, M., Gotlib, I. H., Ma, J., & Williams, L. M. (2024). Personalized brain circuit scores identify clinically distinct biotypes in depression and anxiety. *Nature Medicine, 30*(7), 2076–2087. DOI: 10.1038/s41591-024-03057-9 PMID: 38886626

van Dellen, E. (2024). Precision psychiatry: Predicting predictability. *Psychological Medicine, 54*(8), 1500–1509. DOI: 10.1017/S0033291724000370 PMID: 38497091

van Westrhenen, R., Young, A. H., Heilbronner, U., Juruena, M., Ingelman-Sundberg, M., Jukic, M., Kaprio, J., Kas, M. J. H., Moldovan, R., Nöthen, M. M., Philipsen, A., Shomron, N., Van der Eycken, E., Vieta, E., & Schulze, T. G. (2025). PSY-PGx: A new intervention for the implementation of pharmacogenetics in psychiatry. *World Psychiatry; Official Journal of the World Psychiatric Association (WPA), 24*(1), 141–142. DOI: 10.1002/wps.21289 PMID: 39810666

Wang, P. S., Berglund, P. A., Olfson, M., & Kessler, R. C. (2004). Delays in initial treatment contact after the first onset of a mental disorder. *Health Services Research, 39*(2), 393–415. DOI: 10.1111/j.1475-6773.2004.00234.x PMID: 15032961

Youth Mental Health and Substance Use Task Force. (2025). Redesigning the health care delivery system to better meet the needs of youth. Bipartisan Policy Center. https://bipartisanpolicy.org/report/health-care-redesign-youth/

Section 3
Practices and Applications

Chapter 9
Role Modeling in Medical Education Training

Lawrence Lee
Saint Francis Hospital, USA

Roshini Selladurai
http://orcid.org/0009-0001-7340-508X
Mayo Clinic, USA & Mayo College of Medicine, USA

ABSTRACT

Several reports show a shortage of primary care physicians in the US, and it seems likely to worsen as the population continues to grow and age. Therefore, it is critical to train the next generation of physicians and healthcare providers to effectively meet the needs of the US population. Alongside this structural challenge, the medical profession is also confronting a cultural one—an erosion of professionalism characterized by declining responsibility, integrity, and communication (Foster, 2019). In teaching and training resident physicians and medical students, some of these skills can be taught, but these skills are usually better "caught" than taught. This chapter presents two physicians' personal experiences in medical education. It discusses the significance of role modeling and best practices for effectively transmitting professionalism, competence, and communication to the next generation of resident physicians, medical students, and healthcare providers.

INTRODUCTION

The US healthcare system, one of the largest in the world, continues to face complex and multifaceted challenges. Therefore, these challenges require that the nation's policymakers pursue ongoing reforms to improve access and sustainability

DOI: 10.4018/979-8-3373-2577-4.ch009

of healthcare to all stakeholders. As of 2026, Congress and the administration are focusing on proposals such as the Resident Physician Shortage Reduction Act of 2025 (H.R. 4731) and the $50 billion Rural Health Transformation Program, both designed to address the physician shortage (AAMC, 2024; CMS, 2025; Zucker, 2025). Alongside this structural challenge, the medical profession is also confronting a cultural one—an erosion of professionalism characterized by declining responsibility, integrity, and communication (Foster, 2019).

This chapter draws upon the two authors' experiences to demonstrate how professionalism, competence, and communication can be intentionally cultivated in medical training. Role modeling, an effective teaching strategy in medical education and training, influences the professional attitudes, behaviors, and competence of about 90 percent of medical graduates. Effective mentors integrate and model clinical competence, communication, empathy, teaching skills, and human relations skills, often referred to as the "three Hs": Head, Hands, and Heart (Benbassat, 2014). Continuing to develop highly professional and well-trained resident physicians and medical students would help enhance the quality and delivery of healthcare services provided (including in the much-needed rural areas), improve patient satisfaction, and promote overall sustainability in healthcare. The two authors/physicians share their experiences as role models of best practices for the new generation of healthcare professionals to emulate.

BACKGROUND

Healthcare reform involves challenges and complexities due to the very nature of the subject – ensuring that all people have access to and receive useful, high-quality healthcare, which is an essential part of human life. Key factors in the healthcare providers' ability to provide high-quality healthcare are the preparation and training they have received. Professionalism, competence, and communication are foundational pillars of medical student and resident education and training in the US. They are also considered core competencies for undergraduate medical education. The Accreditation Council for Graduate Medical Education (ACGME) and the Association of American Medical Colleges (AAMC) have established standards for professionalism, competence, and communication in medical training. Medical training is offered by accredited medical schools and residency programs in the US, which teach through explicit curricula (lectures, modules, and essays), faculty role modeling, simulation-based training, feedback and assessment, and faculty development to ensure teaching and assessment are effective. All these core competencies ensure that graduates are knowledgeable and ethical, reliable, and effective in patient care, interactions, and team-based care (ACGME, 2025; AAMC, 2025).

MAIN FOCUS OF THE CHAPTER

The main focus of this chapter is the two authors'/physicians' personal experiences in medical education and training. It discusses role modeling the best practices for effectively transmitting professionalism, competence, and communication to the next generation of resident physicians, medical students, and healthcare providers.

ANALYSIS

Actual conversation from the author, physician Lee (with the patient/s, during hospital rounds accompanied by the resident/s)

(In the following section (s), generic names are used to protect patients' and others' identities).

Dialogues are written (in *italics*) in the first and second person primarily for maximum impact.

Preceptor/physician commentary: Notice how Dr. Lee begins/continues by.... shown in the first two paragraphs and in the rest of the Analysis section.

First encounter at the bedside of a patient already admitted

Preceptor commentary. Notice how Dr. Lee begins by....I knock first, then open the door and place my hand under the hand sanitizer dispenser to show the patient and his/her family that I am washing my hands. Knocking on the door shows respect for the patient's privacy. Showing the patient and family that I washed my hands is better than telling them I did.

Me: "Good morning! I'm looking for Ms. Smith?"

Preceptor commentary. Notice how Dr. Lee continues by.... The salutation and addressing the patient by title and last name are more formal but show respect to someone you may not have met before. By stating who I'm looking for, I avoid talking to the wrong patient when the patient I'm looking for has moved rooms.

Ms. Smith: (nodding) *"You found her."*

Me: "I'm Dr. Lee, and I'm your Hospitalist taking care of you. This is my resident physician, Dr. Jones. Nice to meet you!" While I say this, I am smiling, looking my patient in the eye, and shaking her hand. By introducing ourselves by name, title, and function, I let her know where we fit into the puzzle. A smile, eye contact, and a handshake are social graces that communicate warmth and connection.

Me: "I'm going to pull up your medical chart, and then I'll come and shake all of your hands." I am addressing everyone else who is in the room with the patient. I log in, and while the computer is loading the medical chart, I go around the room and look each person in the eye and shake their hands, and ask, *"And you are...?"* Rather than assuming these people are spouses and/or blood relatives, I ask who they are related to the patient.

Preceptor commentary. Notice how Dr. Lee continues by....By telling everyone what I'm doing and then acknowledging everyone in the room, I show respect to each person and let the patient know I see and recognize the people with them. However, after this, I will primarily be talking with the patient.

Me: "I have looked over your medical chart, and it looks like you have been through the wringer?!"

Ms. Smith: "Yes, it's been a lot!"

Preceptor commentary. Notice how Dr. Lee continues by....Our patients have lives outside of the hospital, and their lives are now on "pause" because of their illness(es). Even taking one sentence to voice sympathy and recognize the humanity of our patients and the fact that their lives have been disrupted by their illness(es) is a worthwhile endeavor. This is one way that you can express to your patients—without actually saying so—that you actually care about them as a person.

Me: "Let's make sure that I have understood correctly what is going on with you, so please let me know if this doesn't match what you've been told. Thus far, it looks like you are being treated for Condition #1, Condition #2, and Condition #3—is that correct?"

Ms.. Smith: "Yep, that sounds right."

Preceptor commentary. Notice how Dr. Lee continues by....It is critical that ascertaining what the patient understands about what is going on is a first step—one cannot always assume that the patient knows and understands what he/she is being treated for. After all, there are times when what concerns the physician is not necessarily what concerns the patient, and vice versa. The invitation to the patient to correct is also important for encouraging two-way communication.

Me: "OK, makes sense. Thus far, I think we are doing Treatment #1 and Treatment #2 for Condition #1, and Management Plan #3 for Condition #2, and Treatment #4 for Condition #3. Does that sound like what you've been told?"

Ms. Smith: "I didn't know about Treatment #2; no one said anything about that."

Me: "OK, you were not aware of Treatment #2. Let me explain why you are on that."

Preceptor commentary. Notice how Dr. Lee continues by....I then proceed to use non-jargon language to explain Treatment #2. It is not always easy to explain things in layman's terms! When my residents use medical terminology, I will often interrupt them and ask the patient, *"Do you know what 'choledocholithiasis' is?"* Some of our patients are very sophisticated and know the medical terminology, but some do not!

Me: "OK, now I have told you what I know about Treatment #2. So now, let's make sure I explained it clearly enough that you can tell me what is going on. True or false: we are giving you a blood thinner for Condition #3—true or false?"

Ms. Smith: "True."

Preceptor commentary. Notice how Dr. Lee continues by....If the patient gets it right, I know they have understood. If he/she gets it wrong, though, I know that I need to explain more.

Me: "Alright! Now, true or false: Being on this blood thinner means that you will never get another blood clot in your legs. True or false?"

Ms. Smith: (grinning) "False."

Preceptor commentary. Notice how Dr. Lee continues by....It is so critical not only to give true statements, but also to throw in some false ones to ensure the patient is listening and truly understands, not just nodding "yes" that they do.

Me: "OK, you are correct. True or false: That blood thinner is going to mean that you are going to be more likely to bleed, so you will have to let your nurse know if you have any pooping blood or bloody pee, or if you are bleeding from anywhere. True or false?"

Ms. Smith: (grinning again) "True."

Preceptor commentary. Notice how Dr. Lee continues by....It is important to ensure that they understand the ramifications, or downstream effects, of the decisions they are making. Again, the quiz method helps us determine whether our patients understand what is going on. If you have any doubt that the patient actually understands what is going on, it would be helpful to ask the question's opposite to ensure they say the opposite answer. For instance, this question's opposite would be, *"True or false: that blood thinner will mean that you are going to be less likely to bleed. True or false?"*

Me: "Great job. Do you have any questions for me?"

Preceptor commentary. Notice how Dr. Lee continues by....By this time, most questions concern the timing of the previously mentioned treatments or diagnostic tests, or when the patient can be discharged from the hospital. Again, I answer these questions in layman's terms (non-jargon language), and I always say, *"The social worker would be the right person to ask that particular question to."* When I'm asked a question about prognosis timelines, I always answer in terms of ranges—*"If I had to venture a guess, I'd be thinking on the order of days to weeks."*

Preceptor commentary. Notice how Dr. Lee continues by....Once we have gone over the patient's active issues in the hospital, my resident or I will inquire about overnight events related to those issues.

Dr. Jones: "Have you had any chest pains?"

Ms. Smith: "Yes."

Dr. Jones: "Oh? Is it new?"

Ms. Smith: "No. I've had it for 10 years now."

Me: (turning to Dr. Jones) "OK! So this is a valuable learning point—Ms Smith did in fact answer your question! But, was the information that she gave you really what you were wanting?"

Dr. Jones: (grinning) "No. OK. Perhaps I could have asked, "Ms. Smith, have you had any NEW chest pain overnight?"

Ms. Smith: (smiling) "No. Not new. This chest pain has been going on for a long time. My heart doctor says it's not my heart, no one knows what it is, so I live with it."

Me: "Not fun. Condolences for that."

Dr. Jones: "Is your breathing improved as compared to when you first came in?"

Ms. Smith: "I think it's a bit better than it was before."

Dr. Jones: "OK, got it. Have you had any other new issues arise overnight?"

Ms Smith: *"I had a really rough night. I felt sick last night and this morning, and I'm also having a severe headache today."*

Me: (furrowing my brow) *"Not Fun. Sorry to hear that you've been feeling sick and having a bad headache. When you say that you felt sick, do you mean that you've been feeling nauseous?"*

Ms. Smith nods, "Yes."

Preceptor commentary. Notice how Dr. Lee continues by....Our patients are human beings, and the symptoms they are experiencing are affecting their lives. As physicians, we are not just vending machines dispensing medicines and diagnostic tests—we are human beings caring for human beings facing a significant trial in their lives. This recognition—and acting upon it accordingly—is what makes this a higher calling than just a regular day job.

Me: "Tell me more about your headache—how would you describe it? Sharp, dull, throbbing...?"

Ms. Smith: "Throbbing and severe, right about here." The patient points to the left side of her head.

Me: "Did it come on suddenly or gradually, would you say?"

Ms. Smith: "Suddenly. I don't normally get headaches, so I thought it was weird."

Me: (turning to Dr. Jones) "OK! Sudden onset headache, severe, doesn't usually get headaches. Give a differential diagnosis for this." (Turning to Ms. Smith) "I'm testing Dr. Jones—she's going to do just fine."

Dr. Jones: "OK. Let's see, Intracranial hemorrhage. Subarachnoid hemorrhage."

Me: "Very good. Very dangerous, we don't want to miss it. What would you do to work that up?"

Dr. Jones: "CT."

Me: "CT of...?"

Dr. Jones: "The head."

Me: "Right! With or without contrast?"

Dr. Jones: “Without contrast.”

Me: “Very good! What else should be on your differential diagnosis, and its matching workup?”

Dr. Jones: “Hmm. Tension headaches. And complicated migraine.”

Me: “Yes, how to work these up?”

Dr. Jones: “History & physical.”

Me: “True. OK, what else is on your differential diagnosis? Don’t forget the matching workup.”

Dr. Jones: “I don’t know.”

Preceptor commentary. Notice how Dr. Lee continues by….Thus far, Dr. Jones has given the most important differential diagnoses for significant headache, but now she has reached a point where she has no further differential diagnoses. This is an important juncture as a teacher—I can either answer my learner or push them further. Whenever possible, I want my learners to make mistakes while on rotation with me, because not only are the stakes zero, but they will remember it better when they get it wrong first, and then get it right afterwards.

Me: “OK, how about if Ms. Smith had a bad fever and neck stiffness as well, then what would you be thinking of?”

Dr. Jones: “Meningitis! I suppose we would have to get an LP if we were worried about that.”

Me: (turning to the patient) “An ‘LP’ is a ‘Lumbar Puncture,’ also known as a spinal tap. Thankfully, in your case, you can probably avoid that! You don’t have other things that would make us be very suspicious of meningitis.”

Me: (Turning to Dr. Jones) “OK! They’re not common, but there are a couple of other things it could be—an acute stroke, or a cerebral venous thrombosis.” (Turning to the patient) “Basically, a blood clot in the veins in your brain. But thankfully, I doubt that you have either of those!”

Dr. Jones: “OK, we’d have to get an MRI of the brain and an MRA for those differential diagnoses.”

Me: “Right! Are we going to order those right now?”

Dr. Jones: “Probably not?”

Me: “Good! The likelihood is low enough that we should probably follow up with a head CT first before doing anything else! Meanwhile, what are we going to do with the headache symptom itself?”

Dr. Jones: “Morphine?”

Me: “So when we talk about medicines, we need to call out the Name, Dose, Route, and Frequency, right? After all, perhaps you meant ‘MS Contin 30 mg PO BID?’

Dr. Jones: (grinning) “No! I was thinking something more like ‘morphine 2 mg IV q2h PRN pain!’”

Me: "Nice! That would be more reasonable! But perhaps before jumping straight to IV opioids, how about a viable PO option?"

Dr Jones: "Tylenol 650 mg PO q6h PRN pain?"

Me: "Very reasonable place to start. What if the pain is not sufficiently controlled with that?"

Dr. Jones: "Norco 5 mg PO q4h PRN breakthrough pain?"

Me: (turning to the patient) "I think Dr. Jones did a nice job, don't you think so too? So we said a lot of things, but in summary, for your severe headache and feeling sick, we're going to check a CT scan of your head so that we can make sure you don't have any bleeding up there. If that comes back clean and your headache is persisting, we will talk again about what else we need to do to check into that condition."

Ms. Smith: (nodding) "OK."

Me: (turning to Dr. Jones) "So, not only did we discuss the differential diagnosis of a sudden severe headache in someone who doesn't usually get headaches, but we also addressed when to think of a differential diagnosis. When the patient presents with a new condition or when things are progressing in a direction different from what you expected, it is important to expand the differential diagnosis and develop appropriate plans. This is how we think critically when we encounter conditions, rather than just aimlessly doing things."

Preceptor commentary. Notice how Dr. Lee continues by....In this back-and-forth with my resident learner, there are a few things we did that are worth noting: first, we kept the patient in the loop and explained anything that could have been misunderstood. Second, I asked my resident to come up with answers before I gave her the answers, and even when she said she had no other answers, I offered clues or prompts to help her arrive at subsequent answers. Third, I want my resident to practice being "put on the spot," because that is real clinical practice—we are always "put on the spot." Also, by getting it wrong first and then getting it right, my learner will remember it better and be more confident next time. Fourth, I explain the point of the exercise—in this case, it was not only to come up with a differential diagnosis for severe headache, but also to learn to recognize the timing and situation that call for one.

Me: *"Is there anything I'm missing that you need me to know?"*

This is a good question to ask, because you never know what the patient wants to know, and it will help you avoid asking a question while you are halfway out the door. If the RN is present with me, I will often ask, *"Is there anything I'm missing from your perspective?"*

Me: *"Ms. Smith, may we do your physical examination?"*

Ms. Smith: (nods)

Me: "Also, as you know, I'm Dr. Johnson's teacher, so I will be pointing things out to her and discussing or correcting her about various things. Would it be OK with you if Dr. Johnson does your physical examination as well?"

Ms. Smith: (nods) "We all have to learn sometimes!"

Preceptor commentary. Notice how Dr. Lee continues by.... These bedside rounds are a terrific opportunity to teach or improve physical examination skills. However, it is critical to let the patient know what you're doing so that he or she won't be baffled by it (and why). If I have not taught this resident before, I will need to assess their baseline physical examination skills. I find it best to give instructions like this: *"Please proceed with showing me the cardiac examination, IPA* (Inspection, Palpation, Auscultation)." In this way, I can know what her routine looks like. If I have taught the resident before, I will invite my resident physician to proceed with the physical examination.

My resident calls out, *"Regular rate and rhythm."*

I respond, *"Are you sure?"*

Preceptor commentary. Notice how Dr. Lee continues by.... This often causes my residents to freeze. They are used to having good roundsmanship, and oftentimes asking something like "are you sure?" is a cue that they have answered incorrectly. However, I am not concerned with good roundsmanship; I am concerned with ensuring that they have listened and examined carefully and long enough to be sure of their findings. More often than not, they hadn't listened or examined long enough to be sure, so they often go back and listen or examine again.

My resident tries again. *"Yes, I'm sure."*

"OK! This one is a bit on the tougher side, but if you feel the pulse on the wrist as you listen, it might be easier to hear (and feel) that the pulse is actually irregularly irregular. Go ahead and try again—do you hear and feel it now?"

Preceptor commentary. Notice how Dr. Lee continues by.... When giving correction, it is often helpful to call it out gently (but never say anything that isn't true!), State the correct answer, then give them another chance to recognize it. Your resident is here to learn, so they need guidance and correction—our job as teachers is to give it to them in a way that will hopefully help them want more of it.

"OK! Just a small thing as well—what is a 'regular' rate?"

"60 to 100."

"That is a normal rate, yes, but it's not a 'regular' rate, right?" This one was harped upon by one of my influential mentors in medical school, who taught me the importance of being precise and accurate in our use of words and language. I usually pass this one along to my residents as well to help encourage them to be accurate and precise in their language.

"OK! Now, does this patient have a cardiac murmur?" I ask.

The resident now shifts uncomfortably, but listens to the patient's heart again. *"Oh. Yes. I hear a murmur."*

"Nice! Is there anything else that you need to tell me about this murmur?"

"Systolic murmur." My resident answers.

"That's correct. Also, we need to include a few other things. Such as...?" I probe further.

"Hmm. Best heard at the Right Upper Sternal Border." My resident answers again.

"Nice! That's good! I also want to know the grade, and if it radiates to the neck or the axilla." After that, I go over grades one (1) through six (6) for grading heart murmurs, explain these points to my resident, and include my patient in the discussion.

Preceptor commentary. Notice how Dr. Lee continues by....After completing the physical exam, we will review the day's plan of action with the patient and family.

Me: *"OK! So, as a recap, for Condition #1, we are doing Treatments #1 and #2. For Condition #2, we are doing Management Plan #3. For Condition #3, we are doing Treatment #4. Is there anything else that we need to discuss further?"*

Preceptor commentary. Notice how Dr. Lee continues by....This recap is extremely brief, just a statement of the active conditions and their matching plans. In this way, we close the loop on communication and let them know we plan to execute on the plan as discussed. If any of the plans involve calling specialists for a consult, I often do so right there in the room so the patient can witness my calling or texting for a consultation. This tells patients that we handle things promptly.

Preceptor commentary. Notice how Dr. Lee continues by....After confirming that they have no further questions, I shake the patient's hand, then the family's hands again, and advise them that I will see them again tomorrow. If my partner will be taking over the next day, I tell them who is coming and write their name on the whiteboard whenever possible.

Discussion

As the dialogue above shows, several important practices can help our residents grow in professionalism, competence, and communication skills.

1) *Being present at the bedside together*. This may seem obvious, but there has been an overall shift away from bedside rounding toward table or hallway rounds (Beigzadeh, 2019).
    a. At the bedside, the physician teacher can demonstrate skilled history-taking, observe the resident's history-taking, offer constructive criticism, and show the resident how he/she might have asked the same question differently to achieve a more effective result.

b. The same can be said for physical examination skills -- and there is no substitute for pointing out and/or corroborating physical exam findings at the same time in the same room. The dialogue above demonstrates this as well. Additionally, if one is doing table rounds and tells the resident or medical student to "check out that murmur later," it can be too easily missed or forgotten.
c. The same can be said for communication skills with the patient and the family—the resident or medical student might think they communicated something a certain way. However, upon direct observation, it turns out they communicated it differently than intended. This type of catch could not have happened if the teaching physician had just been given a report from the resident!
d. Finally, the exhibition of professionalism and critical thinking skills when new or unexpected problems arise is far more accurately observed than reported. When the teacher and learner are together, the teacher can hear directly from the learner what he/she is thinking and would do in real time. It is here that the physician-teacher can help refine the learner's thought processes and critical thinking skills.

2) *Setting a Teachable Attitude as #1 over everything else.* This applies to both teachers and learners! Learning goes both ways, and also with our patients. The authors believe in humility in teaching and learning. This is not about thinking less about oneself. It is not about lacking confidence. It is about understanding where we have demonstrated certain skills and the ability to achieve results, and where we have not yet. The moment we acknowledge that we do not yet have the experience, we move from 'I know it all' to 'I need to learn it' mode. We invest extra time to prepare. We might reach out to others and get their perspective. And through that process, we not only learn but also increase our chances of succeeding with a new task we haven't done before. The execution of this, however, is much easier said than done. It must be modeled by the teaching physician, and must also be expected of the resident physician—after all, our residents will rise or sink to whatever we expect of them and enforce. For best results, the teaching physician must spell it out from the beginning that a teachable attitude of humility is necessary for success on the rotation. If the resident physician is not exhibiting a teachable attitude, then the teaching physician must take note of it and advise the resident as such. Enforcement takes the shape of something like the following:
a. 1st time: (a gentle reminder) "Let us remember the value of humility and teachability, that we may learn and grow in the ways that we need to be our very best."

b. 2nd time: (a firmer reminder, but in the form of a question) "Do you think that you are exhibiting a teachable attitude at this time, which would lead to your fulfilling your full potential as a physician?"
c. 3rd time: (a firmer reminder, this time in the form of a statement) "It seems to me that you are not maintaining the most teachable attitude. I need to see improvement in your attitude toward constructive criticism. If I do not see that, then I may find it increasingly difficult to muster the energy and effort needed to teach you to help you fulfill your full potential as a physician."
d. 4th time: (final reminder) "When you are ready to learn with a teachable attitude, I will be ready to resume teaching you at full tilt."

3) Give direct, real-time feedback.
e. It is important to do this tactfully, especially at the bedside! However, it is equally important to be clear and direct in your feedback. In order to ensure that your learner learned the correct lesson from your feedback, it is helpful to ask him/her to repeat back the corrected version of whatever it is that you gave feedback on right then. That is when it is freshest in his/her mind, helping solidify your feedback and aiding its incorporation into his/her practice.
f. Do not utilize the "Sandwich" model (start with a compliment, then give the correction, and then follow it up with one more compliment). Instead, call out the strengths you see and affirm them, and keep an eye out for 2-3 actionable items they can take on. The more measurable those things are, the better, because you (and your learner) can know if/when your learner has improved. If at all possible, it is important to follow up and praise the learner when he/she has acted on the constructive criticism you gave.
g. The physician teacher might be tempted not to take the time or effort to give meaningful, tactful, constructive criticism, or to decide that he/she would prefer not to hurt the learner's feelings. However, the physician teacher must remember that these learners will someday be our colleagues, our consultants, even our teachers, and (perhaps) our physicians! For that reason, we, as physician teachers, must teach our learners with utmost diligence and professionalism, knowing that our reward will be having done our part to help them be the very best physicians they can be.
h. Follow our own feedback/advice. Our learners will not take us seriously if we are not walking out what we teach.

Application of teachability, feedback, and modeling in practice: Author Lee, a physician, while teaching in the residency program where author RS was then a resident, experienced a teaching moment for both. Lee used to ask the resident (s) on the spot how they would handle a specific situation. RS politely and in private shared with Lee that his direct approach made her nervous and that she learns more effectively by observing his behavior first and then implementing the desired behavior she has seen modeled for her. Seeing the effectiveness of this learning/teaching approach, both agreed to use role modeling with residents (and medical students, when appropriate) who are more comfortable with role modeling as a learning method.

Modeling in all settings:

It is so critical to personally model professionalism, integrity, honesty with patients, effective communication, patient care, and compassion, showing that this is not just a job but a career, and that the physician is passionate about patient care and patient satisfaction (Spaans et al., 2025). Good teaching starts with good practice -- walking the talk, not just talking the talk. The importance of being teachable and of our attitudes is paramount. Shifting an attitude of "how little can I get away with?" to "This is a Sacred Calling," and acting in accordance with that.

The authors also emphasize the importance of an Active Learning model, in which the instructor provides questions and guidance. However, at all times, the learner is expected to be fully engaged, answer questions, and be informed in advance that they will receive both positive and negative feedback. It will be important for the instructor to pay attention to the learner, observe how the learner responds and learns, and adjust accordingly (Sya'ban et al., 2024).

At the bedside:

It is so critical to be present with the learner -- whether the learner is watching the teacher or the teacher is watching the learner-- and, at the beginning of the rotation, have the learner be the shadow. As the rotation progresses, the learner assumes progressively more responsibility for actions/practices until they are independent in the task(s) by the end of the rotation.

The importance of real-time feedback is that it reflects real life, and they need to receive it at the bedside. It needs to be done in a way that is professional (again, modeling professionalism) but is constructive criticism.

It is not the sandwich model; rather, it is identifying strengths, calling them out and affirming them, and then keeping an eye out for two or three actionable items they can take on and measure. It is so critical for it to be direct feedback, not indirect. Also, making sure that the feedback makes sense to the learner! That will require the teacher's time, but it is time well spent because it will ensure we are teaching them effectively and will be worth the investment. The reward will be that these learners will someday be our physicians.

Also, modeling professionalism at the bedside—care and communication with patients and family members, shaking all their hands, etc.—is important to emphasize. Further, talking out loud about what you are thinking and why you are doing it is clearly necessary for making a memorable impression.

In the classroom

Adopting an active learning model in the classroom—knowing your learners' names, making them answer questions, and making that the expectation are all significant behaviors for the preceptor to model. Active learning may be best ilustrated by the following practical applications.

Using repetition

Presenting the facts of the case, presenting decision points, having learners commit to a course of action, and having people vote are all enhancing repetition. Having them split up and debate it! Also, write out the learning points and have them read them out loud in bite-sized chunks. This forces teachers to be sharp and well-prepared. It might be daunting/intimidating to teach in the classroom, but medical teaching is just sharing what was learned.

Being intellectually honest—to say you do not know if you do not know the topic. Lectures are not the best because people can read things on their own. However, you cannot just read decision points; you also need to know how to process and think things through, especially when there is more than one answer. Thus, the classroom should focus on presenting decision points and how to think, rather than just presenting facts or topics.

Learning from experiences

Author Lee says that he will never forget the time that he was a medical student intern and had just completed a week of shadowing a psychiatrist in the psychiatric ward. It had been an eye-opening experience, to be sure, and when he returned to the family practice clinic the next week, he felt like he had returned to a more normal world. During one of those clinic encounters, he made the comment that he was so glad that he was back in the family practice clinic rather than the psychiatric ward because of all of the crazy problems that the patients had. His family practice preceptor immediately said, in an abnormally loud voice, "We all have a lot of crazy in us," then promptly moved on to the next topic, shooting him a look to say no more. It turns out that the patient the author had made that comment in front of was previously hospitalized in that same psychiatric ward. This incident was a significant misstep and led to several important lessons.

The preceptor subsequently emphasized the necessity of recognizing all patients as human beings, each deserving of respect and a commitment to uphold their dignity. This interaction was one of many occasions on which observing the physician preceptor at the bedside proved invaluable. It is believed that such experiences are crucial for fostering professionalism and quality healthcare in future generations. The transmission of lessons learned to upcoming physicians and mid-level providers is essential.

It was a real gaffe —and he learned important lessons from it. And his preceptor took the time to explain the importance of recognizing that all patients are human beings, deserving of respect and of best efforts to uphold their dignity. This was one of many instances in which the author learned from observing his physician preceptor at the bedside. Both authors believe this is a critical way to help develop, optimize, and encourage professionalism and quality health care in the future -- to pass on the lessons they have learned to the next generation of resident physicians, medical students, and healthcare providers.

Verbalizing clinical reasoning at the bedside

One of the most vital practices a preceptor can employ at the bedside is verbalizing his/her clinical reasoning. Learners benefit from hearing the preceptor's thought processes, whether considering differential diagnoses, evaluating the risks and benefits of procedures or medications, or determining the best way to communicate recommendations to the patient. This includes consideration of the complications of adding medications to an already extensive list, the appropriateness of further diagnostic testing, and the cost-effectiveness and patient comfort. While many of these decisions appear automatic to experienced preceptors, they result from years of practice, experience, and iterative learning. Learners, lacking such automaticity, require explicit guidance to develop their clinical reasoning.

For example, it is not yet instinctual for learners to immediately consider scoring systems, assess hemodynamic stability, evaluate renal function, or select appropriate imaging modalities in cases such as acute pulmonary embolism. The bedside environment is where these thought processes are most effectively demonstrated, and when preceptors articulate their reasoning and involve learners in clinical decision-making algorithms, invaluable skills are imparted. Equally important are the "soft skills" inherent to medical practice—greeting every individual present, engaging patients as people rather than problems, maintaining eye contact, communicating in plain language, and actively listening. This includes repeating back patient or family concerns, incorporating their perspectives into management, and ensuring they feel heard before explaining the rationale for clinical decisions. Demonstrating empathy, sitting during difficult conversations, and communicating with clarity and compassion in challenging situations are best learned through observation rather than instruction. Thus, bedside precepting is critical, and skilled preceptors are indispensable. Such proficiency is not innate, but rather cultivated through experience, attentiveness to learners, and a commitment to exemplary practice.

Professionalism extends beyond interactions with patients to the broader clinical environment. It is imperative never to speak disparagingly of a patient's character, even outside the patient's presence, and to treat all staff members with courtesy, regardless of role. Learning staff names, acknowledging their contributions, and expressing gratitude are integral to effective teamwork. Additionally, thorough preparation for consultations—anticipating and addressing consultant questions—demonstrates respect for colleagues' time and expertise. These behaviors are most effectively learned through observation of role models (Spaans et al., 2025).

Role modeling by example

One of the most important things that a preceptor can do at the bedside is to talk out loud. The learner needs to hear what the preceptor is thinking. The preceptor might be considering a differential diagnosis or the risks and benefits of a specific procedure or medication. He or she might be thinking about the ramifications of making one recommendation over another and how best to communicate that to the patient sitting before him or her. The preceptor might be considering the complications that could arise from adding yet another medication to a medication list that already has 20 other medications on it. He or she might be thinking about whether it makes sense to do yet another diagnostic test, whether it would affect management, and whether it would be cost-effective to do one test or another, all the while considering the patient's comfort and ability to tolerate the test. Many of these thought processes may be automatic for the preceptor. However, they are only seemingly automatic because of years of practice and experience, as well as a good amount of trial and error. Our learners do not have these thought processes yet in place, however. For them, it is not automatic to automatically think of the Wells score and to immediately check the Blood pressure to determine if the patient is hemodynamically stable or not, and therefore might require thrombolytics, or to evaluate the renal function and decide whether a CT PE protocol is appropriate or not, and also to obtain an echo to evaluate for right heartstrain. Many of these thought processes occur at the bedside, and the learner whose preceptor spells out what he or she is thinking as he or she is thinking of these things can gain a great deal. If the preceptor takes it to the next level by asking the learner questions, walking them through the decision-making process, and explaining the algorithm for acute pulmonary embolism, the learner will have gained a crucial skill. Equally important are the soft skills that go into being a physician. The importance of greeting everyone in the room upon entry. The importance of smiling and greeting your patients as a human being rather than as a problem to be solved or a number on the list. The importance of looking your patient in the eye while you talk to them, of speaking in plain English only, and never using medical jargon. Also, it is important to listen to the patient and repeat back to them what they have said, or to their family members, and incorporate their input into the decision-making algorithm. Or, at the very least, making sure they feel they have been heard before you explain why what they want may not be in the patient's best interests. Further, it is important to sit down rather than stand the whole time, especially when the patient is sharing difficult things. The importance of sitting down, speaking slowly and clearly, and speaking with compassion in any end-of-life or difficult situation is critical. These are the things that can be taught with words, but are far more effectively caught by observation. This is why precepting at the bedside is so critical and why there is a need for those skilled in this. No one is a skilled preceptor from birth, however. One only becomes a skilled preceptor through trial and error, through a willingness to listen to and learn from their learners, and through doing their best at all times to be the kind of physician their patients want them to be, and their families would want them to be. A preceptor who leads by example but can also spell out what he or she is thinking and doing can offer a tremendous gift to the learner (Spaans et al., 2025).

Another important part of precepting is professionalism outside of the patient room as well. The importance of never speaking ill of a patient's character, even behind his/her back. The importance of treating all of the staff with courtesy, not just the CEO or other physicians, but all of the staff, and trying to learn their names. The importance of looking the staff in the eye and thanking them for their help, after all, we cannot do our job without their efforts. The way to call consults is to gather the information you need to anticipate and answer the consultants' likely questions before calling, and to be prepared so you avoid wasting their time when they ask questions. All of these things are best caught rather than taught (Spaans et al., 2025).

FUTURE DIRECTIONS

Future research could assess the standards of professionalism, competence, and communication in medical training to support continuous improvement, especially in today's AI-driven healthcare environment. Further, research may focus on alternatives and models to manage the physician shortage and medical training, when implemented, to measure their effectiveness and benefits in the short and long term. Research must also evaluate the potential impact on various stakeholders (including patients, physicians, the insurance company, healthcare providers, hospitals, and other healthcare-related organizations) regarding the new solutions and recommendations being more optimal, sustainable, and beneficial to them. Research studies would need to develop strategies to improve existing and proposed healthcare models for medical training, ensuring that all US stakeholders benefit from a comprehensive, sustainable healthcare system.

CONCLUSIONS

In summary, the chapter focuses on strategies for developing, optimizing, and promoting professionalism, communication, competence, and quality in healthcare. They are based on the sharing of the accumulated knowledge and wisdom of the two authors and physicians with emerging resident physicians, medical students, and healthcare providers. Also, best practices for effectively transmitting professionalism and communication have been modeled and discussed. Continuing to develop highly professional and well-trained resident physicians and medical students would help enhance the quality and delivery of healthcare services provided (including in the much-needed rural areas), improve patient satisfaction, and promote overall sustainability in healthcare. The two authors/physicians share their experiences as role models of best practices for the new generation of healthcare professionals to emulate.

REFERENCES

Accreditation Council for Graduate Medical Education (ACGME). (2025). *Common program requirements*. Retrieved from Common Program Requirements.

Association of American Medical Colleges AAMC (2024). *The complexities of physician supply and demand: Projections from 2021 to 2036*. Retrieved from The Complexities of Physician Supply and Demand: Projections From 2021 to 2036.

Association of American Medical Colleges (AAMC). (2025). *Tomorrow's doctors, tomorrow's cures*. Retrieved from Tomorrow's Doctors, Tomorrow's Cures | AAMC

Beigzadeh, A., Adibi, P., Bahaadinbeigy, K., & Yamani, N. (2019). Strategies for teaching in clinical rounds: A systematic review of the literature. *Journal of Research in Medical Sciences : the Official Journal of Isfahan University of Medical Sciences*, *24*(1), 33.

Benbassat, J. (2014). Role modeling in medical education: The importance of a reflective imitation. *Academic Medicine*, *89*(4), 550–554.

Centers for Medicare and Medicaid Services (CMS). (2025). *CMS announces $50 billion in awards to strengthen rural health in all 50 states*. CMS Announces $50 Billion in Awards to Strengthen Rural Health in All 50 States | CMS

Congress.gov. (2025). *H.R.4731 - 119th Congress (2025-2026): Resident Physician Shortage Reduction Act of 2025*. Retrieved from H.R.4731 - 119th Congress (2025-2026): Resident Physician Shortage Reduction Act of 2025 | Congress.gov | Library of Congress

Spaans, I., Verbree, A. R., de Kleijn, R., & Dilaver, G. (2026). Role models in medicine and beyond: A survey study exploring the relationship between role models, academic performance and sense of belonging. *BMC Medical Education*, *26*(1), 5.

Sya'ban, S., Wazir, A., & Horneffer, P. (2024). *Active learning in medical education*. Retrieved from Active Learning in Medical Education | Lecturio

Zucker, H. (2025). Where have all the physicians gone? AARP.org/Bulletin. Retrieved from America Is Facing a Shortage of Doctors

ADDITIONAL READING

Jones, C. & Dalsten, M. (2024). *Healthcare on the brink: navigating the challenges of an aging society in the United States.* Healthcare on the brink: navigating the challenges of an aging society in the United States - PMC

Walensky, R., & McCann, N. (2025). Challenges to the future of a robust physician workforce in the United States. [Challenges to the Future of a Robust Physician Workforce in the United States | New England Journal of Medicine]. *The New England Journal of Medicine, 392*(3), 286–295. DOI: 10.1056/NEJMsr2412784 PMID: 39813651

KEY TERMS AND DEFINITIONS

Challenges: Complex issues, problems, and situations in healthcare that are difficult to manage.

Communication: interpersonal skills including active listening, empathy, clear verbal and nonverbal communication, written communication, shared decision-making, and handling conversations effectively.

Competence: Medical knowledge, patientcare/procedural skills, practice-based learning, and systems-based learning.

Medical training: medical schools and residency programs teach through explicit curricula (lectures, modules, and essays), faculty role modeling, simulation-based training, feedback and assessment, and faculty development to ensure teaching and assessment are effective.

Medical student: A student who is enrolled in a four-year medical program to earn a medical degree and become a doctor.

Physician shortage: Patient demand for physician services exceeds the supply of physicians.

Potential solutions: Possible alternatives, short and long term, to meet the healthcare challenges.

Professionalism: involves ethical behavior, integrity, accountability, respect, and a commitment to excellence.

Resident physician: A physician who, after medical school, undergoes training, usually in a three-year residency program.

Role Modeling: An effective teaching strategy in medical education and training, it influences the professional attitudes, behaviors, and competence of about 90 percent of medical graduates.

Chapter 10
Key Factors, Effective Teamwork, and Healthcare Outcomes:
Mayo Clinic Applications

Raj Selladurai
http://orcid.org/0009-0008-4049-3942
Indiana University Northwest, USA

Tony W. Spaulding
http://orcid.org/0009-0006-4071-9206
Mayo Clinic, USA

Charlie Hobson
http://orcid.org/0009-0001-6520-5002
Indiana University Northwest, USA

ABSTRACT

This chapter focuses on key factors that impact effective teamwork in healthcare organizations, including a case study on the applications of a teamwork model at Mayo Clinic in Rochester, MN. Studies have found positive correlations among effective teamwork, patient care, and provider satisfaction. Key factors such as teamwork training, leaderless online group discussion, servant leadership, and top management support lead to effective teamwork, which would positively impact the quadruple aim—patient experience, high-quality and safe delivery of patient care, lower costs, and provider satisfaction.

DOI: 10.4018/979-8-3373-2577-4.ch010

INTRODUCTION

Teamwork is critical in medicine and healthcare today to provide effective, high-quality patient care at an optimal cost, the ideal goal that healthcare organizations aim to achieve. It involves integrating healthcare professionals from various specialties (physicians, nurses, pharmacists, therapists, administrators, information technology (IT), operations, and other support staff), all working together as a team to achieve common, patient-focused goals. Effective teamwork has been shown to improve patient safety, the quality of patient care, and patient satisfaction. Many research studies have shown a strong correlation between effective teamwork/collaboration and lower medical-related errors, shorter hospital stays, lower mortality rates, reduced nursing turnover, and enhanced overall patient satisfaction (Zajac et al., 2021). The chapter will first provide background information on the significance of teamwork within the healthcare arena. The authors will then analyse the impact of key factors such as teamwork training, leaderless online group discussion, servant leadership, and top management support on effective teamwork, which, in turn, will positively affect the quadruple aims of patient experience, quality of patient care, lower costs, and provider satisfaction. Some strategies to develop effective teamwork in healthcare organizations will be explored and recommended. Next, a case study of Mayo Clinic in Rochester, MN, which shows the application of an innovative teamwork model, will be discussed. Finally, the study will examine areas for future research to determine how teamwork can be most effectively utilized to improve patient experience outcomes, quality of patient care, lower costs, and enhance provider satisfaction.

BACKGROUND

Teamwork is considered a core value in healthcare organizations because it helps deliver excellent patient care. In every healthcare experience with a physician, nurse, or other healthcare professionals, patients, their family members, and friends can see multiple interactions with several healthcare staff across different clinical settings. Recognizing the highest level of coordination and collaboration required among healthcare professionals has driven healthcare organizations to focus on measures and initiatives to foster effective teamwork and continuous improvement (James, 2021). Further, this Harvard Medical School study found that despite developing strong training and development programs to enhance teamwork, including communication, situational awareness, and performance assessment, healthcare organizations often miss a key ingredient, namely collaboration. Effective teamwork needs more than communication skills, mutual goals, and coordination. It needs a collaborative mindset that emphasizes the inherent value of the teamwork model, with professionals working together synergistically, and a strong commitment to building effective relationships among team members (James, 2021).

Several studies have shown that effective teamwork and safety awareness are critically important to the quality of healthcare, ensuring the safe and reliable delivery of services (Weller et al., 2024). In other areas, such as business, education, aviation, and nuclear power/energy, research over the last several decades has shown that effective teamwork is a significant factor in safe, effective performance. In reviewing the extensive literature on teamwork, eight major models that identify essential team-related behaviors/competencies are highlighted. Beginning chronologically in 1950, these include: Bales (1950), Stevens and Campion (1994), Cannon-Bowers, Tannenbaum, Salas, and Volpe (1995), Chen, Donahue and Klimoski (2004), Baker, Horvarth, Campion, Offerman, and Salas (2005), Salas, Sims, and Burke (2005), and Hobson, Strupeck, Griffin, Szostek, Selladurai, and Rominger (2013), and Weller et al., (2024) All these studies have shown the positive effects of teamwork on several variables, including decision-making, job performance, job satisfaction, patient safety, staff well-being, and other related organizational outcomes. Therefore, multiple research studies have shown that enhancing effective teamwork improves the overall quality of patient care and other related outcomes in healthcare organizations.

ANALYSIS

In Figure 1 and the discussion that follows, the authors focus on a conceptual model (KF-ET-QA) of Key Factors and Effective Teamwork, and their synergistic impact on the Quadruple Aim: patient experience, quality of patient care, lower costs, and provider satisfaction.

Figure 1. Key factors, effective teamwork, and impact on the quadruple aim

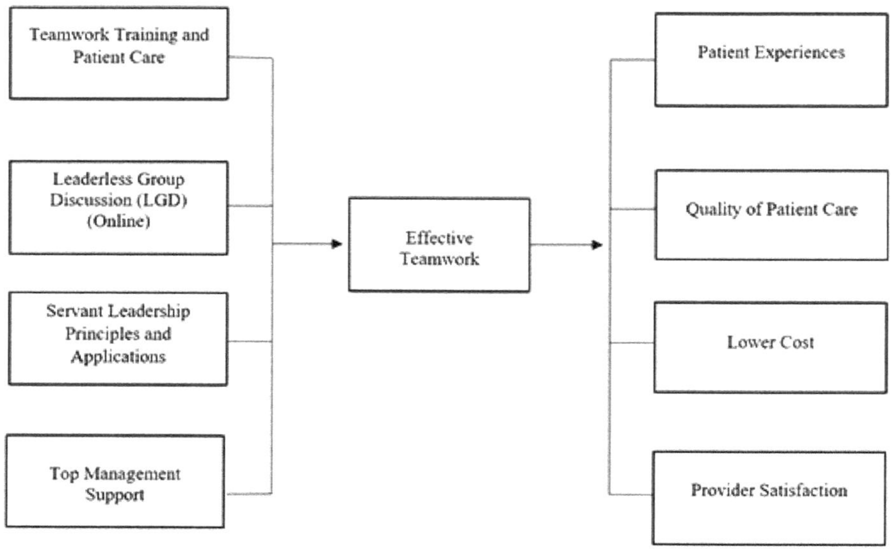

Source: Revised/adapted based on Greer et al. (2020). Effective teamwork and healthcare delivery outcomes." In R. Selladurai, C. Hobson, R. I. Selladurai, & A. Greer. (Eds.) Evaluating challenges and opportunities for healthcare reform. IGI Global, Inc.

The KF-ET-QA model proposes that the teamwork factors of teamwork training and patient care, leaderless group discussion (online), servant leadership principles and applications, and top management support would help enhance effective teamwork, which in turn would positively impact the four critical outcomes of the Quadruple Aim, namely patient experiences, quality of patient care, lower costs, and provider satisfaction. By focusing on achieving the Quadruple Aim's four outcomes, the healthcare organization can work toward providing a more holistic, effective, and sustainable healthcare system that emphasizes both patients' quality of healthcare and providers' satisfaction (Medbridge, 2026).

Teamwork Training and Patient Care

Several structured teamwork training programs may be used to enhance patient care. These include continuous improvement programs focused on teamwork in communication, support, leadership, and situational awareness, which provide strong evidence of improved patient care outcomes. Training in these areas prepares and equips healthcare team members to manage dynamic work environments and multiple healthcare settings and patient care conditions, providing safer, higher-quality, more efficient, and more effective patient care at optimal cost.

However, despite extensive use of teamwork over the years, suboptimal teamwork outcomes and communication-related problems continue to adversely impact patients. Hence, some studies have explored a different, more recent perspective on healthcare team performance by optimizing clinicians' and healthcare professionals' situational awareness, which is a measurable outcome of diagnosis and decision-making (Weller, 2024). Several meta-analyses and studies consistently reveal specific healthcare benefits by using the situational awareness method. Understanding and maintaining situational awareness is essential for providing effective, safe patient care. Situational awareness is the dynamic process of observing the situation, developing diagnoses, and making decisions related to the specific patient condition and situation. Teamwork performance would be enhanced if the entire team were actively involved in monitoring the environment, processing information, and planning decision-making action steps (Weller, 2024). Kelly & Lavelle (2024) reiterate the values of situational awareness and its positive impact on team performance, especially when using artificial intelligence (AI) models. The authors contend that AI can process large datasets and clinical information, and then provide interpretations to improve situational awareness.

Every staff member, in the context of situational awareness, represents another pair of eyes and ears to observe, diagnose, and interpret, and is also a trained mental and psychological resource contributing to the team's performance in this area. Failure to express one's opinions and perceptions may lead to adverse situations related to patient care. The responsibility for ensuring that every team member is actively involved in the situational awareness process must rest with the leadership team. Senior leadership staff can create a safe environment where team members feel valued, respected, and engaged, and included in decision-making, thereby willing to share their observations, ideas, and concerns (Weller, 2024).

Several studies, including three meta-analyses, have provided strong evidence that teamwork training improves team performance, which in turn impacts patient safety, higher-quality, optimal patient care, and related outcomes (Weller et al., 2024). Also, Schmutz et al. (2019) found that teams with effective performance were about three times more likely than ineffective teams to improve patient outcomes, such as mortality and morbidity rates, and closely related outcomes, such as adherence to treatment guidelines. Furthermore, another recent meta-analysis of over 13,000 patients found that measures to improve teamwork performance among multidisciplinary healthcare teams reduced patient mortality by 28 percent (Webster et al., 2023).

Other studies have shown that staff perceptions of teamwork and patient safety are positively associated with significantly lower mortality rates in hospitals with stronger nurse-physician teamwork, and that effective teamwork and communication are associated with greater benefits for staff engagement and patient outcomes (Weller et al., 2024). Further, Spiecher & Francis (2023) contended that positive perceptions of teamwork and communication are strongly related to staff well-being, lower burnout, and lower turnover. Therefore, healthcare organizations must ensure that continuous teamwork training is emphasized and implemented for their patient care teams to improve overall high-quality patient care, patient experiences, and the well-being and satisfaction of their own team members.

Teamwork training has been shown to improve clinical processes, efficiency, and effectiveness in healthcare. Several improvements include shorter hospital stays for many patients, fewer medical and clinical errors, greater decision accuracy, higher patient satisfaction, and enhanced safety culture measures (Haugstetter et al., 2024; Weller et al., 2024). Further, providing strong training for healthcare team members reduces complications and increases patient satisfaction through better coordination and collaboration among team members and perceived care quality (James, 2021). Hospitals and healthcare facilities that foster strong teamwork among their staff often find that patients are more satisfied with their care and are three times more likely to refer the facility to others (AHA, 2026).

Leaderless Group Discussion (LGD)

Online

As everyone knows, the COVID pandemic changed the world dramatically in many ways. Beginning in March 2020 and lasting for several semesters, a mandatory shift from face-to-face college classes to an online format occurred at virtually all higher education institutions. This included the required teamwork classes at our institution, in which we had previously used in-person LGDs at the beginning and end of each semester to assess, develop, and track students' skill development. Let

To conduct our end-of-course LGD assessment in Spring 2020 with existing 5-person teams, we were compelled to use a virtual format. We chose Zoom. This entailed: (1) inviting team members to a scheduled Zoom meeting, (2) explaining the group task for the 20-minute exercise, (3) taping the session, (4) forwarding copies of the taped LGD exercise to participating students for self-assessment purposes, using the same rating scale described above. The instructor also rated LGD tapes and met virtually with students to review their performance and progress.

The sudden transition from face-to-face to fully online classes in March 2020 was not without its challenges. Most of the problems that arose were technology-related (Zoom navigation, insufficient bandwidth, etc.) and were largely resolved in subsequent semesters. It quickly became apparent that telephonic access to competent tech support was essential.

Despite these tech-related challenges, the online LGD continued to provide an excellent, content-valid methodology for assessing and developing teamwork skills. This format would be especially helpful in college courses offered fully online and in those organizations that offer partial or fully remote work options to employees. Bailey-Hughes (2021) offers interesting insights and helpful advice to anyone interested in using online LGDs, based on her academic work with 375 student virtual teams over five years.

Team Leadership

It is important to note that the LGD (either face-to-face or virtual) can also be used to assess team leadership skills. Building upon the early pioneering research on a two-factor theory of team leadership (Stogdill & Coons, 1957; Likert, 1961; Blake & Mouton, 1964) and subsequent meta-analysis by Burke, Stagl, Klein, Goodwin, Salas, and Halpin (2006), Hobson et al. (2014) formulated the following team leadership behavioral roles assessment tool (reprinted with permission):

Table 1. Behavioral Assessment Tool

Task Roles		
1.	Initiator	Proposes tasks, goals, or procedures; defines team problems; begins discussion; restarts discussion during quiet times.
2.	Information Seeker	Asks for factual clarification; requests facts pertinent to the discussion; asks questions of teammates.
3.	Values Seeker	Asks about the values underlying teammate statements or positions; questions values involved in alternative points of view.
4.	Informer	Offers facts related to team's task; gives expression of feelings; gives opinions; answers teammates' questions.
5.	Clarifier	Interprets ideas or suggestions; defines terms; explains complex issues; clears up confusion.
6.	Summarizer	Takes notes on group discussion: pulls together related ideas; restates suggestions; offers summary decisions or conclusions for the team to consider; reviews team progress.
7.	Reality Tester	Conducts critical analyses of ideas; tests ideas against data or experience to see if the ideas would work; shares "real-world" examples to test team ideas.
8.	Orienteer	Keeps the team on track; draws attention to departures from agreed-upon directions or goals; raises questions about the direction pursued in team discussions; refocuses the team when needed; keeps track of time.
9.	Piggy-Backer	Builds on the ideas of others; offers new, creative suggestions, based upon teammate input.
10.	Follower	Allows teammates to participate in leadership roles actively; aligns with the team's movement; accepts others' ideas.
Social Roles		

continued on following page

Table 1. Continued

1.	Harmonizer	Focuses criticism on ideas, not individuals; attempts to reconcile disagreements; reduces tension; helps smooth over minor differences; gets people to explore differences; appropriately uses humor to help keep team relaxed.
2.	Gatekeeper	Helps to keep communication channels open; facilitates the participation of others; suggests procedures that permit sharing remarks; gently calls upon quiet teammates to solicit their input.
3.	Consensus Taker	Asks to see whether the team is nearing a decision; "sends up trial balloons" to test possible solutions; asks if everyone agrees with a proposed decision.
4.	Encourager	Is friendly, warm and responsive to others; indicates by facial expressions or remarks the acceptance of others' contributions; listens attentively; gives positive feedback to teammates; calls teammates by first name.
5.	Compromiser	Proposes solutions that demonstrate flexibility and willingness to "give in" if necessary when his or her own ideas are involved in conflicts; modifies one's position in the interest of team cohesion and/or performance.
6.	Standard Setter	Suggests standards for team interaction and performance; applies these standards to evaluate the quality of team processes and outputs.
Dysfunctional Roles		
1.	Blocker	Blindly and consistently disagrees with and opposes action; stubbornly resists team decisions and thwarts action.
2.	Dominator	Aggressively attempts to force ideas on the team; interrupts others; attempts to manipulate and control team interaction; refuses to compromise; fails to allow others to talk.
3.	Avoider	Withholds involvement from team interaction; fails to contribute to team efforts; refuses to confront important issues.
4.	Clown	Engages in irrelevant, distracting behaviors; seeks team members' attention; tries to show off; inappropriately attempts to create humorous situations; starts side conversations.
5.	Insulter	Attacks other team members in a destructive, personalized manner; sarcastic, pessimistic, and negative.

In conjunction with face-to-face LGDs, this tool has been successfully used for over 20 years with both senior-level undergraduate business and MBA students to assess and improve team leadership skills. Hobson et al. (2014) reported the following results from an anonymous end-of-course survey on the perceived impact of the LGD process among MBA students.

Table 2. MBA Student Survey Item Means[1]– Team Leadership (n = 102)

Items	Means
As a result of participating in the LGD videotaping and coaching in C512…	
1. I have improved my team leadership skills.	4.42
2. I have more confidence in my team leadership skills.	4.40
3. I have become more effective in team leadership activities.	4.30
4. I have a better understanding of my strengths in team leadership.	4.42

continued on following page

Table 2. Continued

Items	Means
5. I have a better understanding of my areas for improvement in team leadership.	4.48
6. I have a better understanding of how to improve my team leadership skills.	4.39

[1] Measurement Scale: 1 = Strongly Disagree, 2 = Disagree, 3 = Neither Agree nor Disagree, 4 = Agree, 5 = Strongly Agree

With minimal effort and few mishaps, this team leadership assessment process was effectively adapted to the online format mandated in March 2020.

Summary

In summary, the LGD offers a proven, content-valid, behaviorally based methodology for assessing individual teamwork/team leadership skills. Given the vital and growing importance of teamwork/team leadership in the provision of patient services, healthcare institutions could utilize the LGD in two major ways: (1) as a screening tool in making hiring and/or promotion decisions to ensure candidates demonstrate high levels of teamwork/team leadership competence and (2) as a framework for assessing and developing teamwork/team leadership skills of current employees. Similarly, schools preparing students for healthcare professions could use the LGD to screen applicants and as a vehicle for assessing and enhancing students' teamwork/team leadership skills. The authors have found that in both business and educational settings, employing the LGD for skill measurement and development is best accomplished by videotaping group interaction and using the tapes to foster self-awareness and motivation to improve.

Servant Leadership

Among the various challenges facing healthcare, one is the need for high-quality, cost-effective patient care. Also, with diverse stakeholder groups operating in the healthcare system, improving the value of healthcare while reducing costs becomes even more complex. A feasible solution is for healthcare providers to learn to adapt to patients' changing needs and effectively lead them and other stakeholders in the organization. Trastek, Hamilton, and Niles (2014) recommended that servant leadership is the best model for healthcare organizations, with its principles and practices focusing on team strengths, fostering trust, and serving patients' needs.

Servant leadership qualities and attributes include listening, empathy, healing, awareness, self-knowledge, persuasion, conceptualization, foresight, vision, and a commitment to people's growth and to building community. These, along with strong moral values, motivate servant leaders to help people achieve their goals and handle challenges (Spears, 2004). Most of these attributes involve a strong passion for people, as well as strong interpersonal interactions and communication, which promote strong relationships and trust between leaders and others in healthcare.

Increasing the overall value of healthcare is another primary challenge for healthcare providers. The value may be measured through an equation that compares the quality of the services provided to their costs, which, over time, best reflects the individual's impact on the healthcare system (Trastek, Hamilton, and Niles, 2014).

In Figure 2, Value is a function of Quality and Cost measured over time.

Figure 2. Value - a function of Quality and Cost

$$\text{Value} = \frac{\text{Quality (outcomes, safety, services)}}{\text{Cost (resources consumed)}}$$

**The value equation measured over time for a patient best reflects the impact of the individual on the healthcare system.*

In the above model, quality focuses on outcomes, safety, and services provided because they are related to an episode of care. The cost of healthcare refers to the resources used for each episode of care and throughout the entire treatment period. Resources used include the costs of a healthcare provider's time, diagnostics, therapeutics, and facility use. Restoring, maintaining, and increasing the sustainability of the healthcare system requires healthcare providers to deliver value by improving service quality—outcomes, safety, and service delivery —while simultaneously lowering costs. The complexity of the challenges facing healthcare, along with the multiple, divergent purposes, goals, and priorities of stakeholders, demands an innovative, unique leadership style. Servant leadership is a unique leadership style that several healthcare experts consider the best solution (Trastek, Hamilton, & Niles, 2014). Therefore, for healthcare leaders to implement effective, sustainable changes that enhance healthcare quality and reduce costs, they require leadership styles that emphasize servant leadership.

Servant leadership integrates well with leadership in healthcare because most healthcare providers' passion, calling, and work are all centered on serving their patients. As servant leaders, healthcare providers are morally and ethically expected to put their patients first in everything - physically, emotionally, and financially. Furthermore, most healthcare providers are trained or possess several key attributes and skills, including listening, empathy, healing, caring, and persuasion, which contribute to the development of a strong provider-patient relationship (Trastek, Hamilton, & Niles, 2014). These strong interpersonal relationships integrate well with patient-centered communication, which has been shown to impact several key outcomes, such as patient satisfaction, adherence, and more favorable health outcomes (Wanzer, Booth-Butterfield, & Grueber, 2014). Servant leadership also fosters strong mutual trust between healthcare providers and patients.

Also, as teamwork is a critical prerequisite for effective healthcare delivery, physicians, nurses, staff, and administrators must work together to provide high-quality care to their patients. Using servant leadership, healthcare leaders can develop a strong community in which team members are committed to placing high value on patients' health and well-being. Healthcare leaders, as dedicated, caring servant leaders, often emphasize and practice sacrificial leadership that puts others above self (specifically patients' needs), thereby enhancing their relationships with patients and ensuring they provide the highest quality of healthcare (Selladurai & Carraher, 2014). Further, by helping healthcare providers become more motivated to achieve their goals, servant leaders can inspire higher performance and the use of new technologies and innovation throughout the organization. And this, in turn, can positively impact safety, outcomes, services, and efficiencies within the healthcare system, increasing the value equation for the patient (Trastek, Hamilton, & Niles, 2014).

At Mayo Clinic, Rochester, MN, servant leadership is practiced among Mayo physicians, administrative staff, and nursing staff throughout the organization according to a senior leadership administrator (T. Spaulding, personal communication, July 9, 2025). In many departments and divisions, new physicians work with senior physicians in a mentorship program to learn to navigate the Mayo system and to develop the Mayo Clinic organization's unique RICH TIES (respect, integrity, compassion, healing, teamwork, innovation, excellence, and stewardship) values and traditions. For those in Administrative leadership roles, there is a rotational model that typically involves 5-7 years within a department or division before rotating to a new area. This rotational model enables the leaders to learn and practice servant-leadership skills across a variety of positions and roles within the Mayo system. Further, each unit and specialty area practices servant leadership principles through participation in a variety of community programs, such as Ronald McDonald House programs, food pantry drives, and drone donations to local police departments, enabling them to become more efficient first responders in the Rochester, MN community.

To enhance the use, impact, and effectiveness of servant leadership in healthcare and to measure various outcomes, several survey instruments may be used, including the two most frequently used: the Global Leadership Scale (Liden et al., 2008) and the Servant Leadership Questionnaire (Barbuto & Wheeler, 2006). Repeated studies using these instruments across the same and different healthcare organizations over time would provide reliability and validity to the results, thereby promoting the benefits of implementing servant leadership in healthcare.

In today's complex healthcare work environment, healthcare leaders must grapple with several major challenges that require strong leadership models to do so. One such leadership model is servant leadership, which is appropriate for healthcare leaders and workers caring for patients and also working closely as a team to deliver high-quality, patient-centered services. Servant leadership emphasizes building trust, empowering patients, and encouraging healthcare providers to work as a team, resulting in high-quality patient care and provider satisfaction.

Top Management Support

Top management support is crucial and plays a decisive role in implementing effective teamwork in healthcare organizations. For any initiative to be successfully implemented, clear, visible, and sustained commitment from top leadership is essential. Senior leadership often sets the precedence, priorities, behaviors, and tone for the organizational culture. Top management is usually responsible for modeling and reinforcing culture. For example, Mayo Clinic's team core values and traditions are the RICH TIES (respect, integrity, compassion, healing, teamwork, innovation, excellence, and stewardship) that the Mayo brothers set, and collaborating with the Sisters of St. Francis, continue to be reinforced by their current management and leadership team (Mayo Clinic, 2026).

Top management leaders display collaborative behaviors – inclusive decision-making, valuing input from all organizational stakeholders, fostering psychological safety, supporting one another, and encouraging the free expression of employees' and team members' ideas, voices, and concerns for the benefit of the organization. Such efforts aim to minimize "us vs them" perceptions among professions (e.g., physicians vs. nurses) and instill a team culture within the organization. Teamwork culture, in turn, helps improve the overall organizational performance, high-quality patient care, patient experiences, employees' and team members' satisfaction, and provides patient care at optimal costs (maximum output per dollar input via providing efficient patient care through effective, integrated, collaborative teamwork) (St. Mary's University, 2026; Medbridge, 2026). Also, lowering healthcare costs is one of the major aims of the current administration's new One Big Beautiful Bill Act (OBBBA), part of the healthcare reform President Trump signed into law in July 2025 (The White House, 2025; The White House, 2026). So, all healthcare policies and guidelines are integrating lower-cost measures and initiatives into current and future discussions, actions, and implementations. Healthcare organizations, along with federal, state, and local governments, are working together to make healthcare more accessible, affordable, and sustainable for all stakeholders in the US.

Top management is mostly responsible for resource allocation and sustainability. Effective training programs require time, training, funding, and integration into the workflow. Top management must provide these by prioritizing budgeting for teamwork training and interprofessional education. This gives credibility and continuity to teamwork training programs, ensuring that all healthcare professionals, especially those involved in patient care, are well trained to provide high-quality, customized patient care. Top management must also encourage and motivate their healthcare professionals, including physicians, nurses, and other related healthcare professionals who provide patient care to focus on achieving measurable outcomes – such as patient safety, lower burnout, higher staff retention, improved satisfaction, and higher clinical results (fewer readmissions, shorter stays, and better chronic care coordination (KiranKumar, 2023).

Mayo Clinic has many strengths, including long-term sustainability as a healthcare organization for over 150 years, a worldwide reputation for excellence, and recognition as a top healthcare organization. It uses several effective teamwork strategies and practices, as well as key servant leadership principles, such as exemplary, sacrificial leadership, strong value for people and productivity, and deep concern for relationships and results (Selladurai & Carraher, 2014; Selladurai et al., 2020). Above all, its strong commitment to patient care and effective organizational teamwork has helped Mayo serve as an excellent healthcare model for other healthcare systems to emulate.

To further illustrate the value of effective teamwork and its impact on critical outcomes, the authors have discussed a case study of Mayo Clinic, a healthcare organization in Rochester, Minnesota. This healthcare organization, as part of its core values (Respect, Integrity, Compassion, Healing, Teamwork, Innovation, Excellence, and Stewardship), enables critical analysis of various situations and encourages the use of specific skills tailored to each, fostering efficient, high-performing teams. High-performing teams impact the four quadruple aims—patient experience, quality of patient care, lower costs, and provider satisfaction.

CASE STUDY: MAYO CLINIC'S ADMINISTRATIVE ROTATIONAL MODEL

Introduction

The Mayo Clinic is internationally recognized for its commitment to putting "the needs of the patient come first." This ethos is embedded in the organization's three-shield practice, which encompasses patient care, research, and education. To support this mission and ensure the highest-quality integrated healthcare delivery,

Mayo Clinic utilizes a unique administrative rotational model, characterized by a triad leadership structure involving physicians, administrators, and nursing leaders (Buell, 2017). This case study analyzes the structure, implementation, and effectiveness of this model, offering insights for healthcare administration and clinicians.

Background: The Three Shields Framework

The three shields of the Mayo Clinic logo represent its core priorities: clinical practice, education, and research (Mayo Clinic, 2025). These three areas are interconnected and work together to improve patient care. Research informs practice, education supports both practice and research, and all three are integrated to ensure the best possible outcomes for patients.

Clinical Practice: The shield for clinical practice encompasses the direct patient care provided by the organization's integrated, multidisciplinary teams.

Education: This shield represents the institution's commitment to educating physicians, scientists, and allied health professionals, including students, residents, and current staff.

Research: The research shield signifies the ongoing work to advance medical knowledge, generate new discoveries, and translate them into therapies that improve patient care.

The integration of these three missions underpins Mayo Clinic's holistic approach to healthcare and is foundational to its success (Mayo Clinic, 2025; Buell, 2017).

Triad Leadership Model

At the core of Mayo Clinic's administrative framework is the triad leadership model. This approach places a physician leader, an administrative leader, and a nursing leader at the helm of each department or clinical unit.

- Physician Leader: Guides clinical decision-making, ensures the highest standards of patient care, and advocates for medical staff. Physician leaders are also key to developing a strategic plan for the department or division, including initiatives to innovate and automate the practice.
- Administrative Leader: Manages operational logistics, financial planning, and strategic resource allocation to help facilitate care delivery while providing support for the development and implementation of strategic objectives.
- Nursing Leader: Oversees nursing practice, patient safety, and quality improvement initiatives, ensuring compassionate, evidence-based care within the nursing team as well as the entire care team.

This triad enables collaborative decision-making, balancing clinical excellence, operational efficiency, and patient experience. By integrating perspectives from each discipline, the model directly supports the patient-centered mission and the three-shield philosophy (Buell, 2017).

Teamwork in Rotational Leadership

Rotational leadership involves periodically changing the person or group responsible for leading a team or project. This model distributes leadership responsibilities among multiple individuals over time, allowing team members to develop their leadership skills and providing fresh perspectives. Teamwork is crucial in this context because:

- Facilitates Smooth Transitions: Team members work collaboratively to support new leaders as they rotate in, reducing disruptions and maintaining continuity while allowing for diverse perspectives.
- Promotes Skill Development: By working together, team members can mentor each other, share knowledge, and build leadership capacity across the group. This also allows all team members to understand each other's roles and expertise.
- Encourages Accountability: Shared responsibility ensures that everyone is invested in the team's success, regardless of who holds the leadership role at a given time. This also helps the rest of the team know that multiple perspectives were considered before a decision was made.
- Enables Diverse Perspectives: Rotational leadership, coupled with teamwork, brings multiple viewpoints to the forefront, helping foster creativity, problem-solving, and sound decision-making.

Teamwork in the Triad Leadership Model

The triad leadership model divides leadership responsibilities among three individuals, each typically representing a different area of expertise or organizational priority (e.g., operations, strategy, and people). Teamwork is essential for the effective implementation of rotational and triad leadership models. It supports leadership transitions, leverages diverse talents, and fosters a culture of shared responsibility. Teamwork is the foundation that allows this model to function effectively:

- Balances Strengths: Each leader in the triad brings unique skills and perspectives. Teamwork ensures these strengths are harmonized for better decision-making.

- Fosters Open Communication: Collaboration within the triad and with the broader team encourages transparency and the sharing of critical information.
- Supports Shared Decision-Making: Teamwork enables the triad to make collective decisions, helping it reach a team decision. This diminishes the risk of bias or blind spots that might arise from a single-leader approach.
- Builds Trust: Regular, honest interactions and joint problem-solving build trust within the triad and the larger team, strengthening overall cohesion (Buell, 2017).

Synergies Between Teamwork and Dynamic Leadership Models

Both rotational and triad leadership models rely on strong teamwork to succeed. Teamwork provides the glue that binds individuals, enabling flexibility, resilience, and shared ownership of outcomes. When teams collaborate openly and effectively, they can adapt quickly to leadership changes, resolve conflicts, and innovate in response to evolving challenges.

Rotational Model Structure

- Cycle Length: Leadership roles rotate every 5–7 years.
- Overlap Period: Incoming leaders shadow outgoing counterparts for several months, facilitating knowledge transfer and minimizing disruption.
- Rationale: This system prevents stagnation, encourages leadership development, and keeps the organization adaptable to evolving healthcare challenges. The rotational model is underpinned by a rigorous selection and onboarding process that ensures each new leader is equipped to uphold Mayo Clinic's standards and mission.

Benefits of Rotational Leadership

The rotational approach offers several distinct advantages:

- Fresh Perspectives: Regularly introducing new leaders brings innovative ideas and strategies, invigorates departments, and promotes continuous improvement.
- Adaptability: Leaders with varied backgrounds and experiences enhance the organization's ability to respond to change and emerging healthcare trends.
- Cross-Disciplinary Collaboration: The triad structure fosters open communication and unified decision-making, reducing silos and enhancing integrated care delivery.

- Leadership Development: Rotational opportunities nurture a pipeline of experienced leaders, supporting succession planning and organizational resilience.
- Cross-Pollination of Best Practices: Rotation across departments and functions enables leaders to share and implement best practices from different areas of the organization. This cross-pollination enhances overall performance and ensures that successful innovations are disseminated throughout Mayo Clinic.
- Rotational leadership also promotes teamwork amongst the triad. This allows others to assist their colleagues when making decisions across divisions and departments.

Supporting Data: Effectiveness of the Model

Evidence from Mayo Clinic and industry research demonstrates the effectiveness of the rotational triad model:

- A Mayo Clinic internal survey (2022) reported a 15% increase in employee engagement scores and reduced burnout in departments with recent leadership rotations compared with those with static leadership (Weineke, 2025; Kruse, 2022).
- A study published by the American College of Education (2021) found that organizations with rotational leadership structures reported higher rates of innovation adoption and better cross-functional collaboration than those with traditional, static leadership (Hiatt, 2021).
- Mayo Clinic's patient satisfaction scores (HCAHPS) consistently rank in the top 5% nationally, a testament to its patient-centered, collaborative leadership approach (HCAHPS (2025)); Mayo Clinic, 2025).
- A study published by MEDI leadership (2025) based on an MGMA poll found that 77% of healthcare organizations use a physician-administrator dyad leadership model. When implemented effectively, these models can enhance decision-making, streamline operations, and improve patient outcomes (Angus, 2025).

These data points highlight the model's positive impact on organizational performance, patient outcomes, and staff engagement.

Clinical Scenario: Triad Model in Action

Consider a scenario in which Mayo Clinic's Cardiology Department undergoes a scheduled leadership rotation—the outgoing triad, Dr. Smith (physician), Ms. Lee (administrator), and Mr. Patel (nursing leader)—initiates a structured handover to the incoming triad.

During the overlap period, the new physician leader, Dr. Martinez, works closely with Dr. Smith to review ongoing quality improvement initiatives, such as reducing heart failure readmissions. The new administrator, Ms. Johnson, shadows Ms. Lee to understand operational priorities, including resource allocation for new telemedicine services. The incoming nursing leader, Ms. Green, collaborates with Mr. Patel on patient safety protocols and nurse training programs.

As the new triad assumes full leadership, they leverage insights gained during the transition to introduce an integrated care pathway for heart failure patients. Drawing on their diverse backgrounds, they streamline communication between cardiologists, nurses, and administrative staff, leading to improved patient outcomes and higher satisfaction scores in subsequent months.

Challenges and Lessons Learned

While the Administrative Rotational Model offers numerous advantages, it is not without challenges:

- Continuity vs. Change: Frequent leadership transitions disrupt the continuity of long-term initiatives. Thorough documentation, robust handover processes, and clear strategic planning are essential to maintain momentum.
- Learning Curves: New administrators may require time to acclimate, potentially slowing progress in the early months of their tenure. Ongoing mentorship and support structures help minimize these effects.
- Balancing Roles: Leaders must balance administrative responsibilities with clinical, research, or educational duties, which can be demanding. Clear role definitions and workload management are crucial.

Nevertheless, Mayo Clinic's experience underscores that, with careful planning and commitment to shared values, these challenges can be effectively managed.

Mayo Clinic's administrative rotational model, anchored by the triad leadership structure, is a powerful mechanism for ensuring that "the needs of the patient come first." By systematically rotating leadership roles and fostering collaboration among physicians, administrators, and nursing leaders, the organization maintains a dynamic, patient-centered culture. Supporting data and clinical experience underscore the model's effectiveness in enhancing engagement, quality, and adaptability, offering a blueprint for integrated healthcare delivery in complex environments.

SOLUTIONS AND RECOMMENDATIONS

Several potential solutions may be derived from the above analysis of teamwork. The healthcare sector can learn from extensive research on teamwork in organizational behavior, which has proven effective in increasing employee satisfaction, improving efficiency, and enhancing quality. Implementing what organizational research has already revealed in the healthcare sector can be achieved through screening applicants for essential characteristics of high-functioning team members during the hiring process. Part of the interview could include incorporating the applicant into an already established, high-functioning team. For current employees, the Leaderless Group Discussion (Online) method described above can be used to evaluate established team members, and feedback is provided to help increase their impact. These could even be incorporated into existing performance reviews (Greer et al., 2020).

Also, servant leadership survey instruments may be used to measure servant leadership attributes among team members and identify potential servant leaders appropriate for various roles in the organization. Further, the surveys may be used to assess the impact of servant leadership applications on effective teamwork and the quadruple aims of patient experience, quality of patient care, lower costs, and provider satisfaction.

Several evidence-based strategies to develop and strengthen teamwork include team training programs such as TeamSTEPPS, which teach strategies in communication, leadership, and mutual collaboration and support (Team Strategies and Tools to Enhance Performance and Patient Safety) (AHS, 2025). Also, strategies focused on training in clear roles and responsibilities to reduce overlap may be beneficial for healthcare organizations. Training students and team members in interpersonal and interprofessional skills to build trust and a collaborative, working-together mindset would enhance teamwork. Leadership and culture-related training would also instill strong teamwork and collaboration skills among healthcare professionals. Regular reflection and feedback-related strategies, including team huddles, constructive performance reviews, and coaching, would help improve teamwork effectiveness (AHS, 2025).

Several approaches can be explored to promote effective teamwork in healthcare in the future. The existing research on teamwork in healthcare demonstrates strong results in increased efficiency and patient satisfaction, but could be strengthened by a greater focus on patient-oriented outcomes. Such a focus would require lobbying Congress for increased NIH research funding. Professional organizations, such as the

AMA (American Medical Association), AAP (American Academy of Pediatrics), ACP (American College of Physicians), and ABMS (American Board of Medical Specialties), among others, can provide professional development opportunities that promote the importance of teamwork. Allowing physicians currently in practice to obtain CME in this important area could greatly benefit the teams they already serve. A valuable current resource is the AAPL (American Association for Physician Leadership), which offers physician-targeted education on teamwork. Another strategy could be to incorporate teamwork into current accreditation standards and into medical school and residency program education. Allowing students and residents to participate in interdisciplinary teams early will help them function more effectively throughout their professional careers (Greer et al. 2020).

FUTURE DIRECTIONS

Several directions may be explored in the realm of teamwork and its impact on healthcare outcomes. One such study could empirically test the conceptual model (KF-ET-QA) discussed in this chapter to evaluate it and measure its outcomes at a healthcare organization. Further, the study could be replicated to assess the reliability and validity of the research results in other healthcare organization settings, benefiting all stakeholders.

Also, future research will focus on multidisciplinary teams and teamwork, the application of servant-leadership principles in healthcare, shared leadership, and programs such as TeamSTEPPS as healthcare becomes increasingly technology-based and AI-driven. Moreover, studies will continue to explore evidence of positive correlations between teamwork and reduced mortality, fewer clinical and medical errors, a better safety culture in patient care, and other improved outcomes. Many studies have already shown that effective teamwork is essential for achieving the goals of the quadruple aim. However, more research is needed to demonstrate a correlation between the quadruple outcomes and the medical school education and professional training opportunities offered by medical schools and healthcare organizations.

Other studies would examine the impact of AI, telemedicine, predictive analytics, virtual reality for teamwork training, situational awareness, and the use of simulations and models via digital platforms. Research needs to continue exploring longitudinal studies on retention during crises (like post-COVID lessons and takeaways), patient safety metrics, and the effects of condition- and situational-specific awareness in healthcare.

Further, research could examine the impact of patient/family perspectives on teamwork and collaboration regarding patient-focused priorities. Although evidence for teamwork benefits is extensively documented in several studies, future research should emphasize the sustainability of these benefits beyond initial teamwork training, including continuous reinforcement, top management collaboration, and systemic support.

CONCLUSION

Effective teamwork will remain critical to healthcare reform now and in the future. Many studies have already shown that effective teamwork is essential to achieving the goals of the quadruple aim. This study focused on key factors—teamwork training, leaderless online group discussion, servant leadership, and top management support—that lead to effective teamwork and would positively impact the quadruple aim—patient experience, high-quality and safe patient care, lower costs, and provider satisfaction. Also, the Mayo Clinic case study discussed the effective teamwork within its organization with a focus on its administrative rotational model, anchored by the triad leadership organizational structure. Mayo Clinic has integrated effective teamwork models, including the administrative rotational model and the triad leadership structure, which have contributed to its excellence in organizational healthcare performance, making it one of the premier healthcare organizations in the world (Kayser, 2025). Further, teamwork will remain a key component of healthcare reform debates, discussions, policies, and guidelines in 2026 and beyond, as the US continues to formulate, refine, and implement policies to build an optimal, sustainable healthcare system for all its stakeholders.

REFERENCES

American Hospital Association (AHA). (2026). *Improvements in safety culture linked to better patient and staff outcomes*. Retrieved from Improvement in Safety Culture Linked to Better Patient and Staff Outcomes | AHA

Angus, L. (2025). *Healthcare executive coaching - MEDI Leadership*. MEDI Leadership. Retrieved from https://medileadership.org/beyond-role-clarity-unlocking-excellence-in-healthcare-dyad-and-triad-leadership-teams/

Bailey-Hughes, B. (2021). A communication audit exercise to enhance virtual team and individual communication skills. *Management Teaching Review*, *6*(4), 298–308. DOI: 10.1177/23792981211001527

Baker, D. P., Horvath, L., Campion, M. A., Offermann, L., & Salas, E. (2005). The ALL Teamwork Framework. In Murray, T. S., Clermont, Y., & Binkley, M. (Eds.), *International Adult Literacy Survey, Measuring Adult Literacy and Life Skills: New Frameworks for Assessment*. Ministry of Industry.

Bales, R. F. (1950). A set of categories for the analysis of small group interaction. *American Sociological Review*, *15*(2), 257–263. DOI: 10.2307/2086790

Barbuto J., & Wheeler, D. (2006). Scale development and construct clarification of servant leadership. *Group Organization Management,* 31(3):300–326. Retrieved from Scale Development and Construct Clarification of Servant Leadership - John E. Barbuto, Daniel W. Wheeler, 2006.

Blake, R. R., & Mouton, J. J. (1964). *The managerial grid*. Gulf Publishers.

Buell, J. (2017). The Dyad Leadership Model: Four case studies. Retrieved from PRMT-Mod3-CreateChange-CaseStudies_1_.pdf

Burke, C. S., Stagl, K. C., Klein, C., Goodwin, G. F., Salas, E., & Halpin, S. M. (2006). What type of leadership behaviors are functional in teams? A meta-analysis. *The Leadership Quarterly*, *17*(3), 288–307. DOI: 10.1016/j.leaqua.2006.02.007

Cannon-Bowers, J. A., Tannenbaum, S. I., Salas, E., & Volpe, C. E. (1995). Defining competencies and establishing team training requirements. In Guzzo, R., & Salas, E. (Eds.), *Team effectiveness and decision making in organizations* (pp. 333–380). Jossey-Bass.

Chen, G., Donahue, L. M., & Klimoski, R. J. (2004). Training undergraduates to work in organizational teams. *Academy of Management Learning & Education*, *3*(1), 27–40. DOI: 10.5465/amle.2004.12436817

Greer, A., Selladurai, R. I., Pfeifle, A., Selladurai, R., & Hobson, C. (2020). Effective teamwork and healthcare delivery outcomes. In Selladurai, R., Hobson, C., Selladurai, R. I., & Greer, A. (Eds.), *Evaluating challenges and opportunities for healthcare reform*. IGI Global, Inc. DOI: 10.4018/978-1-7998-2949-2.ch004

Haugstetter, M., Hines, S., Sousane, Z., & Mossburg, S. (2024). *Revising TeamSTEPPS: The evolution of patient safety teamwork training*. Retrieved from Revising TeamSTEPPS: The Evolution of Patient Safety Teamwork Training | PSNet

Hiatt, G. (2021). *A phenomenological study of rotational leadership experiences' potential influence on promotability within organizations*. Retrieved from A Phenomenological Study of Rotational Leadership - ProQuest.

Hobson, C. J., Strupeck, D., Griffin, A., Szostek, J., & Rominger, A. S. (2014). Teaching MBA students teamwork and team leadership skills: An empirical evaluation of a classroom educational program. *American Journal of Business Education*, *7*(3), 191–212. DOI: 10.19030/ajbe.v7i3.8629

Hobson, C. J., Strupeck, D., Griffin, A., Szostek, J., Selladurai, R., & Rominger, A. (2013). Facilitating and documenting behavioral improvements in business student teamwork skills. *Business Education Innovation Journal*, *5*(1), 83–95.

Hospital Consumer Assessment of Healthcare Providers and Systems (HCAHPS). *CAHPS Hospital Survey*. Retrieved from https://hcahpsonline.org/en/summary-analyses/

James, T. (2021). *Teamwork as a core value in health care*. Retrieved from Teamwork as a Core Value in Health Care | Harvard Medical School Professional, Corporate, and Continuing Education

Kayser, A. (2025). *World's best hospitals 2025 – United States of America*. Retrieved from World's Best Hospitals 2025 - United States of America

Kelly, R., & Lavelle, A. (2024). *Teamwork matters: team situation awareness to build high-performing healthcare teams*. Retrieved from Teamwork matters: team situation awareness to build high-performing healthcare teams.

KiranKumar, Y. (2023). *Role of management in healthcare*. Retrieved from Role of Management in Healthcare

Kruse, K. (2022). *How Mayo Clinic develops leaders who drive engagement and reduce burnout*. Retrieved from How Mayo Clinic Develops Leaders Who Drive Engagement And Reduce Burnout.

Liden, R., Wayne, S., Zhao, H., & Henderson, D. (2008, April). Servant leadership: Development of a multidimensional measure and multi-level assessment. [Retrieved from Servant leadership: Development of a multidimensional measure and multi-level assessment - ScienceDirect]. *The Leadership Quarterly*, *19*(2), 161–177. DOI: 10.1016/j.leaqua.2008.01.006

Likert, R. (1961). *New patterns of management*. McGraw-Hill.

Mayo Clinic. (2025). "*The Mayo Effect*:" *Ten things you may not know about Mayo*. Retrieved from https://share.google/ZqnWlKFoTzFDKXSk2

Mayo Clinic. (2025). *Why Mayo Clinic*? Retrieved from https://executiveeducation .mayo.edu/catalog?pagename=why-mayo-clinic

Mayo Clinic. (2025). *How Mayo Clinic measures patient experience*. Retrieved from Patient Experience - Mayo Clinic.

Mayo Clinic. (2026). *Mission and values*. Rerieved from Mission and values - Mayo Clinic

Medbridge (2026). *Why the Quadruple Aim matters for healthcare systems today*. Retrieved from Quadruple Aim in Healthcare: 4 Key Goals | Medbridge

Salas, E., Sims, D. E., & Burke, C. S. (2005). Is there a "Big Five" in teamwork? *Small Group Research*, *36*(5), 555–599. DOI: 10.1177/1046496405277134

Schmutz, J., Meier, L., & Manser, T. (2019). *How effective is teamwork really? The relationship between teamwork and performance in healthcare teams: A systematic review and meta-analysis*. Retrieved from Schmutz: How effective is teamwork really? The relationsh... - Google Scholar

Selladurai, R., & Carraher, S. (2014). Lead like the greatest leader! Case Study. In Selladurai, R., & Carraher, S. (Eds.), *Servant leadership: Research and Practice* (pp. 350–355). IGI Global. DOI: 10.4018/978-1-4666-5840-0.ch026

Selladurai, R., Hobson, C., Selladurai, R. I., & Greer, A. (2020). *Evaluating challenges and opportunities for healthcare reform. IGI Global, Inc.*

Spears, L. C. (2004). Practicing servant leadership. *Leader to Leader*, *34*(34), 7–11. DOI: 10.1002/ltl.94

St. Mary' University. (2026). *Exploring effective leadership and team management in healthcare*. Retrieved from Exploring effective leadership and team management in healthcare - Blog

Stevens, M. J., & Campion, M. A. (1994). The knowledge, skill, and ability requirements for teamwork: Implications for human resource management. *Journal of Management, 20*(2), 503–530. DOI: 10.1177/014920639402000210

Stogdill, R. M., & Coons, A. E. (1957). *Leader behavior: Its description and measurement.* Ohio State University, Bureau of Business Research.

The White House. (2025, July 4). *The One Big Beautiful Bill.* Retrieved from The One Big Beautiful Bill – The White House

The White House. (2026). *President Trump unveils the Great Healthcare Plan to Lower Costs and Deliver Money Directly to the People.* Retrieved from President Trump Unveils The Great Healthcare Plan to Lower Costs and Deliver Money Directly to the People – The White House.

Trastek, V. F., Hamilton, N. W., & Niles, E. E. (2014). Leadership models in healthcare – A case for servant leadership. *Mayo Clinic Proceedings, 89*(3), 374–381. DOI: 10.1016/j.mayocp.2013.10.012 PMID: 24486078

Wanzer, R., Booth-Butterfield, M., & Grueber, K. (2014). Perceptions of healthcare providers' communication: Relationships between patient-centered communication and satisfaction. *Health Communication, 16*(3), 363–383. DOI: 10.1207/S15327027HC1603_6 PMID: 15265756

Webster, C., Coomber, T., Liu, S., Allen, K., & Jowsey, T. (2023). *Interprofessional learning in multidisciplinary healthcare teams is associated with reduced patient mortality: A quantitative systematic review and meta-analysis.* Retrieved from Webster: Interprofessional learning in multidisciplinary... - Google Scholar

Weineke, K., Berkland, B., Kruse, G., Priestly, M., Teal, D., & West, C. (2025). *Charting a New Path Forward in Addressing Employee Well-being in Health Care.* Retrieved from Charting a New Path Forward in Addressing Employee Well-being in Health Care -. *Mayo Clinic Proceedings, 100*(3), 501–513. DOI: 10.1016/j.mayocp.2024.11.018

Weller, J., Mahajan, R., Fahey-Williams, K., & Wesbster, C. (2024). "*Teamwork matters: team situation awareness to build high-performing healthcare teams, a narrative review.*" Retrieved from Teamwork matters: team situation awareness to build high-performing healthcare teams, a narrative review - ScienceDirect

Zajac, S., Woods, A., Tannenbaum, S., Salas, E., & Holladay, C. (2021). "*Overcoming Challenges to Teamwork in Healthcare: A Team Effectiveness Framework and Evidence-Based Guidance,*" Retrieved from Frontiers | Overcoming Challenges to Teamwork in Healthcare: A Team Effectiveness Framework and Evidence-Based Guidance

ADDITIONAL READING

Baek, H., Han, K., Cho, H., & Ju, J. (2023). *Nursing teamwork is essential in promoting patient-centered care: a cross-sectional study.* Retrieved from Nursing teamwork is essential in promoting patient-centered care: a cross-sectional study | BMC Nursing | Springer Nature Link

Bodenheimer, T., & Sinsky, C. (2014). From triple to quadruple aim: Care of the patient requires care of the provider. *Annals of Family Medicine*, *12*(8), 573–576. DOI: 10.1370/afm.1713 PMID: 25384822

Institute for Healthcare Improvement (IHI). (2025). *Improve topic: Quintuple aim.* Retrieved from Improvement Topic: Quintuple Aim | Institute for Healthcare Improvement

KEY TERMS AND DEFINITIONS

Effective Teamwork: Two or more people working together synergistically to accomplish more than the sum of individuals alone.

Lower Costs: Financial sustainability for every healthcare system – the goal is to provide higher quality outcomes for every dollar spent/optimal cost. Reducing the per capita cost of healthcare.

Quadruple Aim: Patient care that encompasses four overarching goals of enhancing the patient experience, improving patients' health, reducing costs, and improving provider satisfaction.

Patient Care: Healthcare organizations are looking to manage patient care beyond the individual to the entire community, providing high-quality, safe healthcare delivery.

Patient Experiences: Do patients feel they are heard, respected, and supported throughout? Healthcare providers deliver high-quality care that builds trust and promotes patient satisfaction.

Provider Satisfaction: improving healthcare workforce well-being – training and development, reduced burnout, feeling supported, and leading to improved organizational results.

Sacrificial Leadership: A type of leadership where the leader sacrifices his/her own interests, time, efforts, and sometimes his/her own life for the sake of others. Examples include: Jesus Christ, Dr. Kent Brantly (the American doctor who first contracted the deadly disease Ebola in Liberia in 2014), the Mayo brothers, Drs. William James Mayo and Charles Horace Mayo (founding pioneers of Mayo Clinic organization), and business leaders Dan Cathy (Chick-fil-A) and David Green (Hobby Lobby).

Servant Leadership: A new type of leadership gaining momentum in recent years, where serving others takes precedence over all other tasks. Includes attributes of empathy, humility, compassion, caring, listening, respect, concern for others' growth, and raising one's team members to a higher level of performance.

Chapter 11
Supply Chain Leading Practices:
The Mayo Clinic Journey.

Joe Dudas
http://orcid.org/0009-0004-6225-1849
Mayo Clinic, USA

James R. Francis
Mayo Clinic, USA

ABSTRACT

This chapter provides an overview of Mayo Clinic's history, achievements, and supply chain management (SCM) strategies. As a prominent academic medical center in the United States, Mayo Clinic operates major campuses in Minnesota, Florida, and Arizona. The organization manages an annual supply expenditure of $6.8 billion and employs approximately 1,300 SCM staff. Mayo Clinic SCM leading practices encompass a vision, mission, and strategic plan; active engagement of senior leadership; clinical practice–supply chain integration; talent recruitment, development, and retention; partnerships (strategic) and supplier relationship management; commitment to service excellence and continuous improvement; digital information technology (IT) platform and strategy; innovation and automation; benchmarking; and business continuity.

INTRODUCTION

Supply Chain consists of the movement of all products, information, and associated financial transactions, from raw materials to the end customer. In healthcare,

DOI: 10.4018/979-8-3373-2577-4.ch011

the end customer is the patient. As a result, the healthcare supply chain is indispensable and critical to the provision of safe, high-quality patient care. The lack of an effective supply chain can often result in the opposite. This chapter provides an in-depth overview of this important function and how Mayo Supply Chain Management (SCM) supports healthcare professionals and clinical staff in the provision of direct patient care. Additionally, the chapter will showcase one of healthcare's top-performing supply chains through an overview of its history, achievements, strategies, and tactics.

Mayo Clinic is the first and largest integrated, not-for-profit medical group practice in the world. Mayo's mission is to inspire hope and promote health through integrated clinical practice, education, and research. Its vision is to transform medicine by connecting and curing, as the global authority in the care of serious or complex diseases. As a prominent academic medical institution in the United States, Mayo Clinic operates major destination medical center campuses in Minnesota, Florida, and Arizona. Mayo Clinic is widely recognized for its excellence and consistently ranks among the best hospitals in the nation, with more #1-ranked specialties than any other healthcare institution (US News, 2026). Net revenues from operations and other sources exceed $19 billion annually (Mayo Clinic Finance, 2025)

Similarly, Mayo Clinic's SCM has been recognized by Gartner (an industry research firm) as one of the top 25 supply chain organizations in healthcare every year since the ranking list's inception in 2009 (Gartner, 2024). In 2018, Mayo Clinic's SCM moved into Gartner's Master's category and has remained there every year since its initial designation (2018-2025). For the benefit of its patients and staff, Mayo Clinic expends more than $7 billion annually on supplies, drugs, services, and capital medical equipment. Some 1,300 staff from the SCM organization provide support to Mayo (Mayo Clinic Supply Chain, 2025a). Typical supply chain functions include sourcing and contracting; procurement; accounts payable; and receiving, inventory management, distribution, and replenishment services. Depending upon the sophistication and resource capabilities of an organization's supply chain, it may provide other services, including healthcare technology management (also known as biomedical engineering), sourcing in multiple categories (e.g., pharmacy, laboratory, facilities), third-party risk and supplier management, business continuity, clinical support services, auditing, customer support, travel management, and information technology (IT) systems support.

Like other prominent healthcare systems, Mayo Clinic has dramatically improved its supply chain performance over the past two decades. These efforts have been achieved through the deployment of people, processes, and technology focused on the complete end-to-end supply chain. As the name implies, a supply chain consists of interconnected links of relationships between trading partners. A break in the chain or lack of a comprehensive focus on the entire process will result in suboptimal outcomes or, worse, supply disruptions. As the supply chain has evolved, Mayo Clinic has attributed several practices to its successful performance. Some of these leading practices include a vision, mission, and strategic plan; active engagement of senior leadership; clinical practice–supply chain integration; talent recruitment, development, and retention; partnerships (strategic) and supplier relationship management; commitment to service excellence and continuous improvement; digital IT platform and strategy; innovation and automation; benchmarking; and business continuity. Business continuity is a more recent leading practice that involves risk monitoring and maintaining risk mitigation plans. Achieving supply resiliency and assurance has become increasingly significant in recent years, amid environmental factors (e.g., natural disasters) and geopolitical developments (e.g., tariffs).

Mayo Clinic's supply chain, like those of other healthcare institutions and industries, faces challenges. These challenges include ever-changing technology, lack of data standards and single sources of truth, cybersecurity vulnerabilities, labor shortages, and supplier risks. In the face of challenges, focus must be on lessons learned and a strong commitment to continuous improvement and adaptation through leading practices, benchmarking, and the successful execution of strategies and tactics.

While all healthcare supply chains, including those of leading institutions such as Mayo Clinic, need improvement, many healthcare systems still lack supply chain excellence. This deficiency results in unnecessary costs and risks for many patients who depend on their healthcare providers to live as healthily as possible.

MAYO CLINIC HISTORICAL BACKGROUND AND GROWTH

What began as a small medical practice on the prairie, today Mayo Clinic represents 22 hospitals and more than 70 healthcare practice locations in five states. Outside of the destination medical centers, Mayo Clinic operates a community-based health system_the Mayo Clinic Health System. The phrase "Category of One," coined by Mayo Clinic, describes its care philosophy. This approach emphasizes Mayo Clinic's ability to serve as the global authority in the treatment of serious or complex disease and to deliver an unparalleled experience with the most-trusted clinical expertise and knowledge.

Efforts to integrate nonlabor expense management activities across Mayo Clinic began in earnest in 1999. Mayo's leadership team identified inconsistencies in supply chain performance and reliability, but what really triggered change was the recognition of the significant potential to leverage its collective buying power to reduce costs. Before this time, each Mayo Clinic location had its own supply chain operations, enabling decentralized, direct negotiations with suppliers and service providers. It was not uncommon to have multiple agreements with the same supplier for the same product with different pricing, terms, and conditions. Multiple group purchasing organization (GPO) memberships, enterprise resource planning (ERP) systems, and distributor relationships existed. In short, there was no single, integrated strategic plan guiding Mayo Clinic's supply chain. The launch of a single SCM function began with a focus on leveraging the organization's aggregated spend and delivery of a value proposition (i.e., better pricing, terms, and conditions). Following the launch of an overarching strategic plan (now updated annually) and the demonstrated value creation from various initiatives, Mayo Clinic fully integrated all SCM functions and operations.

MAYO CLINIC SUPPLY CHAIN MANAGEMENT OVERVIEW

Mayo Clinic's Supply Chain Management Office (SCMO) now operates as a shared service, delivering services, information, and solutions that support the organization, provide higher-value healthcare, and improve performance. As a division within the Department of Finance, SCM provides services to all clinical practice, education, research, and diversified activity locations. Mayo Clinic's SCM strategic plan is updated and revised annually to ensure alignment with Mayo Clinic's overall strategic plan and the Department of Finance's desired future state.

The vision of SCM is, "To excel at supply chain management that enables a transformative and sustainable focus on meeting the needs of patients."

The mission of SCM is, "To be a trusted partner for services and innovative solutions that improve performance."

To achieve the mission and vision of SCM, the strategic intent is "To transform healthcare delivery by building an agile, digitally empowered supply chain and biomedical ecosystem. We are committed to fostering resiliency, driving synergistic collaborations, and achieving self-sufficiency to ensure access to vital resources and technologies. We will enable staff to adapt, thrive, and deliver exceptional care" (Mayo Clinic Supply Chain, 2025d)

The SCM plan succinctly articulates key priorities for both current and upcoming fiscal years. The plan also lists the critical initiatives that tie to the Mayo Clinic strategic plan and identifies key supply chain priorities. To ensure the SCM maintains its position as a Category of One, SCM identifies key priorities and tactics. SCM's top initiatives are technology enabled and drive the five-year financial macro model, with significant scope and outcomes. The planning process integrates the strategic approaches of Mayo Clinic practice, Department of Finance, and SCM, and ensures key priorities cascade for the benefit of patients. The planning process is managed (both internally, with Mayo Clinic stakeholders, and externally, with supply partners), to ensure the SCM continues to meet and exceed the expectations of its patients. SCM's current priorities include the following:

- Building a more resilient network that responds to supply disruptions
- Delivering high-quality products and services
- Embracing innovation and automation
- Enabling a highly productive and diverse long-term workforce
- Delivering significant operational and financial value
- Scaling what we do through commercialization and self-sufficiency

The pursuit of self-sufficiency (commercialization of SCM capabilities) began with intensity a few years ago, but its history dates to 2008. As a shared service, SCM's operating expenses are allocated to the various operating entities of Mayo Clinic. This allocation is based on each entity's percentage share of total spend for supplies, pharmaceuticals, purchased services, and capital medical equipment. The allocation of operating costs comes with its share of scrutiny from leaders across the organization. During annual budget planning and preparation, SCM is queried to identify opportunities to improve efficiency and cost-effectiveness. As most organizational leaders know, when asked to reduce operating costs, there is another alternative: create revenue-producing opportunities. All well-run businesses must maximize revenue, reduce and manage expenses, generate an adequate return, and invest wisely for future success. The road to a more cost-effective SCM operation (which is largely personnel- and technology-driven) is to become a revenue/profit center; most healthcare systems fail to invest in this important function. A common theme in SCM is the need for scale, which often cannot be achieved independently. SCM leaders need to be aware of this limitation and be open to solutions that allow similar parties to pool their resources (collaborating with those that are well aligned outside of their own enterprise).

Although Mayo Clinic and its associated operations are clearly SCM's primary focus, SCM began building revenue-producing supply chain operations in 2008. Today, eight commercial services are operated by SCM. These include sourcing and contracting services for the largest national aggregation group in the United States; a freight management company; a national, high-committed program offered in partnership with a group purchasing organization; a pharmacy benefit management company; a collaboration offering co-management of supply chain operations with other healthcare providers; a provider of supplies and durable medical equipment, with 22 retail locations and an e-commerce site; sourcing and contracting consulting with healthcare providers in the Asian marketplace; and provision of service and maintenance to mobile medical devices. Through these commercial efforts, SCM effectively offsets approximately 55% of Mayo Clinic's supply chain operating costs.

This reduces the allocation to the operating entities and allows for investments that might otherwise be deprioritized—and now it is not only Mayo Clinic that benefits.

LEADING PRACTICES IN SUPPLY CHAIN MANAGEMENT

Most everyone assumes that supply chain is like a utility. If you flip the light switch and the light comes on, all is well—at least, that was the assumption until early 2020 when a worldwide pandemic wreaked havoc on supply chains. In a very short period, the entire world came to recognize the importance of the supply chain, especially in healthcare. Hospitals scrambled to find necessary personal protective equipment so that staff could care for patients with COVID-19. While COVID-19 was an immense challenge and an illumination of just how important the supply chain is to healthcare, many of the risks existed prior to the pandemic and remain today. Other global risks include those related to the economy, environment, geopolitics, society, and technology (e.g., cybersecurity threats). Knowing how to identify such risks, prevent or mitigate them, and improve supply chain practices and processes has become increasingly important to healthcare executives post-2020.

Managing supply disruption requires mature processes, technology, and subject-matter experts from multiple SCM functions to effectively and proactively identify risks, communicate them throughout the organization, determine alternative products, source those products, and monitor supply utilization until the disruption is over. Such work can be complex but achievable if the organization has learned from past disruptions, developed automation to monitor inventory and replenishment activities, and advanced capabilities through leading or best practices to improve overall performance.

Mayo Clinic has systematically learned from each disruption from the last two decades, including the Ebola outbreak in 2014, Hurricane Maria in 2017, the COVID-19 pandemic from 2020 to 2023, and Hurricane Helene in 2024. Mayo Clinic SCM reviewed lessons learned, developed recommendations, and implemented necessary improvements, resulting in meaningful changes to enhance resiliency and supply assurance. The largest changes were a result of the COVID-19 pandemic. Mayo Clinic switched its distribution method from just-in-time to warehouse inventory; consolidated and increased its supply inventory; changed distribution partners and channel sources for product movement; opened two new warehouses; and expanded IT systems, automation, reporting tools, and data analytics for monitoring.

Despite these efforts, further improvements are necessary to continue the journey toward greater supply resiliency. Only through adopting leading practices has Mayo Clinic positioned itself as a leader in resiliency efforts.

Often used interchangeably, *best practice* and *leading practice* both refer to effective methods but differ slightly in meaning. Best practice would indicate the most effective approach, whereas a leading practice is one that produces a more effective or efficient method to produce an outcome. At Mayo Clinic, it is preferable to use leading practices because of the pursuit of more innovative and efficient methods is constantly evolving and serves as the basis for continuous improvement in supply chain. In today's global, dynamic, and financially constrained healthcare environment, effective SCM is crucial for hospitals and health systems to stay competitive and achieve sustainable success. A well-managed supply chain can help hospitals reduce costs, improve efficiency, and enhance patient satisfaction, ultimately leading to greater financial and operational performance.

Mayo Clinic's SCM journey has involved developing, implementing, and refining many leading practices over the years. The success of the SCM and its progress and performance are the result of many leading practices, including the following:

1. *Vision, mission, and strategic plan.* As mentioned, Mayo Clinic SCM has been guided by a strategic plan for many years. Establishing a vision (an aspirational or ideal state desired), mission (why an organization exists), and strategic plan (processes and tactics with key performance metrics to monitor progress) are all critical components of this leading practice. The strategic plan should be developed collaboratively and involve key stakeholders. Such stakeholders will be important to plan alignment and, in many cases, are responsible for its successful execution. An SCM plan must be in sync with and supportive of the entity's overall strategic plan and direction. The SCM plan should clearly detail how it contributes to achieving the entity's strategies, goals, and objectives. Senior leadership should endorse the plan and be vocally supportive of it. Significant communication across the organization and with key departments is necessary to increase understanding and support for the plan. Plans should be reviewed and updated annually. If executed well, a plan will guide an organization's SCM to successful results and advance its overall performance to even higher levels.
2. *Active engagement of senior leadership.* SCM executives need clear, unwavering commitment from senior leadership (e.g., chief executive officer, chief financial officer, chief nursing officer) to implement the changes needed to advance the organization's supply chain. This support will be needed as the organization reacts and adapts to the changes. Given environmental and market fluctuations, the plan and staff responsible for its implementation will need to be agile enough to pivot to other tactics to address challenges and issues as they arise. An organization's commitment to SCM is key to success. It is equally important to an SCM executive as it is to the organization.

3. *Clinical practice–supply chain integration.* At Mayo Clinic, clinical practice–supply chain integration is part of the culture and has been the modus operandi since Mayo began managing a single, enterprise-wide supply chain. Working closely with the clinical practice is not only an expectation but a requirement. Mayo Clinic is a physician-led organization. In accordance with the bylaws of the organization, the chief executive officer must be a physician. In addition, Mayo Clinic has found that having a medical director that works closely with SCM and engages with physicians directly can garner many positive results. Physician-to-physician dialogue can likely overcome barriers or obstacles to progress. The close working relationships among SCM, healthcare, and allied health professionals enable the achievement of strategic goals and objectives, facilitating smooth, transparent changes. Trying to initially develop these relationships at the time of a disaster or significant supply chain disruption is not productive and can lead to erosion of trust.
4. *Talent recruitment, development, and retention.* Talent is the lifeblood of any organization. Recruiting, developing, and retaining staff are major contributors to success. Any good leader should surround themselves with the best talent available, provide the tools to succeed, and offer support as necessary. Leaders should not be intimidated by those who are smarter than them. Rather, leaders should support staff in meeting their developmental needs to achieve career goals and plan for appropriate succession. Key team members are often the first line of defense to address customer-related issues. Staff satisfaction can significantly impact how the supply chain is perceived across the organization.
5. *Partnerships (strategic) and supplier relationship management.* The words *partners* or *partnerships* are often overused in most organizations and frequently erroneously. Most transactions in the supply chain are just that: transactional. Very few relationships with suppliers rise to the level of a partnership. A partnership is characterized by a shared understanding of strategic plans, commitment of resources and capabilities, shared risk and reward, and potential financial investment. Partnerships are usually affected by a written agreement. In today's environment, hospitals and health systems are relying more on collaborations with suppliers and/or service organizations to realize their strategic goals and objectives. Understanding relationships with key suppliers and segmenting them into specific categories is a leading practice to organize and manage collaborations effectively.
6. *Commitment to service excellence and continuous improvement.* Commitment to service excellence and continuous improvement is a foundational principle that guides work in SCM. Every SCM employee must demonstrate an excellent service attitude. Policies and procedures must reflect this behavioral requirement: regardless of whether one *owns* an issue (meaning it is a direct responsibility or

function), an employee must take ownership of it, refer customers to the individual who can resolve the issue, and follow up to ensure it has been resolved to the customer's satisfaction. Knowing when to escalate an issue to SCM leadership is also critically important. Procedures must indicate when leadership is required for awareness, further escalation, and deployment of mitigation strategies, as necessary. Such processes have been used to address disasters and disruptions, preventing delays in patient care.

7. *Digital IT platform and strategy.* It would be difficult to identify an area that has seen more change and development than overall IT and IT systems in the healthcare supply chain. SCM IT has evolved from manual systems and processing to full automation with integration between systems (ERPs, electronic health records, and warehouse management systems). Advancements in automation are ongoing and include replenishment technology, machine learning, robotic process automation, artificial intelligence (AI), and advanced ERP systems. The industry has moved from being largely dependent on an ERP to one that functions as a platform with various interfaces, enabled by application programming interfaces that enable integration and the benefits they bring to a supply chain. All these enhancements have increased SCM capability and revolutionized the industry, and they continue to hold great promise. Further, developments in reporting tools and data analytics have brought much-needed improvements in keeping key leaders informed about supply chain performance and related financial results.
8. *Innovation and automation.* A commitment to innovation through the adoption of leading practices or new investments will result in improved performance. Innovation is a key strategic priority for Mayo Clinic SCM. Opportunities for innovation must be planned and eventually incorporated intoan organization's business strategy. Before that can happen, an organization must dedicate time to discussing innovative ideas or ways to improve a leading practice. It is easy to fall short of time to discuss opportunities, as most SCM staff are very busy. But time must be allocated to develop creative, new approaches and improvements. Given advancements in IT, as previously noted, many innovative improvements will be driven by automation. Significant dialogue currently circles AI. Whether augmenting human intelligence or advancing natural language comprehension and text processing, AI will likely have a significant impact on the effectiveness and efficiency of SCM as it evolves.
9. *Benchmarking.* Benchmarking (comparing key metrics on SCM performance with those of similar hospitals and health systems) is a method of learning from other organizations, potentially leading to the implementation of a new best practice or the improvement of existing ones. Unfortunately, benchmarking in healthcare SCM has been elusive over the years. Clean, accurate data are often

not accessible or comparable between one hospital and another. Uniformity in benchmarking formulas and resulting metrics has historically been suspect in terms of comparability accuracy. Progress is being made, though. It is important that organizations first begin by benchmarking internally. If the organization is a multihospital system, comparing one hospital to another within the system can often afford insights into areas of opportunity or improvement.

10. *Business continuity.* Many factors contribute to supply disruptions. Such factors have given rise to the focus on business continuity and the importance of supply resiliency. Business continuity is a relatively new development in SCM. However, other industries have used backup suppliers for some time, particularly for raw materials used in manufacturing.

It is essential to keep in mind that although the leading practices listed here are deemed the most important at Mayo Clinic, they may not be applicable to other healthcare organizations. The key to success is remaining nimble and adaptable and, adopting the practices best suited to a specific organization, and effectively implementing them to continuously elevate SCM performance. The following sections go into more detail.

Elevating the Supply Chain

Elevating the SCM is critical to any healthcare organization that seeks to provide efficient and effective care. To successfully advance Mayo Clinic's strategic plan to cure, connect, and transform healthcare, SCM assists by building an agile, digitally empowered supply chain and biomedical ecosystem. SCM is committed to fostering resiliency, driving synergistic collaborations, and achieving self-sufficiency to ensure access to vital resources and technologies. The strategic intent is to enable staff to adapt, thrive, and deliver exceptional care.

To accomplish this strategic intent, SCM must position itself as a trusted partner and as indispensable to its customers. The supply chain is the lifeblood of many industries, especially healthcare, where equipment, pharmaceuticals, implants, and basic supplies are crucial. However, for historical and cultural reasons, executives are often slow to appreciate the importance of the supply chain. To be successful, the supply chain must be elevated to a position where it is viewed as excellent—or in a Category of One. As noted, Mayo Clinic SCM has pursued many leading practices guided by a strategic plan with a continuous improvement philosophy.

According to the Oxford Dictionary, *excellence* is "the quality of being outstanding or extremely good." But how does an organization know if a function or discipline has reached the pinnacle of excellent performance? Is the achievement of excellence defined and recognized uniformly across healthcare? It is probably safe to say that it is not. Excellence can be both an objective and subjective journey. Excellence is objective, in the sense that most organizations know what they need to improve and which strategies and tactics they need to develop. Organizations typically have clear performance metrics and, ultimately, know when they have made progress. Excellence is also subjective because areas of improvement are at the discretion of the SCM executive and team. The pace of improvement and the practices deemed leading vary; thus, the strategic priorities for healthcare organizations vary. Achieving excellence is a marathon and not a sprint (though a sense of urgency varies widely as well). Excellence is not necessarily a destination but rather the achievement of milestones and successes, with a commitment to continuous improvement. In essence, elevating the SCM is a never-ending journey. Ultimately, supply chain excellence means doing many things right, not just excelling in one area.

Unifying the Voice of the Supply Chain

"A chain is only as strong as the weakest link" is a common saying that suggests an organization's strength is limited by its least capable members. This saying applies to many situations, including teams, organizations, and businesses. This is especially true for the SCM, where each interconnected function serves as a link to the next. The lack of a single, consistent voice in the supply chain can significantly weaken any function and, by extension, the entire chain.

Having a unified voice within an organization and throughout the market is a crucial component of Mayo Clinic's SCM strategy. A unified voice means providing sellers with the same message from all levels of an organization, including from senior leaders, physicians and clinical staff, and the SCM organization. Without a consistent message, the chances increase that the SCM will be significantly disadvantaged. Although Mayo Clinic SCM strives for positive, win-win (where mutual value is achieved) relationships, buyer-side chaos significantly weakens the buyer's position, making it highly likely that the supplier will exploit this weakness. Most modern supply chain literature suggests that win-win negotiations are the only way to seek an agreement. However, organizations should recognize that win-win negotiations are not always possible or in the organization's (or the supplier's) best interest. In negotiations, it is crucial to recognize when leverage is unbalanced, and when one side realizes they have an advantage, they will likely seek to move to a WIN-win or even a win-lose result (O'Brien, 2024).

For this reason, a uniform strategy with supporting policies and procedures, as well as a team-based culture, is critical. For example, the Mayo Clinic Supply Chain Contracting and Competitive Bid Requirements Policy outlines the guidelines and requirements for contracting and competitive bidding within the organization. The following are key points:

- Role of SCM: SCM must be contacted and will aid with the competitive bidding process. A written request for proposal is typically used.
- Compliance: All contracts and acquisitions must comply with Mayo Clinic policies, standards, and legal terms.
- Contract review: Perpetual agreements will be reviewed by SCM every 6 years to determine whether a competitive bid is needed. Overall value must be benchmarked and adjusted with the supplier, consistent with what could be achieved in a competitive bid.
- Exceptions: Requests for exceptions to the competitive bidding requirement for new or renewed contractual agreements must be filed with SCM.
- Procurement: Purchase orders must be issued by an SCM Procure to Pay agent, who will act in accordance with the Procurement Policy.
- Authorization: Only corporate officers or approved delegates who are authorized to sign contracts on behalf of the organization have execution authority. The individual signing a contract is responsible for confirming that all such policies and procedures are fully compliant.

A unified voice does not start and stop at sourcing and contracting but should continue throughout ongoing and subsequent activities, such as purchasing, receiving, payments, inventory management, and supplier management. The Supply Chain Management Office aids the organization in varying degrees with each of these functions, in accordance with the Contract Lifecycle Management Policy. Such coordination requires that stakeholders outside SCM work together to ensure speed, efficiency, and effectiveness. At Mayo Clinic, the organization emphasizes the need for a culture of teamwork. Theteam approach means that staff never have to search for answers alone, and this applies to SCM. The cross-functional, interdisciplinary teams are handpicked and include specialists with the common value of "the needs of the patient come first."

Many supply chain professionals outside of healthcare advocate for demand sensing and shaping, as do we. Demand shaping actively influences and aligns demand and supply rather than passively reacting to them. Typically, these activities involve leveraging various demand and supply signals. Healthcare clinicians sometimes find it perplexing as to why we (SCM) discuss demand shaping with them. After all, the impacts that they have on demand shaping is often not their primary concern. However, clinicians are directly impacted if planning is not done well and together. Clinicians have a crucial role; without their engagement, the SCM is only half of a solution. All parties must ensure that supplies are available when patients need them.

Thus, demand-shaping decisions cannot be made in isolation. To avoid doing so involves identifying supply issues (such as inventory or supply shortages or surpluses), any new technologies that are available and desirable, and any significant service line and practice change that may affect demand for certain products or services. It is essential that this planning occur regularly but also, even more critically, during sourcing and contracting meetings. All plans need to be vetted to determine whether they align. Improving the alignment of end-to-end demand with supply eliminates waste, enhances service, and leads to increased value.

Lastly, a cohesive, robust, and highly integrated technology strategy produces the transparency needed to manage at an enterprise level. Teamwork, leadership, and data are critical. In healthcare, people work in an environment where science is respected. The same applies to SCM. Data are generally not biased one way or another and aid in seeing what is not often apparent until it is too late. The significance of supply chain visibility cannot be overstated in achieving a unified voice of supply chain. Real-time tracking enhances coordination, reduces delays, and is essential for identifying and addressing disruptions. When used effectively, real-time tracking significantly enhances teamwork.

Product Standardization

Stock-keeping unit (SKU) rationalization is the practice of analyzing and streamlining a company's product portfolio by eliminating unnecessary or redundant SKUs (Science Direct, 2013). This practice originated from the increasing complexity of product offerings in retail environments, particularly as companies sought to cater to increasingly specific customer preferences. This is akin to what the healthcare supply chain has experienced over the past decade with a proliferation of "new and improved" or "preferred" products. Consequently, businesses of all sorts have been driven to actively identify and remove low-performing SKUs to optimize inventory and profitability. In the context of the Association for Operations Management standards, SKU rationalization involves analyzing a company's product portfolio and deciding which SKUs to retain, eliminate, or add.

Key Points of SKU Rationalization

- Goal: The primary objective is to reduce the number of SKUs by identifying and removing products with low utilization, high carrying costs, or duplicate functionalities. This process aims to improve operational efficiency and maximize value.
- Analysis process: This involves reviewing product specifications, utilization data (current as well as projected), inventory levels, value metrics, and market trends, to determine which SKUs should be discontinued or adjusted.

- Benefits: The benefits of SKU rationalization include reduced inventory costs, improved space utilization, increased value, better forecasting accuracy, and enhanced customer experience.

We have all experienced SKU rationalization as patients within the healthcare system if we are currently or have ever been prescribed a pharmaceutical. Pharmacy formularies have existed for years. A pharmaceutical formulary is a list of generic and brand-name prescription medications covered by health insurance plans.

A health plan's formulary is divided into tiers based on drug type. Prescription medications in a lower tier cost less. If medications are not included in an insurance plan's formulary, patients may be responsible for paying for them out of pocket. The reasons for a pharmacy formulary align with the SKU rationale stated previously (i.e., formularies ensure the necessary drugs for treatment are available while keeping costs as low as possible).

The idea of formularies of various products within a hospital setting has also been around for some time (albeit behind the scenes). Product formularies are managed by a critical team within the SCM organization called Clinical Quality Value Analysis (CQVA). Among other things, this team facilitates supplier and product standardization efforts. They strive to make the best products available while also minimizing redundancy and waste.

Historically, product standardization has been highly valued in healthcare, with the question being, "Why would you not want to standardize, given the value that could be achieved?" However, due to current supply chain instability, Mayo Clinic has slightly adjusted its position on the degree of standardization. Significant global disruptions continue to impact the U.S. healthcare supply chain and providers are still experiencing hundreds, if not thousands, of different product shortages. For this reason, one of the tactics to improve supply chain resiliency has been to move away from sole source (single) suppliers for critical products. SCM may standardize to two or three suppliers while maintaining a justified, rational formulary of products.

Within Mayo Clinic SCM, the CQVA work unit manages product issues and recalls and provides additional supply chain resources for clinical staff. Embedded within the CQVA work unit are product review teams (PRTs). PRTs provide clinical input on the product review process, participate in product trials, and communicate outcomes to clinical work groups. PRTs are facilitated by a clinical value analyst nurse. Other members include clinical experts, contract portfolio managers, and SCM staff. PRTs are divided into categories, such as surgical; medical; respiratory and anesthesia; wound, ostomy, and orthopedic; general; and laboratory. The Mayo Clinic Commodity Committee serves as the enterprise approval committee for commodities and clinical preference products.

CQVA PRTs implement a systematic, five-step, value analysis process to product management (Mayo Clinic Supply Chain, 2025b). The CQVA process is as follows:

1. Initiative: Generated by expired contracts; practice, standards, and regulatory changes; department and/or clinical practice goals; and product discontinuation.
2. Data gathering: Involves collecting product usage and spend data, conducting supplier meetings, requesting cross-references, benchmarking, and reviewing supplier questionnaires.
3. Analysis and recommendation: Includes final review by PRTs, financial and nonfinancial information analysis, product validations, and recommendations for awarded suppliers.
4. Implementation: Comprises a 90-day conversion window after contract launches, assigning formulary flags, and communicating contract details to each campus.
5. Compliance: Includes product-level reporting, communication to end users if non-approved products are still in use, and compliance checks 180 days after conversion.

Leadership emphasizes results —outcomes and costs —and recognizes that some level of standardization is necessary to achieve them. Mayo Clinic's approach to standardization is not one size fits all and flexes to the specific needs of the practice.

Value-Based Reimbursement

Value-based reimbursement programs are designed to incentivize healthcare providers to deliver high-quality, cost-effective care by linking payments to performance and outcomes, rather than merely the volume of services under a typical fee-for-service model (Nadeau, 2019).

Examples of these programs include:

- Population health management: This approach involves caring for a broad population, often at a capitated rate, or implementing highly targeted programs that address care for specific diseases (such as diabetes) or life stages.
- Bundling: Providers receive a single payment for an entire episode of care, covering all services within that period. An example of this is a joint replacement.
- Targeting known patient quality concerns: Providers receive payments based on meeting specific quality and efficiency benchmarks (e.g., hospital readmissions, hospital-acquired conditions).

- Incentivized cost reduction: Providers participate in shared savings programs (i.e., share in the savings generated by delivering high-quality, cost-effective care).

The shift toward value-based reimbursement has had a profound impact on how organizations view their supply chains, elevating their importance and adherence to leading practices. Broadly, the following examples of SCM functions that have undergone change illustrate this point:

Procurement: Analyzing data on supply usage, patient outcomes, and costs helps identify opportunities for value. Streamlining the supply chain by using fewer, higher-quality suppliers can reduce waste, improve efficiency, and enable a higher level of service. Optimizing performance and negotiating committed contracts leads to significant savings.

Inventory Management and Logistics: Accurate forecasting of supply needs helps avoid shortages and excess inventory, reducing waste and costs (Harvard Business Review, 2021). Implementing strategies to reduce waste and improve supply utilization saves money and improves patient care. By ensuring that the right supplies are available at the right time, healthcare organizations can improve patient outcomes and reduce complications.

Transparency: Building strong relationships with suppliers leads to better pricing, improved service, and greater resilience to disruptions. Sharing information and data across the supply chain can improve efficiency and collaboration.

Importantly, beyond having an impact to these functions, value-based reimbursement has necessitated a more holistic approach to supply chain, compelling SCM professionals to consider the entire episode of care and the total cost of the procedure rather than focusing solely on the price of a single device or piece of equipment. In some cases, value-based reimbursement has shifted the conversation to value generation and innovation. Additionally, value-based reimbursement has changed the scope of their logistics, as many procedures have transitioned from hospital settings to outpatient care or even home care. They are prompted to rethink postdischarge care strategies and the reach of the supply chain in this context. The move away from fee-for-service models has affected supply chain dynamics similarly to its effects on the broader system, where costs are not transferred onward. Mayo Clinic SCM has responded to these changes by adopting different sourcing strategies, enhancing inventory management and logistics, and implementing e-commerce solutions that provide direct access to the supply chain, which is connected to the electronic health record database. This shift has allowed us to focus on what is truly needed —the value provided, the delivery method, and reasonable pricing—all of which result in a more comprehensive package.

However, not everything has worked seamlessly. Attempting to integrate supplies too extensively into reimbursement processes has proven challenging. For example, integrating supply chain contracting with payer contracting has not gone well because payers have often tried to dictate specific supplies to clinicians. It is essential to maintain choice (to standardize) through consensus. Simplicity remains key.

The concept of total cost of ownership (TCO) has also become increasingly important. TCO is a financial estimate that helps companies determine the direct and indirect costs of a product or system. It goes beyond the initial purchase price or implementation cost and additionally considers the full cost of an asset over its useful life. Some buyers may be coerced by suppliers who offer discounted or free capital, requiring the purchase of their disposables at noncompetitive prices. Often, the capital cost is recouped multiple times through supplies, service, and maintenance costs. Future contract negotiations may also pose risks because initial pricing may be competitive—but subsequent negotiations, particularly when conversion is difficult, can be costly. To avoid being misled, it is crucial to exercise caution. Suppliers are becoming increasingly creative with their pricing strategies, so if an offer seems too good to be true, it likely is not. Conducting a TCO analysis and comparing alternative options is essential. Engaging cross-functional experts from SCM, finance, facilities, and clinical practice ensures a comprehensive evaluation.

Digital Strategy

Supply chain technology, often underappreciated (and vastly underfunded), operates in the background of every healthcare system; in fact, supply chain IT is most noticeable when it fails to function as expected, leading to disruptions and lack of visibility. IT is widely regarded as the heart of the supply chain and critically important. The supply chain system, or systems, execute the decisions made by healthcare leaders with precision, ensuring that the correct product is available at the right time, place, and price so that healthcare practitioners can care for their patients effectively.

Supply chain systems not only perform much of the work but also provide invaluable information. These data help organizations identify which products are performing well and which are not. The insights phase of the sourcing and contracting process focuses entirely on gathering and analyzing data to prepare for an appropriate event. Data are also used to determine which products to order, when to order them, and how much to stock. Additionally, data guide staff on which orders to fulfill and where to deliver them. Supply chain systems enforce corporate policies and procedures related to acquisition decision-making and authorization. They impose limitations that prevent fraud by controlling access to cash and payments to third parties. These systems ensure that sourced and delivered products are approved and safe to use, among other functions.

Modern healthcare providers typically leverage ERP systems, comprehensive software platforms that streamline and automate core administrative functions within hospitals or clinics. ERP systems generally support functions such as finance, accounting, human resources, and SCM. They collect organizational data from multiple sources, ensuring data integrity and eliminating duplication. ERP systems support real-time reporting tools and data analytics, which are crucial for decision-making and enhancing operational efficiency.

Within an ERP system, there are generally two critical applications: the procurement system and the inventory management system. The procurement system consists of tools and processes that allow buyers to identify, evaluate, and select the best available supplier or service provider, helping to reduce costs by streamlining the procurement process. The inventory management system ensures that purchased products are received, delivered, and stocked at the point of care. These systems are vital for reducing shipment delays and other disruptions by providing critical insights into SCM processes, enhancing transparency, decreasing inventory write-offs, and lowering inventory holding costs.

Beyond the ERP system, best-of-breed tools provide specialized functionality, such as recall management, sophisticated inventory monitoring, e-commerce, supplier authentication and risk management, contract administration, and analytics. These systems integrate with the ERP to create a seamless workflow for all staff across the supply chain and for those who interact with it daily.

Mayo Clinic's Digital Supply Chain Program aims to modernize and transform its IT infrastructure beyond traditional systems to improve efficiency and agility and to generate cost savings. The primary objective is to enable better integration and data access. Utilizing Amazon's "working backwards" methodology, the Program emphasizes collaboration across diverse teams to achieve its goals. Emphasizing the importance of technology ownership and proactive partnerships with IT, the Digital Supply Chain Program highlights the need for a skilled workforce and self-service tools. It is driven by investments in AI and a transformative approach similar to Uber's impact on transportation.

Like traditional systems, the digital supply chain system focuses on procurement (source to settle) and inventory management (operations management). However, it repositions processes as secondary to data with the addition of an information management platform. This platform allows ERP and ancillary systems to integrate and orchestrate work without being constrained by ERP rigidity. It also allows information beyond the supply chain system to be joined, aggregated, and shared, enabling alignment with newer reimbursement programs, better product standardization, synchronization and visibility with suppliers, and even the detection of world events that might disrupt the supply chain. In fact, although not fully deployed at the time, notable advancements in the Mayo digital supply chain system enabled early detection of the COVID-19 pandemic and the securing of critical inventory before shortages occurred. Most importantly, the digital supply chain enables SCM staff to manage and configure the system rather than being constrained by often-limited IT resources. These are just examples of the program's potential and value.

The next generation of the program integrates generative AI, robotics, and autonomous transportation, such as drones for delivery. For example, orders in the Mayo Clinic warehouse will be received by robots that will go to the precise location, pick the order, and deliver it to the requester with some human assistance. It is also envisioned that voice (as opposed to traditional input devices such as keyboards) will be used to interact with the system, and cameras will be the eyes of the supply chain. These advancements will further enhance the speed, agility, and resiliency needed to care for patients while improving efficiency and control.

Many healthcare institutions fail to proactively invest in supply chain systems, making the systems the weakest link in their organizations. In fact, it is common for organizations to focus mainly on the cost of their SCM operations, rather than the overall spend the operation supports, which is orders of magnitude larger. These organizations lack the systems to act quickly and the data to do so efficiently and effectively. Mayo Clinic has always been a leader in advancing healthcare supply chain IT and is recognized by Gartner, reflecting the success of its digital initiatives and its fearless investment in technology.

Inventory Management

Inventory management is a crucial aspect of understanding the allocation of resources at an enterprise level. This function encompasses inventory centers, points of use, and distribution and supplier partnerships. Built on full automation, scalability, and management science, inventory management must be dynamic and regularly adapt to the practice's needs. For instance, during the COVID-19 pandemic, Mayo Clinic established a fully operational personal protective equipment inventory center (80,000 square feet) within just two weeks.

Many view SCM services as excellent when clinicians get what they want when they ask. Mayo'sSCM takes this to the next level and operates under the fundamental principle: "The best supply service for the practice is when clinicians have what they need without having to ask." This means SCM staff must be able to anticipate demands and position needed supplies so that they are available when and where they are needed (as opposed to requested)—allowing clinicians to focus their time on patient care rather than on chasing supplies.

Mayo's enterprise SCM functions include several key areas. Demand planning involves monitoring and tracking inventory levels, establishing policies to replenish stock before it depletes, and balancing that with costs and waste (such as excess freight and obsolescence). Points of use as well as its inventory centers are included in demand planning, which involves strategically stocking critical supplies to buffer against risk. Inbound logistics, a function of managing inventory centers, ensures orders are fulfilled and delivered according to the demand plan. Outbound logistics focuses on managing points of use and ensuring stock is accurately accounted for and put away as orders are received from the inventory center. Automation, data visibility, and unrestricted access to information are crucial. The systems and analytics team addresses this need by managing the information systems that support various inventory management functions and ensuring end-to-end visibility.

Over the past decade, the inventory management function at Mayo Clinic has undergone significant changes. The prior distribution model was overly complex and lacked scalability. Additionally, the function was largely outsourced and built on a just-in-time model with a distribution partner. Service levels had deteriorated to a point of intolerable risk. Factors like COVID-19 further exposed vulnerabilities in the healthcare supply chain, not only at Mayo Clinic but worldwide. Unfortunately, many of these issues have not gone away. For example, shortages are now commonplace, and back orders have increased significantly since 2019. To an outsider's eye, supply chain may seem "back to normal," but service level rates have not been restored to anywhere near what would have been considered acceptable in the past. For this reason, Mayo Clinic SCM now plays a more active role in managing the end-to-end inventory management function.

The new strategy aims to optimize and expand Mayo Clinic's distribution facilities and capabilities, streamline operations, and enhance control over inventory and demand planning. More importantly, we are far less reliant on a single distribution partner and instead provide just-in-time services from its own inventory centers to the practice (or points of use). This strategy also includes product and location layout standardization across the enterprise and the integration of technology for better visibility. For example, at the point of use, we now have shelves outfitted with high-precision scales that register depletions and put aways in real time. This ensures that no person must scan at the point of use, inventory counts are accurate, and information is collected in real time. Although this may sound extreme, it ensures that those providing care can focus 100% of their time on patients. Current leading practice necessitates that the provider SCM transition from an orchestrator of services to an active operator and manager. This ensures risks are properly managed and allows more direct and transparent relationships with manufacturers. Improving safety stock management is critical because out of stocks can result in cancellation of critical patient procedures, not to mention significant cost increases in substitution products, labor, and freight.

Mayo Clinic's strategy for enhancing its distribution network was developed largely in response to evolving healthcare challenges, such as the degradation of basic service levels (failure to supply from the suppliers). This vulnerability highlighted the need for a simplified, resilient, and agile supply chain that can adapt to changing demands and risks. This was particularly evident during the COVID-19 pandemic. The new distribution network comprises three core functions: point of use, inventory center, and network center, each designed to enhance efficiency and service delivery. The strategy emphasizes the importance of a digital supply chain that acts as a “digital twin” for the entire network, enabling better data integration and operational efficiency. Using a phased implementation roadmap, Mayo Clinic isfocusing on consolidating operations and strengthening partnerships to optimize the distribution network.

Business Continuity and Risk Management

In an increasingly interconnected global landscape, supply chains are subject to numerous disruptions (Business Continuity Institute, 2025). At Mayo Clinic, the healthcare physicians and staff have recognizedthe critical importance of maintaining a proactive stance. Although they may not always identify specific risks, the organization remains vigilant, andits ability to respond has significantly improved. To effectively address risks and proactively meet the patients' needs, they must look beyond the organization's confines. They regularly monitor various risks, including those related to geopolitics, the economy, trade barriers and regulations, the environment and weather, cybersecurity, plant closures, and the availability of common or critical raw materials.

Business continuity planning (BCP) at Mayo Clinic involves monitoring internal and external risks and taking proactive, preemptive actions. In essence, BCP is preparing strategies to help the organization avoid crises and quickly return to “normal” when they occur. BCP encompasses two distinct processes:

1. Planning: This involves bringing attention to factors, which many others often overlook, that could affect the ability to supply critical products to the clinical practice.
2. Management: After a risk is identified and it becomes clear that there will be some impact, they develop management plans and execute them to avoid the risk.

The planning process involves three key steps: risk identification, risk prioritization, and risk monitoring. Mayo Clinic proactively evaluates potential risks and vulnerabilities, prioritizing them on the basis of their likelihood and impact on the enterprise. They continuously monitor trends and market insights. Although much emphasis is placed on the planning function, the management of risks sets the best programs apart. In many organizations, BCP fills gaps in supply chains by providing a clear overview of the overall organization, its structures, dependencies, suppliers, and stakeholders. Although the organizational owner of BCP may be a single department, the planning and management process involves cross-functional, interdisciplinary teams.

A key component of the management process at Mayo Clinic is the Supply Shortage Oversight and Management (SSOM) team. This team comprises representatives from various SCM functions. They meet regularly to review current constraints and impending risks. Team members coordinate with each other and their respective departments to execute agreed-upon plans and address related issues collaboratively. These staff ensure that not only tactics (e.g., procuring and stockpiling substitutions) are implemented but also that the practice is engaged in decision-making and practice changes, including conservation, if that is an agreed-upon tactic.

BCP also involves assessing organizational culture and fostering a climate where all employees are aware of everyday risks and their responsibility to report, manage, and mitigate them. The ADKAR (Awareness, Desire, Knowledge, Ability, and Reinforcement) model is an essential part of the goal-oriented, change management approach that focuses on facilitating change at the individual level (Prosci, 2025). The words that form the acronym ADKAR represent the five key stages individuals must go through to adopt and sustain change successfully.

The following is an example of how the Mayo Clinic SSOM team managed a significant supply chain disruption that occurred in early 2024 when a hurricane hit the coast of North Carolina. Baxter International, a major manufacturer of intravenous fluids, experienced a significant impairment. Hurricane Helene caused extensive damage to the manufacturing facility, leading to nationwide disruptions in production. The SSOM team determined there could be a risk when the storm first surfaced in the Atlantic Ocean and immediately contacted Baxter International. The teams collaborated to assess and prepare for a potential disruption. However, the storm and subsequent disruption were worse than expected. The SSOM team enhanced communications, collaboratively identified alternative products as well as conservation leading practices, developed inventory-tracking dashboards, and launched a website that included a list of all affected products, with instructions, contacts, and frequently asked questions. This all occurred in days. Although the supply chain was severely constrained, it did not break—and, most importantly, patient care continued.

Every crisis is a learning experience, and many new lessons are learned as we "return to normal." Various supply chain leading practices are not only desirable but necessary to sustain the healthcare system. However, one pressing issue remains: end to end visibility and automation. Challenges related to automation and data are now being addressed but will take some time to resolve. While their systems have advanced (as mentioned previously), each major stakeholder (consumers, suppliers, manufacturers, etc.) largely operate within their own siloed systems and the visibility and automation across stakeholders is very limited. As a result, various management strategies are valuable but they require significant effort and a lot of manual work-arounds. In the future, Mayo Clinic SCM intends to address automation and data challenges with a new AI-enabled platform that can utilize predictive insights to detect constraints, assist the end-to-end supply chain in addressing them, and learn from actions taken so that future events can be handled automatically.

Where to Begin "The Roadmap"

Where does one begin this journey? Consistent with the identification and adoption of leading practices, most SCM executives begin with an assessment of an organization's supply chain. In fact, newly hired supply chain executives should conduct a thorough assessment of a supply chain to establish baseline performance metrics. Assessing the supply chain can help determine where to begin improvement efforts. This assessment will also allow for the ongoing measurement of progress and serve as a basis for the development of a strategic plan that will serve as the roadmap to financial and operational performance improvements. Typical areas of assessment and questions to consider include:

1. Overview of the supply chain organization: A review of the organization's basic building blocks, such as organizational structure, job descriptions, policies, and procedures. Does the organization have an existing strategic plan for SCM? Review key performance metrics and agreements with third parties that support the supply chain or a particular function, if outsourced. What is the operating budget and plan for SCM? What is the current financial performance for SCM? What investments has the organization made in SCM?
2. Relationship management: One of the most important areas that should be part of any supply chain assessment is that of its' relationships. What is the current state of relationships between SCM employees and the organization's senior leadership, physicians, and professional staff, as well as other key stakeholders? What is their unbiased opinion of the SCM currently and desires for the future? The importance of relationship management cannot be stressed enough for the future success of a supply chain executive and the strategy they seek to

implement in the organization. Relationships require work, initially focused on trust and mutual respect. SCM executives would be well advised to deliver on promises.

3. Sourcing and contracting: A thorough and systematic review of staff involved with sourcing and contracting should be done. A review of span of control or how much of the nonlabor spend is managed by SCM. Included in the review are agreements for group purchasing affiliations or other sources of contracts with suppliers available to the organization. Do contractual templates exist? Are policies and procedures pertaining to sourcing and contracting, such as conflict of interest, authorization levels, and signature authority in place? How does the organization assess the overall value of the sourcing and contracting unit? Is benchmarking widely endorsed? How do they know whether the pricing is competitive or best in the marketplace?
4. Procure to pay or source to settle: An integrated purchasing and payable department has been recognized as a leading practice. Does the organization embrace this approach? Does appropriate segregation of duties exist? How automated are the processes and opportunities for improvement? Overall, the objective would be to have supplies and products available on an automated replenishment basis rather than to have staff complete a requisition. How sophisticated is the function? Do they have favorable payment terms? Do they practice dynamic discounting? Do they leverage credit cards and/or procurement cards?
5. Distribution, logistics, and inventory management: What is the distribution model? If third-party logistics are relied on, how competitive is the agreement? How are they performing? What are the inventory management policies and procedures? How does the distribution function perform overall (e.g., fill rates). Are the replenishment areas capable of producing a demand signal? Is the organization able to share this demand signal with key suppliers to smooth out supply and ensure on-time, in-full delivery?
6. IT systems and strategy: Is there an overall strategy for IT that supports the supply chain from end to end? How current is the strategy, and does it include the latest technology to advance supply chain performance in terms of efficiency and cost effectiveness? How up to date is the ERP system, and are there necessary integration interfaces?
7. Data governance and management, spend analytics, and reporting: This area has undergone significant change and improvement. Understanding an organization's data governance and management model is ultimately the key to the efficiency and success of all products, cash, and information flows in the supply chain. Corrupt or bad data produce bad outcomes and make it nearly impossible to know what is happening in the supply chain. Having a single source of truth that feeds data into the SCM IT systems is critical. Interfaces that enable these data

to seamlessly move from technology to technology will facilitate automation of information capturing, manage inventory, and ease and enable replenishment while minimizing the need for requisitioning.

8. Legal, risk management, and financial departments: What is the state of SCM's relationships with the organization's legal, risk management, and financial departments? Are there landmines lurking that would come as a surprise? Is SCM currently engaged with any legal challenges, audits, or other risks? What has been the focus of past internal audits, and have they been resolved? What is the level of engagement with these key areas, and how much professional discretion does SCM exercise in securing contracts and other agreements? What are the supply chain's most significant risks, and what mitigation strategies exist (e.g., cybersecurity)?
9. Service level agreements: Does SCM have service level agreements with operating entities? Are performance metrics mutually agreed upon between SCM and the entities? As a shared or business service organization, how well is SCM performing? What areas for improvement are needed, and what opportunities exist? If service level agreements do not exist, does SCM conduct customer service satisfaction surveys?
10. Business integrity and continuity: How well is the supply chain financially performing? Does SCM have an audit and recovery unit? Has it adopted internal controls? What are the disaster recovery plans? What are SCM's strategies to ensure supply chain resiliency and business continuity?
11. Organizational commitment to supplier diversity and sustainability: What policies and business processes exist to support the use of diverse suppliers and the advancement of sustainability? What is the organization's commitment to these areas of focus?

The previous information is not intended to be an exhaustive list of all areas or functions in need of an assessment but can serve as a good place to start. If done thoroughly, an assessment will provide significant insight to the supply chain and identify opportunities for improvement. Such information can be incorporated into a new, overall strategic plan and prioritized roadmap for SCM to elevate its performance.

CONCLUSION

This chapter has provided an overview of one of the healthcare sector's leading supply chains, highlighting its historical development, notable accomplishments, strategies, and operational tactics. As outlined in the introduction, the ultimate customer in healthcare is the patient. Effective supply chain management (SCM) is essential to delivering safe and high-quality patient care, making it a central consideration for anyone pursuing healthcare transformation and reform with a patient-centric approach. As emphasized previously, achieving excellence necessitates consistently strong performance across multiple dimensions, making it an ongoing process. Additionally, reaching this level of excellence is not an individual endeavor; leveraging scale through partnerships and collaboration is vital. In this context, the analogy of a relay race may more accurately represent the collective journey toward excellence.

FUTURE DIRECTIONS

Recent progress is expected to continue, with innovation accelerating due to new technologies and a skilled workforce. Artificial intelligence could likely automate up to 70% of core supply chain tasks (Mayo Clinic Supply Chain, 2025c). Advances in robotics, analytics, and agential AI are emerging, but broad implementation is just beginning. As experienced professionals retire, a new generation with strong data science and AI expertise is taking on leadership roles is emerging and they are prepared to tackle the future.

REFERENCES

Business Continuity Institute. (2025). Business continuity and risk management. https://www.thebci.org

Gartner. (2024). Gartner Announces Ranking of the Gartner Healthcare Supply Chain Top 25 for 2024. https://www.gartner.com/en/newsroom/press-releases/2024-11-13-gartner-announces-ranking-of-the-gartner-healthcare-supply-chain-top-25-for-2024

Harvard Business Review. (2021). A simpler way to modernize your supply chain. Harvard Business Review. https://hbr.org/2021/09/a-simpler-way-to-modernize-your-supply-chain

Mayo Clinic Finance. (2025). Mayo Clinic Financial Operating Budget. [Unpublished].

Mayo Clinic Supply Chain. (2025a). Mayo Clinic 2025 Operating Budget. [Unpublished].

Mayo Clinic Supply Chain. (2025b). Mayo Clinic Five Step CQVA Process. [Unpublished].

Mayo Clinic Supply Chain. (2025c). Mayo Clinic Supply Chain Automation Assessment. [Unpublished].

Mayo Clinic Supply Chain. (2025d). Mayo Clinic Supply Chain Strategic Plan. [Unpublished}. Nadeau, K. L. (2019). Value-based care: The role and impact of healthcare supply chains. https://www.ghx.com/the-healthcare-hub/role-supply-chain-management-healthcare/

O'Brien, J. (2024). *Category Management in Purchasing*. Kogan Page.

Prosci. (2025). ADKAR model. https://www.prosci.com

Science Direct. (2013). Product Variety Management. https://www.sciencedirect.com/science/article/pii/S0007850613001972

US News. (2026). America's Best Hospitals: 2025-2026 Honor Roll and Overview. America's Best Hospitals: The 2025-2026 Honor Roll and Overview I U.S. News

Section 4
Strategic Process: Foundations and Practices in Healthcare

Chapter 12
Healthcare at Its Foundations:
Recovering Purpose and Meaning

Barry A. Doublestein
http://orcid.org/0009-0009-8994-2611
Regent University, USA

Walter T. Lee
http://orcid.org/0000-0002-5487-3603
Duke University School of Medicine, USA

Richard M. Pfohl
Belhaven University, USA

ABSTRACT

This chapter argues that meaningful healthcare reform requires returning to foundational questions about purpose and structure rather than incremental system adjustments. Three critical fractures impede reform: eroding public trust (declining from 51% to 32% between 2020-2025), failure to progress beyond goods and services delivery to patient transformation, and consolidation-driven system design that undermines patient-centered care while fueling physician burnout. Before proposing solutions, the authors insist healthcare leaders must address five worldview questions: What is healthcare for? What is a patient? What good are we pursuing? What does it mean to be a healer? What system best serves human dignity? Only then can leaders effectively apply the six-component Strategy Development Process: Strategic Foresight, Strategic Thinking, Strategic Innovation, Strategic Planning, Strategic Implementation, and Strategic Analysis and Assessment. This framework enables continuous adaptation in an era of exponential change while maintaining moral clarity and operational excellence.

DOI: 10.4018/979-8-3373-2577-4.ch012

INTRODUCTION

Before beginning to offer this perspective on post-2020 healthcare reform, it has been difficult to offer a fresh perspective which would be meaningful and impactful to readers. While the authors have a combined total of nearly eighty years of healthcare experience spanning patient care as a physician, leadership in various healthcare insurance organizations, pre- and post-graduate medical education programs, and even public policy advocacy, from time to time they truthfully struggled with whether healthcare, as it presently exists, can be saved.

Their struggle boils down to one simple question: What is it that is attempting to be reformed; the system that is the result of decades of previous reforms, one built upon the previous, or one that returns to the very basic foundational purpose for its existence; patient-care? The system, as it is today, is the product of compromising interests from competing stakeholders instead of a consensus of purpose around giving patients what they simply seek; transformation (Pine & Gilmore, 2020). How one answers this question determines its structure, focus, capital investments, and its success. One might consider that this approach is rather simplistic, naïve, or reductionistic, but the future of healthcare depends on its answer. How one answers this question determines their view of reality and stands as the basis for all their future actions and decisions.

How does one even expect to discuss necessary reforms to healthcare without first looking into the foundations upon which it is built and stabilized? Some might think that a few simple tweaks here or there might suffice, but reality contradicts that thinking while gaping cracks in the foundations are being ignored, even while they widen before one's eyes.

Consider the NFL's Green Bay Packers coach Vince Lombardi's famous approach in 1961, precipitated by a loss in the previous season's championship game, he walked into the next season's training camp with a renewed dedication to starting from scratch, holding up a football and stating: "Gentlemen, this is a football" (Maraniss, 2000). This return to fundamentals, though seemingly simplistic, represented a profound understanding that excellence requires mastery of the basics. Similarly, healthcare reform demands a return to foundational questions before any sustainable solutions can be built.

The basis of this chapter is to focus upon assessing the foundations undergirding the healthcare industry, expose the cracks that impede reforms, and provide a strategy development tool that will aid in uncovering driving trends that often go unnoticed, which ultimately could lead to disaster or irrelevance for the organization.

CRACKED FOUNDATIONS

Loss of Trust

While much of the erosion of trust has deeper historical roots, the last five years provide a concentrated window in which the consequences of earlier reforms have become unmistakably visible. This period is not the origin of the problem, but the clearest manifestation of long-developing fractures within the system; so, reference to this timeframe is intended to highlight the most recent cycle of reform efforts and their outcomes, not to suggest that the challenges began within that period. While the astute observer of social media finds the loss of trust palpable, polling confirms the extent of this distrust; with 51% of Americans having a great deal or quite a lot of trust in the medical system in 2020, however, by 2025, that number had declined to 32%; a full 19% loss of trust, representing the lowest level since 2007 (Gallup, 2025a). Similarly, another Gallup poll on views of the healthcare industry reveals a dramatic shift; in 2025, 51% expressed very negative or somewhat negative views compared to only 36% with very positive or somewhat positive views. This represents a stark reversal from 2020, when 51% held very or somewhat positive views against 31% holding negative views (Gallup, 2025b).

Public trust in medicine is not necessarily related to individuals' perception of the quality of care they receive (Blendon & Benson, 2022), because 82% of respondents rated the quality of healthcare they receive as excellent or good, with only 16% rating it as only fair or poor. On the other hand, when it comes to one's own physician, the numbers are even more favorable, with 76% rating their care as excellent or very good and 16% rating it as good. This data suggests that factors other than personal care experiences drive public distrust of the leaders of medicine.

Trust varies significantly depending on the healthcare entity in question; while 85% of respondents trust doctors completely or somewhat, and hospitals garner 72% complete or somewhat complete trust, pharmaceutical companies fare far worse with only 34% trust and a mere 3% complete trust. Health insurance companies perform similarly poorly with 33% trust and only 4% reporting complete trust. Perhaps most concerning is that only 34% rated the public health system as excellent or good; leaving 65% at fair to poor ratings (Blendon & Benson, 2022).

Some Reasons for This Decline in Trust are Multifaceted

The retraction of ten thousand peer-reviewed articles in 2023 due to faulty study design and ethical conflicts has significantly undermined confidence in medical research (Van Noorden, 2023). This unprecedented wave of retractions raises fundamental questions about the integrity of the scientific publishing process and the reliability of research that informs clinical practice. When the foundational research upon which medical decisions are made proves unreliable, public confidence inevitably erodes.

A perceived lack of informed consent associated with the COVID-19 mRNA vaccines has created lasting concerns about transparency in public health decision-making (Bardosh, et al, 2022). This, combined with what many perceive as a lack of transparency related to adverse vaccine injury reports (Flint, 2024), has contributed to a growing skepticism about the authenticity of health authorities' communications. The gap between official messaging and individual experiences has led many to question the credibility of healthcare institutions.

The lack of institutional transparency is not limited to the public health sector for it thrives in the greater pharmaceutical industry which is being exposed as hiding known adverse drug complications in patients during clinical trials and after governing authority approvals are given (Miller, et al, 2017; Jutley, G.S. et al, 2024; B. Cassie, 2025), lacking of biotech-safety concerns for those who are responsible for research and development in working with pathogens, and the prevalence of negligence, corruption, and conflicts of interest between governing oversight agencies and those financially benefitting from approvals. Transparency is suppressed often because of the fear of exposing 'trade secrets' could undermine institutional property rights and potential future profits (McClain, 2025). Even when adverse drug reactions are uncovered by healthcare providers, they experience barriers in reporting their findings because there is an absence of access to a professional and trustworthy reporting system (Ali, et al, 2021).

The credibility crisis extends into healthcare insurance practices as well. For example, recent whistleblower allegations supported by internal documents and former Cigna executives revealed that insurance claim-reviewing physicians reject claims without even opening patient files. Over a period of two months, Cigna doctors denied over 300,000 requests for payments using this method by spending less than 1.2 seconds on each case (Rucker, et al, 2023). These accusations fundamentally call into question the objectivity of medical review processes and suggest that financial incentives may be misaligned with patient welfare.

Perhaps most damaging to healthcare's scientific credibility has been the "science-is-settled" attitude that dominated discourse during the recent pandemic (Porterfield, 2021). Science-fiction author, Michael Crichton (2003) speaks to the problem inherent with this perspective:

"Historically, the claim of consensus has been the first refuge of scoundrels; it is a way to avoid debate by claiming that the matter is already settled. Whenever

you hear the consensus of scientists agrees [sic] on something or other, reach for your wallet, because you're being had.

Let's be clear: the work of science has nothing whatever to do with consensus. Consensus is the business of politics. Science, on the contrary, requires only one investigator who happens to be right, which means that he or she has results that are verifiable by reference to the real world. In science consensus is irrelevant. What is relevant is reproducible results. The greatest scientists in history are great precisely because they broke with the consensus. There is no such thing as consensus science. If it's consensus, it isn't science. If it's science, it isn't consensus."

The 'science-is settled' stance is directly contradictory to Thomas Kuhn's seminal work, *The Structure of Scientific Revolutions* (1962), which offers that science advances through paradigm shifts rather than linear accumulation of settled facts. "Normal science" operates within accepted paradigms, but revolutionary advances occur when anomalies force the scientific community to reconsider fundamental assumptions. Many refused to consider exposed anomalies in the pandemic science because they were heavily invested in the process, that to them, was an absolute conclusion beyond question. Science is a method, not a conclusion (Kuhn, 1962).

For example, the story of Barry Marshall and Robin Warren exemplifies why science must never be considered settled. In 1982, Marshall and Warren proposed that peptic ulcers were caused by *Helicobacter pylori* (H. pylori) bacteria, directly challenging the longstanding belief that stress and lifestyle factors were the primary causes. The medical community initially rejected their findings, with their first paper submission rated in the bottom 10% of submissions that year…surely, they said, no bacteria could survive in the acidic conditions of the stomach and duodenum. So convinced was Marshall of his hypothesis that in 1984 he deliberately infected himself with *H. pylori*, developed gastritis, and then cured himself with antibiotics. Despite intense criticism from the established medical community, Marshall and Warren persisted, and in 2005 they were awarded the Nobel Prize in Physiology or Medicine for their discovery; which is now the standard of care (Ahmed, 2005). This paradigm shift transformed treatment for millions of patients, replacing lifelong medications with short courses of antibiotics. The moral is clear; science is never settled, and today's 'heresy' may become tomorrow's standard of care.

Finally, the democratization of news through social media and alternative information sources means that people are no longer willing to accept information filtered exclusively through traditional media outlets. Individuals can now access unfiltered information, compare sources, and discern for themselves. While this creates challenges around possible misinformation, it also reflects a healthy skepticism about centralized control of information flow.

Economic-Value Disconnect

Healthcare has not kept pace with the macroeconomic trends that predominate in successful and desirable organizations and industries. It is as if healthcare is collectively unaware of the *Progression of Economic Value* (Pine & Gilmore, 2020) as it is viewed from the vantage point of late 2025. In the past, the drivers of economic growth centered around extracting commodities that would make goods which would then be delivered to customers in the form of services. Today, however, the focus of value is in staging experiences that bring about transformation (Pine & Gilmore, 2020).

Healthcare has honed its skills, predominantly over the last four decades, in providing excellent quality goods and services, however, in the progression of this provision, it has built an entrenched system that promotes and protects its ends. But it has failed to take the next step in economic value: creating experiences that bring about transformation in their stakeholders. One of the major reasons why healthcare has not progressed to this level is that in order for this to happen, customization is foundational to success (Pine & Gilmore, 2020). Healthcare has built an infrastructure that promotes the provision of goods and services, but is not even remotely focused on experiences and transformations. Healthcare's intense focus on technology and capital improvements, without considering the human-capital training to put those things into play, exacerbates the 'good and services' focus instead of what patients really want. Technology, capital, and infrastructure offer only inert potential…but nothing improves patient satisfaction until that potential is put into play by some human, regardless of their position within the organization. This can only happen when people are exposed to these skills and supported throughout the organization in the form of culture. This cannot be faked, rather it must become part of the very fabric of an institution; practiced in a habitual way until they become part of the character of the organization (Greenhalgh, et al, 2020).

People desire experiences that lead to transformation, and when their care falls short of these expectations, they seek alternatives. One part of the healthcare industry that is finding some success in creating experiences and transformations in patients is the medical tourism industry. Aside from affordable excellent care from well-trained practitioners in high-quality facilities, patients find comfort as they are empowered and cared for by dedicated care coordinators that take the worry away from procedures and healing. The difference between these entities and the current industry standard is found in the focus moving from the process (institution-centered) to the patient (Christensen, 2003).

Patients across the board are serious about the importance of their healthcare experience, with 95% of those surveyed stating that it is extremely or very important to their overall health and well-being. When asked about the reasons for the experience being so important to them, the top six comments are related to personal transformation: (1) personal importance of health and wellbeing (68%), (2) knowing that their physical needs are taken seriously (62%), (3) good patient experiences contribute to healing/good outcomes (51%), (4) they deserve to be treated with respect (47%), (5) being treated as a person, not as a symptom, diagnosis, or disease (44%), and (6) it will influence how future healthcare decisions are made (39%) (The Beryl Institute, 2023).

On the other hand, patients generated underwhelming scores related to four core areas of their experience: (1) cost of care and billing concerns, as they are not getting proper information regarding what they need to pay and what their insurance will cover; (2) care-team communication, as they are not getting proper or complete information about prescriptions, pain management, and discharge guidelines; (3) access-to-care and wait times, as patients cited obstacles to easy scheduling of appointments, getting stuck on phone holds, waiting for extended periods of time for a visit, or transportation/parking logistics; and, (4) missed expectations of care, as feeling rushed by their physicians, being interrupted during discussions, being ignored by reception staff, and a lack of empathy from physicians (Physicians Practice, 2024).

System Design and Focus

Healthcare is becoming more consolidated as physicians are leaving private practice to join hospitals, health insurers, and private equity firms (U.S. Government Accountability Office, 2025). Nearly a decade ago, 60% of physicians were in private practice; now that number has dropped to 42% (U.S. Government Accountability Office, 2025). This consolidation trend has profound implications for how healthcare is delivered and experienced.

As healthcare systems have consolidated, care has shifted from personal, relationship-based practice to standardized processes governed by the priorities of large organizational owners. Consolidation introduces new rules, metrics, and workflows that operate at the level of systems rather than persons. These structures privilege efficiency, throughput, and risk-avoidance, often at the expense of presence, listening, and individualized care. The system becomes calibrated to the "average patient" (a statistical abstraction) resulting in greater patient sacrifice and diminished patient satisfaction (Pine & Gilmore, 2020). When the structure of healthcare no longer supports clinicians in practicing relationship-based care, both patients and physicians experience a loss of meaning. The system grows more efficient, but less humane.

Herein lies a major concern for leaders of healthcare organizations: what is it that patients truly desire? Many might state that their marketing departments delve into the specifics of patient expectations through patient-satisfaction surveys, which are valuable tools for gaining understanding, but a major question asks what is being surveyed? Are the right questions being asked? Are surveys structured in a way that assess what the institution is providing, or do they dig more deeply to uncover patients' true desires/expectations?

Patient satisfaction is the product of 'what a customer expects to get' *minus* 'what a customer perceives he gets.' These surveys often focus on understanding and managing customer expectations of what companies already do, as compared to gaining an understanding of what customers really want (Pine & Gilmore, 2020). It is critical that healthcare leaders design their surveys in ways that do not seek confirmation bias, which is about procuring information that confirms their hoped-for outcomes as opposed to determining their actual standing.

A more helpful tool would be to understand the nature of customer sacrifice, which is the product of 'what a customer wants exactly' *minus* 'what a customer settles for.' When leaders truly understand this concept of customer sacrifice, they are able to more fully discern the difference between what patients accept and what they really need; something that is possible to discern by the astute leader, even if the customer doesn't know what they need or be able to articulate it (Pine & Gilmore, 2020). But, there are difficulties for organizational leaders in solving this dichotomy:

"While companies employ total quality management (TQM) techniques to drive up customer satisfaction, they must employ Mass Customization techniques to drive down customer sacrifice. And while TQM programs help reduce the waste associated with mass produced goods and services—by eliminating redundancies, bottlenecks, and other inefficiencies—focusing on customer sacrifice eliminates the waste that occurs whenever a business performs an activity or expends a resource that a particular customer does not want. Indeed, because TQM programs often result in new features (of a good) or dimensions (of a service) geared to improving the satisfaction of the average customer, the solution to effect increased satisfaction becomes the source of additional sacrifice. No matter how many improvements are made, the offering remains uniform for all customers. But individual customers differ in the exact combination of features or benefits they desire. They constantly face trade-offs, trying to decide if enough beneficial components exist to tolerate the marginal and offset the detrimental. Rarely do wants and needs match exactly the one bundle that constitutes a company's product, so whenever a customer buys any mass produced offering, he accepts the undesired components along with the desired, and this means that the company wasted resources in production or delivery" (p. 105).

They continue:

"Designing for the average is the root cause of customer sacrifice; every mass produced product comprises a bundle of take-it-or-leave-it features or dimensions offered to all customers. The more features bundled, the greater the like-

lihood of introducing an element that disqualifies the product with a particular buyer (either because the buyer flat doesn't want the element or doesn't want to incur the perceived higher price for a marginal element). Similarly, talk about 'designing for the customer' in many organizations really means designing for 'the average customer'—who doesn't really exist. Unless people keep particular customers—real, specific, and known individuals—in view, such efforts only trigger initiatives to perform activities and expend resources without knowing the individual levels actually required" (p. 106).

If the intended outcome of our consolidated system is cost-savings and efficiencies, the threat of increasing the customer-sacrifice gap threatens patients' expectations and desires. If leaders dismiss or diminish the impact of a widening gap or even take on an attitude of 'they won't mind,' patient satisfaction will decline.

Consider how physicians themselves feel about working in this system. Physician burnout has reached crisis levels. In a survey of nearly 9,000 physicians, 78% reported experiencing burnout in their medical practices (The Physicians Foundation, 2018). The survey revealed that one of the chief culprits contributing to physician burnout is the frustration physicians feel with the inefficiency of electronic health records (EHRs). Physicians report that what attracts most of them to medicine is the unique nature of the physician-patient relationship, yet they find themselves increasingly unable to focus on this core calling.

The challenges healthcare providers face are numerous, but burnout from administrative burdens and dealing with insurers and their complexities for prior authorizations, are among the most egregious factors stressing them. At least, excessive charting paperwork is being minimized with the availability of new AI tools that use advanced algorithms and machine-learning techniques to translate natural conversations into pertinent medical documentation (Ulrich, 2025). While beneficial in helping to mitigate a major challenge, providers find little hope for relief simply because of the intense intransigence on both sides, providers and insurers, who are unwilling to change their views, agree, or even come to the table to listen to varying public-policy possibilities. This unwillingness emboldens stubbornness and inflexibility, which certainly fuels the perspective that any attempts to negotiate would be a waste of time. Based on experience as a healthcare policy lobbyist, one of the authors has witnessed firsthand how this intransigence perpetuates systemic dysfunction.

The move away from patient-centered care is particularly concerning. The concept of the Patient-Centered Medical Home, which gained prominence about 15 years ago, as a proposed solution, is now in jeopardy as more and more private practices are sold to hospitals and health systems. This consolidation threatens the personalized, relationship-based care that is fundamental to the patient-centered care movement.

Marketing changes that ignore people's preferences spell disaster, as evidenced by recent high-profile corporate missteps made by consumer brands: Bud Light, Target, and Cracker Barrel (Accelerant Research, 2025). Instead of asking customers what they want, these companies told them what they were going to get, resulting in significant backlash. Healthcare leaders would do well to learn from these cautionary tales.

The reputation of medicine has been damaged through inauthenticity. Once an organization has lost authenticity, it is generally conceptually unrecoverable, however, those institutions that recognize the loss of purpose at the core of their problems can recover, but it will take a major effort (Pine & Gilmore, 2007). With the rapid adoption of artificial intelligence and deep fakes (voices, videos, and pictures that are created artificially), more and more people are questioning authenticity. This is a problem for 76% of Americans say that it is important to be able to tell the difference between AI- and human-generated content, but few feel confident that they can (Pew Research Center, 2025). Exacerbating the issue is that AI-text generating tools have been found rewriting scientific papers that produce ‘copycat’ versions that are passed off as new research (Naddaf, 2025; Spredemann, 2025). Now that these papers are being uncovered in scientific-literature databases a question begs an answer; can one of the most important and basic structures that supports healthcare, scientific research, be trusted? Can the industry recover when it has allowed corruption of truth in its underpinnings? Distrust in competence and authenticity is growing widely as previously trusted institutions revel in irrelevance and incompetence on a level unseen in the last century (Howe, 2023).

Fundamental Questions That Must Be Answered

Before healthcare leaders can develop meaningful strategies for reform, they must first address fundamental questions about the nature and purpose of healthcare itself. These questions operate at the worldview level, which is the set of basic assumptions that defines one’s reality and offers a blueprint for making decisions. Without this basic underpinning, relevant plans cannot be carried out effectively and efficiently. If the industry does not go back to these basics, it cannot effectively accomplish its purposes.

Worldview serves as the lens through which all strategic decisions are filtered. It determines not only what one sees as problems but what they consider valid solutions. Two healthcare organizations may look at the same data and arrive at completely different conclusions based on their foundational assumptions about the purpose of healthcare, the nature of the patient, and the role of the healer. Understanding and articulating these foundational assumptions is therefore not an academic exercise but a practical necessity for effective leadership.

The Teleological Question: "What is Healthcare's Purpose?"

Every reform must begin with *telos* (purpose). This foundational question asks what healthcare is ultimately meant to accomplish. Is healthcare about prolonging life, or promoting wholeness? Is the aim efficiency and cost control, or human flourishing and dignity? Is the focus on treating disease, or is it on healing persons? Who defines health, is it the patient, the practitioner, the state, or a moral framework rooted in truth about the human person?

This question is foundational because the system's ends determine its ethics. If the purpose is profit or compliance, then compassion becomes incidental. If the purpose is healing, then technology and policy become instruments of that higher good. Consider how differently a healthcare organization will operate if it views its purpose as maximizing shareholder value versus maximizing patient wellbeing. Both may use similar language about "quality care," but their decision-making frameworks will lead to vastly different outcomes when conflicts arise between profitability and patient benefit.

For emerging healthcare leaders, clarifying this teleological question means examining every strategic initiative through the lens of ultimate purpose. When evaluating whether to implement a new electronic health record system, the question is not merely whether it will save time or reduce costs, but whether it will ultimately serve the healing purpose of healthcare. When considering organizational restructuring, leaders must ask whether the changes bring the organization closer to or further from its core purpose.

The practical implications are significant. An organization that clearly articulates healthcare's purpose as promoting human flourishing will make different decisions about everything from facility design to staffing ratios to technology investments. It will measure success not merely in throughput metrics or financial performance, but in the degree to which patients experience genuine transformation and healing. This clarity of purpose provides the North Star by which all other decisions can be oriented.

The Anthropological Question: "What is a Patient?"

Medicine's anthropology, its understanding of what a human being is, fundamentally shapes how care is defined. Are human beings machines to be repaired, or souls embodied? Are patients consumers, or persons bearing inherent dignity and worth? Is suffering merely a pathology to eliminate, or also a mystery to accompany? What does human flourishing mean when healing, in the traditional sense, is not possible?

When medicine loses a coherent anthropology, it devolves into biological reductionism where measuring what can be counted takes precedence over what counts most. A mechanistic view of the patient leads to care that focuses exclusively on fixing broken parts while neglecting the person's emotional, spiritual, and relational needs. Conversely, a holistic anthropology recognizes that patients are complex beings whose physical ailments cannot be separated from their psychological state, social connections, and sense of meaning and purpose.

Consider the practical difference this makes in end-of-life care. A purely mechanistic anthropology might view a terminally ill patient as a failing system to be maintained as long as possible, deploying every available technology regardless of the patient's suffering or wishes. A more holistic anthropology would recognize that sometimes the most healing act is not to prolong biological function but to honor the person's dignity, manage their pain, and support their emotional and spiritual wellbeing in their final days.

For healthcare leaders, this anthropological question has immediate practical implications. How patients are viewed determines how staff is trained, care processes are designed, how resources are allocated, and success is measured. An organization that views patients primarily as consumers will design experiences optimized for satisfaction and efficiency. An organization that views patients as persons with inherent dignity will design experiences that honor autonomy, provide genuine presence, and attend to the whole person.

This question also challenges leaders to consider how their organizational culture reflects their anthropology. Do staff members see patients as room numbers or as individuals with names, stories, and relationships? Are care protocols designed with statistical averages in mind, or with the recognition that each person's needs are unique? The answers to these questions flow directly from foundational beliefs about human nature.

The Moral Question: "What is the Good We Are Pursuing?"

Healthcare decisions nearly always imply moral judgments, whether acknowledged or not. What constitutes good care, is it defined by outcomes, patient satisfaction, or integrity of process? How are truth, autonomy, and compassion weighed when they conflict? Can medicine be morally neutral, or must it be morally formed? Who decides what is right when moral frameworks diverge?

Without moral clarity, organizations trade ethical formation for regulatory compliance and call it virtue. They confuse legal permissibility with moral rightness. They measure success by whether they avoided lawsuits rather than whether they acted with integrity. This confusion is particularly dangerous in healthcare, where life, death, and human dignity hang in the balance.

Consider the moral complexity of truth-telling in medicine. When a patient has a terminal diagnosis, what constitutes "good care"? Is it providing complete, unvarnished information regardless of the patient's emotional state? Is it framing the information in a way that maintains hope? Is it deferring to family members who request that certain information be withheld? Different moral frameworks will answer these questions differently, and leaders must be equipped to navigate these complexities.

For emerging leaders, this moral question demands the development of practical wisdom, which is the ability to discern the right action in complex, ambiguous situations where rules and guidelines provide insufficient guidance. It requires cultivating moral imagination to see beyond the immediate tactical decision to its broader implications. It necessitates the courage to make difficult choices that may be unpopular but are morally necessary.

Organizations must also grapple with moral questions at the systems level. How should scarce resources be allocated? What obligations do profitable healthcare systems have to serve unprofitable populations? When financial sustainability conflicts with optimal care, where should the balance be struck? Leaders who have clarity about the moral goods they are pursuing will be better equipped to navigate these difficult trade-offs with integrity.

The Vocational Question: "What Does it Mean to Be a Healer?"

The question of vocation requires healthcare leaders to ask whether clinicians are merely providers of technical services, or whether they are moral agents entrusted with the well-being of persons. The system's dominant incentives have increasingly trained physicians to operate as technicians (efficient, standardized, compliant, and legally protected) rather than as healers who accompany patients through suffering with wisdom, compassion, and integrity. Yet if physicians are viewed only as technical experts, the moral dimensions of care become incidental rather than essential. A healthcare culture that reduces clinicians to measurable outputs inevitably diminishes the very relationships that make healing possible. To reform healthcare, we must recover the understanding that clinicians are not only skilled professionals but also bearers of a vocation grounded in moral responsibility.

Before systems can be reformed, the self-concept of those who lead them must be considered. Is the physician a technician, or a moral agent? What virtues define a good clinician, is it competence alone, or compassion, humility, and justice as well? What does moral courage look like in a system that rewards efficiency over empathy? How do we form not just skilled professionals, but wise healers?

This question moves from policy to personhood. It calls healthcare leaders to cultivate character as deeply as they cultivate knowledge. The vocational question recognizes that one must understand the role of the healer fundamentally in shaping the culture of healthcare organizations. If healers are viewed primarily as technical experts who apply evidence-based protocols, systems optimized for efficiency and standardization will be stressed and created. On the other hand, if healers are viewed as moral agents called to accompany patients through suffering, systems must be built that allow for presence, relationship, and personalization.

Consider the difference between a physician who sees herself as a technician applying medical science and one who sees herself as a healer accompanying patients through illness. Both may prescribe the same medications and order the same tests, but the quality of the encounter will be fundamentally different. The healer will attend not only to the disease but to the person experiencing the disease. She will recognize that her presence itself is therapeutic, that her words can heal or harm, and that her role extends beyond the purely technical to encompass the emotional and existential dimensions of illness.

For healthcare leaders, this vocational question has profound implications for recruitment, training, and organizational culture. Are hiring and promotion based solely on technical competence, or are character, compassion, and commitment to service being considered? Are training programs focused exclusively on clinical skills, or do they also address moral formation and the cultivation of healing presence? Does the organizational culture reward solely productivity metrics, or does it also recognize and celebrate exemplary care relationships?

The vocational question also challenges leaders to consider their own calling. What does it mean to be a healthcare leader? Is leadership primarily about managing resources and optimizing processes, or is it about creating conditions where healing can flourish? Leaders who understand their role as a vocation, in which they feel called to serve others, will lead differently than those who view it as merely a job or career advancement.

The Structural Question: "What Kind of System Best Serves Human Dignity?"

Leaders must ask how organizational forms reflect moral commitments. Do their structures prioritize the patient, or the payer? Are metrics and data tools used for the purpose of gaining wisdom, or substitutes for it? How are systems designed that embody trust, equity, and compassion and not just compliance? What would a healthcare culture look like if its foundation were virtue rather than volume?

This structural question recognizes that systems are not morally neutral. The way healthcare delivery is organized, the incentives created, the processes designed, and the metrics measured all reflect and reinforce particular values. A system built primarily around maximizing revenue will inevitably create pressures that compromise care. A system built around honoring human dignity will make different structural choices.

Consider how different reimbursement structures shape care. Fee-for-service incentivizes volume over value, potentially leading to overtreatment. Capitation models can incentivize withholding care to reduce costs. Value-based care attempts to align incentives with outcomes, but defining and measuring "value" remains challenging. Each structure reflects different assumptions about what constitutes good care and creates different pressures on providers. Leaders must understand these dynamics and work to align structural incentives with the organization's stated values.

The structural question also addresses issues of access and equity. Does the system serve all members of the community, or only those who can pay? Are facilities located conveniently for vulnerable populations, or only in affluent areas? Are services offered in multiple languages and with appropriate cultural sensitivity? These are not merely operational questions but moral ones that reflect the level of commitment to human dignity.

For emerging leaders, this structural question demands a systems thinking approach. It requires understanding how organizational design, incentive structures, technology choices, and cultural norms interact to create the actual experience of care. It calls for the courage to redesign systems that may be profitable or efficient but fail to serve human dignity. It necessitates working across traditional boundaries to create structures that truly support the healing mission of healthcare.

THE STRATEGY DEVELOPMENT PROCESS

Now, having answered these fundamental worldview questions, which serve as governing boundaries for all strategic decisions, healthcare leaders can begin the actual work of strategy development. These foundational answers provide the framework within which strategic choices are made which govern operations that maximizes the potential of hoped-for outcomes. Without this framework, strategy becomes rudderless, pulled by competing pressures without a clear sense of direction.

However, strategy development is no longer a "one-and-done" activity that occurs during annual strategic planning retreats. The speed of change in healthcare has accelerated dramatically. Rapidly advancing technologies (artificial intelligence, robotics, 3D printing, nanotechnology, genomics, and others) are transforming healthcare at an unprecedented pace (Diamandis & Kraft, 2025). What once took months or years to accomplish can now be made obsolete within a few hours or days.

Healthcare leaders must commit to a continuous Strategy Development Process that is in constant review and reconsideration. This requires changing one's mindset from seeking a static plan to one that embraces change and eschews the status quo. This is particularly difficult for large organizations that find themselves caught in a "sunk-cost fallacy" in which so much capital, time, and systems have been invested that even when the world has changed, they double-down and plod forward without considering that they may be fortifying their position of irrelevance.

The Strategy Development Process is comprised of six-interconnected components, each building upon the others. While presented sequentially, in practice these components operate in a continuous cycle, with insights from later stages informing earlier ones.

Strategic Foresight

Strategic Foresight is the beginning of strategy development for it provides an understanding of the present conditions surrounding an organization. It looks outward at the driving trends across various industries (not just healthcare) recognizing that if these trends continue unabated, they will create problems or, on the positive side, unforeseen opportunities for the organization. This is not an exercise in prediction but in preparation. The goal is not to forecast the future accurately but to be ready for multiple possible futures.

Trends are uncovered through environmental scanning using the STEEPLE model, which examines Social, Technical, Economic, Environmental, Political, Legal, and Ethical sector trends. For each sector, leaders must ask: What are the major shifts occurring? What forces are driving these shifts? What would happen if current trajectories continue? What disruptive changes might alter these trajectories?

This is where the concept of signals becomes critical. In strategic foresight, a signal is any sign that something might be changing, as an early indicator of a potential shift in how the world works, even if that change is still emerging on the fringes of awareness (Hiltunen, 2008; Sarpong, Maclean, & Davies, 2013). Signals can be technological, social, cultural, or behavioral. The important thing is not their intensity, but what they reveal about what might be forming just over the horizon.

Some signals are loud and easily recognized. Others are faint, ambiguous, and easy to overlook. Both, however, offer insight into where the future might be headed. Organizations often fail not because they don't see change coming, but because they filter out signals that don't fit their current mental models (Day & Schoemaker, 2005). Listening to both strong and weak signals is essential for navigating uncertainty wisely.

- *Strong signals* are the trends that are clearly visible and widely acknowledged. For example, healthcare leaders today are all aware of the growing cost of care, widespread workforce shortages, and the surge in digital health tools designed to increase efficiency or expand access (Bates et al., 2018; Shanafelt et al., 2022). These signals show up in board reports, executive dashboards, and national headlines. They are the symptoms of the present and often the drivers of short-term strategic plans.

- *Weak signals*, by contrast, are quieter. They are the early signs of change that often go unnoticed because they don't yet have mass visibility or clear data attached to them (Ansoff, 1975; Hiltunen, 2008). Yet, they can be far more powerful. Consider the subtle trend of patients avoiding formal healthcare channels, not out of convenience, but due to distrust or fatigue; or the rise of informal peer-support groups in underserved communities; or the quiet departure of young clinicians who choose not to renew their contracts, not due to burnout alone, but because they feel disillusioned with the very structure of care delivery. These are weak signals. But taken together, they suggest deeper shifts in values, expectations, and legitimacy. Sometimes, weak signals come from sources that a leader might ignore simply because they originate outside of their usual mainstream communication networks. Failing to consider signals from these sources could result in unmitigated disaster for an organization. Leaders who fail to do this as part of their environmental scanning processes, must consider unorthodox sources with as much interest as those commonly found. This means that a competent strategist must seek out sources that might herald views contrary to their own.

Unfortunately, many health systems are structurally attuned to manage strong signals while ignoring weak ones. Recent data suggest that around 70 percent of healthcare leaders recognize that their sector faces major disruption and future-oriented challenges, yet fewer than 10 percent believe their organizations are adequately equipped or have embedded foresight in their strategic processes (Softheon, 2025; Meskó, et al., 2024). One reason foresight remains underutilized in healthcare leadership may be that many executives are struggling even with short-term strategic alignment in the face of volatility, in fact, 61% of healthcare executives are actively rethinking their short-term strategies due to ongoing market, regulatory, and policy uncertainty (PwC, 2025). This instability is compounded by a high rate of leadership turnover. In 2024 alone, nearly 18% of hospital CEOs left their positions, reflecting an erosion of organizational continuity and long-range planning capacity (American College of Healthcare Executives [ACHE], 2024). These patterns underscore a broader reality; healthcare operates within a VUCA environment (volatile, uncertain, complex, and ambiguous) which challenges traditional linear planning models and requires more adaptive, responsive leadership practices (Syamsir et al., 2025). Without the capacity to plan beyond immediate crises, many organizations miss the early signals of transformation, focusing instead on reactive strategies that may no longer be sufficient.

Foresight, at its core, is not about predicting the future, it's about preparing for it. It invites leaders to notice small changes before they escalate, to ask deeper questions before disruptions take hold, and to build adaptive capacity instead of relying solely on reactive mechanisms. In doing so, it transforms uncertainty from something to fear into something to engage. To rebuild trust and navigate a healthcare environment marked by complexity and fatigue, leaders must tune their attention to the margins. Weak signals are not distractions, rather, they are invitations. Yet these weak signals often provide the earliest warning of transformative shifts. They whisper that *something new is happening*. And if one listens carefully, they may have a better chance to shape that future, before it crashes into the present. The most skilled foresight specialists have finely-tuned abilities to distinguish meaningful signals from noise.

Strategic Foresight is not a one-time activity but requires constant assessment. Trends emerge regardless of organizational awareness. Ignorance is no excuse when a trend that was foreseeable disrupts operations. Leaders must establish processes for continuous environmental scanning, dedicating time and resources to looking beyond the immediate operational horizon.

Example: Rural Healthcare Access

A rural hospital system conducts a STEEPLE analysis and identifies several converging trends: (1) Social: increasing preference for care delivery in home settings; (2) Technical: maturation of telehealth platforms and remote monitoring devices for both chronic- and acute-care management in the home setting through hospital-at-home programs (AHA, 2025); (3) Economic: continued reimbursement challenges for rural hospitals; (4) Environmental: improving broadband infrastructure even in rural areas; (5) Political: growing state and federal support for telehealth; (6) Legal: relaxation of interstate licensing requirements for telemedicine; (7) Ethical: recognition that health equity includes access to specialty care. These trends suggest that traditional models of hospital-based care may face increasing pressure, while new models of distributed care could become viable.

Strategic Thinking

The next step in the process is Strategic Thinking; where the organization considers the impact of a particular trend on its present operations. It personalizes the problem caused by a driving trend to the organization specifically. This phase deals with problems from a 360-degree perspective, considering the negative outcomes if no strategies are implemented that will confront the trend from wreaking havoc on the organization's future.

Strategic Thinking also considers the possible alternative futures that a trend might create for the organization. This is where leaders look for opportunities to operate in spaces that no competitor has considered. It requires being very aware of how the organization currently produces its goods, services, experiences, and transformations, as well as understanding how competitors operate.

This phase demands rigorous honesty about organizational vulnerabilities. Leaders must ask: If this trend continues, how specifically will our operations be affected? What revenue streams might be threatened? What capabilities might become obsolete? What new needs might emerge that the organization is not currently equipped to meet? The goal is not to generate anxiety but to create clarity about the stakes involved.

Equally important is opportunity identification. What advantages might the organization have in addressing this trend? What unique capabilities or relationships could be leverage? What new value could be created that competitors cannot? Where might this trend take the organization that could be better than where they are now?

Example: Rural Healthcare Access (Continued)

The rural hospital system realizes that if current trends continue, their inpatient volumes may decline as patients increasingly access care through telehealth or travel to urban centers for non-emergency care. Emergency department visits may remain stable, but profitable elective procedures could decrease. On the other hand, the organization recognizes an opportunity: they have deep community trust, existing relationships with local patients, and physical infrastructure that could be repurposed. They could potentially become the local hub for coordinating distributed care rather than the sole provider of centralized care.

Strategic Innovation

Strategic Innovation is where solutions to the problems identified in the Foresight stage are developed. This phase requires a curious mind willing to explore unconventional approaches. It demands listening carefully to the needs, desires, and hopes of customers; in this case, patients and communities. It requires an inquisitive mindset that is unwilling to be controlled by fear of failure and is willing to take calculated risks.

Innovation in healthcare is not merely about adopting the latest technology. It is about fundamentally rethinking how value is created and delivered. The most significant innovations often come from applying insights from other industries or recombining existing capabilities in new ways. Leaders must create environments where experimentation is encouraged and failure is treated as a learning opportunity rather than a career-limiting event.

Also of importance is how innovation gets diffused into the market. Not all innovations succeed, regardless of their merit. Understanding adoption patterns, identifying early adopters, and designing implementation strategies that account for organizational and market readiness are all crucial to successful innovation.

Example: Rural Healthcare Access (Continued)

The rural hospital system develops an innovative "hub-and-spoke" model. The main hospital becomes a hub coordinating a network of care delivery points including: (1) community care coordinators embedded in local churches and community centers; (2) home-based monitoring for chronic disease patients using connected devices; (3) mobile clinics for preventive care and routine follow-ups; (4) partnerships with retail pharmacies for basic health screenings; (5) telehealth connections to specialist networks in urban centers. This model flips the traditional paradigm of patients traveling to care; instead, care travels to patients.

Example: Academic Medical Center Addressing Clinician Burnout: Recognizing that EHR burden is a major driver of clinician dissatisfaction, an academic medical center innovates by creating a team of "medical scribes 2.0," trained personnel who not only document visits but also handle pre-visit chart review, post-visit orders and referrals, and patient communication. Additionally, they implement AI-powered clinical decision support that reduces rather than increases clicking. The innovation is not just technological but also workflow-based, fundamentally redesigning how clinicians interact with documentation systems.

Strategic Planning

The fourth element of strategy development is Strategic Planning, where the strategist provides a concrete plan for making a particular innovation happen. This is where vision becomes operational. The plan must answer: Who will do what? What resources are required? What is the timeline? What milestones will indicate progress?

This phase requires a SWOT analysis (Strengths, Weaknesses, Opportunities, Threats) to determine whether the organization has the resources to bring about the innovation, and to be aware of possible opportunities or threats if the innovation is brought to market. Not all innovations can or should be pursued; as Strategic Planning requires making difficult choices about where to invest limited resources for maximum impact.

The plan must be both ambitious and realistic. It should stretch the organization's capabilities without breaking them. It must account for resistance to change, resource constraints, competing priorities, and the inevitable obstacles that will arise during implementation. A good plan includes contingencies and decision points where leaders can reassess and adjust course as needed.

Example: Rural Healthcare Access (Continued)

SWOT Analysis reveals: Strengths include community trust, existing infrastructure, and committed staff. Weaknesses include limited capital, no experience with distributed care models, and inadequate IT infrastructure. Opportunities include state grant funding for rural health innovations and partnerships with technology vendors. Threats include resistance from staff accustomed to traditional models and potential pushback from referring physicians who fear losing patients.

The plan includes: Phase 1 (Months 1-6): Pilot program in two communities with 100 patients. Phase 2 (Months 7-12): Expand to five communities with 500 patients. Phase 3 (Year 2): Full deployment across service area. Specific responsibilities are assigned: Chief Medical Officer leads clinical protocol development, Chief Operations Officer manages infrastructure and logistics, Chief Financial Officer secures funding and develops financial models, Chief Nursing Officer trains community-care coordinators.

Example: Specialty Clinic Addressing Appointment Access: A specialty clinic frustrated by 90-day wait times conducts SWOT and realizes its strength is its highly-skilled specialists but its weakness is the assumption that specialists must see every patient. The plan: create an advanced practice provider (APP) team trained to handle routine follow-ups and uncomplicated new referrals, reserving specialist time for complex cases. Implementation over six months will involve APP recruitment and training, protocol development with specialist input, and phased introduction of the new model, with success measured by reduced wait times and maintained quality metrics.

Strategic Implementation

Next in the process is Strategic Implementation; where plans become reality. At this stage when and specifically how the innovation will be implemented is determined. Implementation requires careful attention be paid to change management, communication, training, and continuous problem-solving.

Leaders must recognize that implementation is never a straightforward process of executing a plan, because unexpected obstacles will arise; as resistance will emerge from unexpected quarters, technology will not work as advertised, and people will need more support than anticipated. The key to successful implementation is to maintain flexibility while staying committed to the core objectives.

Effective implementation requires creating quick wins that build momentum and credibility. It demands over-communication about why changes are being made, what is expected of people, and how success will be measured. It necessitates supporting front-line staff through the turbulence of change and celebrating early successes to maintain morale.

Example: Rural Healthcare Access (Continued)

Implementation begins with intensive training for community-care coordinators, including two weeks of clinical protocols and three weeks of field experience with preceptors. Technology infrastructure is deployed to pilot sites with redundant systems to prevent failures. Weekly huddles with pilot teams identify and resolve problems in real-time. Monthly town halls communicate progress to the broader organization, and offer real stories of improved patient access that are shared to build broader support within the organization and the broader community. Physicians rotate through community sites to understand the model firsthand and provide clinical guidance.

Strategic Analysis and Assessment

The final step in the process is Strategic Analysis and Assessment; where the strategist considers the success (or lack thereof) of the implemented innovation and determines what tweaks to the system will make the product better or more effective. This phase requires intellectual honesty and the willingness to admit when something is not working.

The most dangerous trap in this phase is the "sunk-cost fallacy," which is the tendency to continue investing in a failing initiative because of the resources already expended. Leaders must be willing to pivot or even abandon initiatives that are not working; freeing resources for more promising opportunities. The question is not "How much have we invested?" but rather "Given what we now know, what is the best path forward?"

Assessment should be both quantitative and qualitative; because metrics matter as do the stories and experiences of those involved. Leaders should ask: Are we achieving the intended outcomes? What unintended consequences have emerged? What is being learned that should inform our next steps? How has this initiative changed the organization's capabilities and capacities?

Example: Rural Healthcare Access (Continued)

After six months, assessment reveals: Patient access has improved significantly with average time to first appointment dropped from 45 days to 10 days. Patient satisfaction scores increased by 18 points. However, some challenges emerged: community coordinators feel isolated and would benefit from more peer support; some patients prefer in-person hospital or office visits despite longer waits; technology reliability in remote areas remains problematic; and, specialist physicians worry about liability for care delivered by coordinators.

Based on assessment, refinements include: monthly in-person gatherings for community coordinators to reduce isolation and share best practices; offering patients choice between community-based and hospital-based care; investing in better cellular-based backup systems; and, implementing structured supervision protocols between specialists and coordinators with clear delegation of authority. The core model is sound and should be expanded, but modifications as proposed should be implemented.

Example: Specialty Clinic (continued): Assessment after six months shows wait times reduced from 90 to 45 days; a solid improvement but not within the target range of 30 days. Patient outcomes remain excellent; however, specialists report that many patients that are being triaged to APPs actually need specialist evaluation; resulting in the creation of inefficiencies. Refinement: enhance referral screening protocols, add a brief specialist phone consultation before appointment scheduling to improve triage accuracy, and expand APP team by two more providers. With these adjustments, the model can achieve its goals.

FUTURE DIRECTIONS

Healthcare leaders who hope to bring about flourishing organizations that truly usher in patient-centered transformation, must develop internal strategy development teams who are dedicated to continual environmental scanning. Putting the strategy development process into practice will broaden understanding as to how reforms should be considered and implemented. Great organizations are those that have eyes to see what lies ahead and just over the horizon. Practice makes perfect.

CONCLUSION

The Strategy Development Process provides healthcare leaders with a complete roadmap for actionable reform. Through this structured approach, leaders can transform theoretical insights into tangible strategies that not only address current pain points but also anticipate future challenges. What makes this process so powerful is that when used properly, it can uniquely position an organization for success in an increasingly complex and rapidly changing environment.

However, the process cannot function effectively without the foundational work of answering the five fundamental worldview questions. These questions; about purpose, anthropology, morality, vocation, and structure, provide the governing framework within which all strategic decisions must operate. Attempting to develop strategy without this structure is like trying to build a house without first laying a solid foundation. The structure may stand temporarily, but it will ultimately fail under pressure.

The integration of worldview clarity with strategic rigor creates a powerful approach to healthcare leadership. Leaders who understand why their organizations exist, what they believe about patients and healers, and how their systems should reflect these values will make fundamentally different decisions than those who focus solely on operational efficiency and financial performance. Both groups may succeed in the short term, but only the former will build organizations capable of sustained excellence and meaningful impact.

Fulltime strategy development engagement provides opportunities to truly solve problems that never get resolved. By maintaining constant vigilance through Strategic Foresight, leaders can identify emerging trends before they become crises. Through Strategic Thinking, they can understand implications specific to their organizations; coupled with Strategic Innovation, they can develop creative solutions. Strategic Planning ensures these solutions are grounded in operational reality. Strategic Implementation brings them to life. And Strategic Analysis closes the loop, ensuring continuous learning and improvement.

The practice of strategy development brings awareness to leaders of driving trends even when signals are weak. This allows leaders to, in part, create futures of their own determination rather than being bound to pre-determined paths. In an era of exponential change, where Dr. Diamandis and Dr. Kraft have shown that technologies are advancing at unprecedented rates, this proactive stance is not optional, rather it is essential for survival.

For emerging healthcare leaders, the task ahead is both daunting and exhilarating. The healthcare system faces genuine crises: eroding trust, misaligned incentives, burned-out clinicians, frustrated patients, and unsustainable costs. Yet these challenges also represent opportunities for transformative leadership. Leaders who are willing to return to first principles, who have the courage to ask fundamental questions, and who commit to rigorous and continuous strategy development can chart new paths forward.

The choice facing healthcare leaders is clear; continue with incremental reforms that address symptoms while leaving fundamental structures unchanged, or commit to the more difficult task, but ultimately more rewarding work, of building reform upon strong foundations. The former may offer the comfort of familiarity and the appearance of progress, but the latter offers the possibility of genuine organizational and patient transformation.

As Vince Lombardi understood, excellence begins with mastery of fundamentals; as Barry Marshall demonstrated, transformative breakthroughs often require challenging conventional wisdom; as Kouzes and Posner have shown, credibility is the foundation of effective leadership; and, as Pine and Gilmore have articulated, true value is created through transformation, not merely transactions.

Healthcare reform built upon strong foundations is not easy, but it is necessary. It demands intellectual rigor, moral courage, and practical wisdom. It requires leaders who are willing to think deeply about fundamental questions while also attending to operational details. It necessitates organizations that can hold together clarity of purpose with flexibility of approach.

The path forward begins with each leader making a personal choice to answer some critical questions: Will I invest the effort to understand and articulate my organization's foundational assumptions? Will I commit to continuous strategic development rather than episodic planning? Will I have the courage to make decisions based on core values even when they conflict with short-term pressures? Will I create environments where innovation can flourish and where people can reconnect with the healing purpose that drew them to healthcare in the first place?

These questions cannot be answered abstractly. They require concrete actions and sustained commitment. But for leaders who are willing to engage in this work, the rewards extend far beyond organizational success; for they include the satisfaction of building something genuinely valuable, the joy of creating environments where healing can flourish, and the knowledge that their leadership has made a meaningful difference in the lives of patients and communities.

In the end, healthcare reform built upon strong foundations is not merely a professional obligation for healthcare leaders it is a moral imperative. Patients deserve systems that honor their dignity, providers deserve work environments that allow them to practice their calling, and communities deserve healthcare organizations that genuinely serve rather than merely extract value. Building such systems requires returning to first principles, thinking strategically about the future, and leading with courage and integrity. The work is difficult, but it is precisely the work that this moment demands.

REFERENCES

Accelerant Research. (2025, September 2). *Branding backlash: What Cracker Barrel, Target, and Bud Lite can teach us about the power of market research*. https://www.accelerantresearch.com/articles/branding-backlash-what-cracker-barrel-target-and-bud-light-can-teach-us-about-the-power-of-market-research

Ahmed, N. (2005). 23 years of the discovery of *Helicobacter pylori*: Is the debate over? *Annals of Clinical Microbiology and Antimicrobials*, *4*(1), 17. Advance online publication. DOI: 10.1186/1476-0711-4-17 PMID: 16262889

Ali, I., Ahmad, W., Ullah, A. R., Khan, F., Ijaz, M., Khan, S., & Khan, T. M. (2021). Knowledge, attitude, and barriers toward ADRs reporting among health-care professionals at tertiary care health settings in Peshawar, Pakistan: A web based study. *Hospital Pharmacy*, *56*(4), 384–391. DOI: 10.1177/0018578720910401 PMID: 34381279

American College of Healthcare Executives. (2024). *Hospital leadership crisis 2025: CEO action plan*. https://www.thehealthcareexecutive.net/blog/blog-hospital-leadership-crisis-2025

American Hospital Association. (2025, July). *Fact sheet: Extending the hospital-at-home program*. https://www.aha.org/fact-sheets/2024-08-06-fact-sheet-extending-hospital-home-program

Ansoff, H. I. (1975). Managing strategic surprise by response to weak signals. *California Management Review*, *18*(2), 21–33. DOI: 10.2307/41164635

Bardosh, K., De Figueiredo, A., Gur-Arie, R., Jamrozik, E., Doidge, J., Lemmens, T., Keshavjee, S., Graham, J. E., & Baral, S. (2022). The unintended consequences of COVID-19 vaccine policy: Why mandates, passports and restrictions may cause more harm than good. *BMJ Global Health*, *7*(5), e008684. Advance online publication. DOI: 10.1136/bmjgh-2022-008684 PMID: 35618306

Bates, D. W., Saria, S., Ohno-Machado, L., Shah, A., & Escobar, G. (2018). Big data in health care: Using analytics to identify and manage high-risk and high-cost patients. *Health Affairs*, *33*(7), 1123–1131. DOI: 10.1377/hlthaff.2014.0041 PMID: 25006137

Blendon, R. J., & Benson, J. M. (2022). Trust in medicine, the health system & public health. *Daedalus*, *151*(4), 67–82. DOI: 10.1162/daed_a_01944

Cassie, B. (2025, September 4). *Big Pharma's worst nightmare? FDA now exposes drug harms in real time.* https://www.newstarget.com/2025-09-04-big-pharma-nightmare-fda-drug-harms.html

Christensen, C. M. (2003). *The innovator's dilemma.* HarperBusiness Essentials.

Crichton, M. (2003, January 17). *Aliens cause global warming* [Caltech Michelin Lecture]. https://stephenschneider.stanford.edu/Publications/PDF_Papers/Crichton2003.pdf

Day, G. S., & Schoemaker, P. J. H. (2005). *Peripheral vision: Detecting the weak signals that will make or break your company.* Harvard Business Review Press.

Diamandis, P. H., & Kraft, D. (2025). *Exponential medicine* [Conference]. https://danielkraftmd.net/exponential-medicine

Flint, A. (2024, October 22). *Avoiding discussion of vaccine side effects isn't pro-vaccine. It's anti-science.* https://harvardpublichealth.org/policy-practice/vaccine-side-effects-are-real-we-should-talk-about-them/

Gallup. (2025a). *2025 confidence in institutions poll.* https://news.gallup.com/poll/1597/confidence-institutions.aspx

Gallup. (2025b). *2025 healthcare system poll.* https://news.gallup.com/poll/4708/healthcare-system.aspx

Greenhalgh, T., Wherton, J., Papoutsi, C., Lynch, J., Hughes, G., A'Court, C., Hinder, S., Fahy, N., Procter, R., & Shaw, S. (2020). Beyond adoption: A new framework for theorizing and evaluating nonadoption, abandonment, and challenges to the scale-up, spread, and sustainability of health and care technologies. *Journal of Medical Internet Research, 19*(11), e367. DOI: 10.2196/jmir.8775 PMID: 29092808

Hiltunen, E. (2008). The future sign and its three dimensions. *Futures, 40*(3), 247–260. DOI: 10.1016/j.futures.2007.08.021

Howe, N. (2023). *The fourth turning is here.* Simon & Schuster.

Jutley, G. S., Pucci, M., Ferner, R. E., & Coleman, J. J. (2024). Adverse drug reactions and interactions. *Medicine, 52*(1), 15–22. DOI: 10.1016/j.mpmed.2023.10.006 PMID: 38221612

Kouzes, J. M., & Posner, B. Z. (2011). *Credibility: How leaders gain and lose it, why people demand it* (2nd ed.). Jossey-Bass. DOI: 10.1002/9781118983867

Kuhn, T. S. (1962). *The structure of scientific revolutions.* University of Chicago Press.

Maraniss, D. (2000). *When pride still mattered: A life of Vince Lombardi*. Simon & Schuster.

Marshall, B. J., & Warren, J. R. (2005). *Helicobacter pylori and peptic ulcer disease* [Nobel Prize in Physiology or Medicine]. https://www.nobelprize.org/prizes/medicine/2005/marshall/facts/

McClain, C. R. (2025). Trade secrets and transparency in medical research. *Journal of Healthcare Ethics*, *14*(2), 112–128.

Meskó, B., Kristóf, T., Dhunnoo, P., Árvai, N., & Katonai, G. (2024). Exploring the need for medical futures studies: Insights from a scoping review of health care foresight. *Journal of Medical Internet Research*, *26*, e57148. DOI: 10.2196/57148 PMID: 39383528

Miller, J. E., Wilenzick, M., Ritcey, N., Ross, J. S., & Mello, M. M. (2017). Measuring clinical trial transparency: An empirical analysis of newly approved drugs and large pharmaceutical companies. *BMJ Open*, *7*(12), e017917. Advance online publication. DOI: 10.1136/bmjopen-2017-017917 PMID: 29208616

Naddaf, M. (2025, September 23). Journals infiltrated with 'copycat' papers that can be written by AI. *Nature*. https://www.nature.com/articles/d41586-025-03046-z

Pew Research Center. (2025). *How Americans view AI and its impact on people and society*. https://www.pewresearch.org/wp-content/uploads/sites/20/2025/09/PS_2025.9.15_AI-and-its-impact_report.pdf

Physicians Practice. (2024, April 23). *What over 2 million patients say about their healthcare experiences*. https://www.physicianspractice.com/view/what-over-2-million-patients-say-about-their-healthcare-experiences

Pine, B. J., & Gilmore, J. H. (2007). *Authenticity: What consumers really want*. Harvard Business Review Press.

Pine, B. J., & Gilmore, J. H. (2020). *The experience economy*. Harvard Business Review Press.

Porterfield, C. (2021, December 21). Dr. Fauci on GOP criticism: 'Attacks on me, quite frankly, are attacks on science.' *Forbes*. https://www.forbes.com/sites/carlieporterfield/2021/06/09/fauci-on-gop-criticism-attacks-on-me-quite-frankly-are-attacks-on-science/

PwC. (2025, May 29). *Healthcare execs rethink strategy amid market and policy volatility*. Fierce Healthcare. https://www.fiercehealthcare.com/providers/healthcare-leaders-rethinking-short-term-strategy-amid-market-policy-volatility-pwc

Rucker, P., Miller, M., & Armstrong, D. (2023, March 25). How Cigna saves millions by having its doctors reject claims without reading them. *ProPublica*. https://www.propublica.org/article/cigna-pxdx-medical-health-insurance-rejection-claims

Sarpong, D., Maclean, M., & Davies, C. (2013). A matter of foresight: How practices enable (or impede) organizational foresightfulness. *European Management Journal*, *31*(6), 613–625. DOI: 10.1016/j.emj.2013.03.004

Shanafelt, T. D., West, C. P., Dyrbye, L. N., Trockel, M., Tutty, M., Wang, H., Carlasare, L. E., & Sinsky, C. (2022). Changes in burnout and satisfaction with work-life integration in physicians during the first 2 years of the COVID-19 pandemic. *Mayo Clinic Proceedings*, *97*(12), 2248–2258. DOI: 10.1016/j.mayocp.2022.09.002 PMID: 36229269

Softheon. (2025, September). *Strategy in action healthcare executive survey: 4 key insights for health plans*. https://www.softheon.com/blog/strategy-in-action-healthcare-executive-survey-4-key-insights-for-health-plans

Spredemann, A. (2025, November 9). How AI is supercharging scientific fraud. *The Epoch Times*. https://www.theepochtimes.com/article/how-ai-is-supercharging-scientific-fraud-5937211

Syamsir, S., Saputra, N., & Mulia, R. (2025). Leadership agility in a VUCA world: A systematic review, conceptual insights, and research directions. *Cogent Business & Management*, *12*(1), 2482022. Advance online publication. DOI: 10.1080/23311975.2025.2482022

The Beryl Institute. (2023, January). *Consumer perspectives on patient experience in the U.S. PX Pulse*. https://theberylinstitute.org/wp-content/uploads/woocommerce_uploads/2023/02/PXPulse_Q1_Jan2023-nc4w5c.pdf

The Physicians Foundation. (2018). *2018 survey of America's physicians: Practice patterns and perspectives*. https://physiciansfoundation.org/wp-content/uploads/2018/09/physicians-survey-results-final-2018.pdf

Ulrich, A. (2025, July 8). *8 best AI medical documentation tools for healthcare in 2025*. https://austinulrich.com/best-ai-medical-documentation-tools-for-healthcare

U.S. Government Accountability Office. (2025, September 25). *Healthcare is becoming more consolidated—including physicians. What effect is it having?* https://www.gao.gov/blog/health-care-becoming-more-consolidated-including-physicians.-what-effect-it-having

Van Noorden, R. (2023, December 12). More than 10,000 research papers were retracted in 2023—a new record. *Nature*. https://www.nature.com/articles/d41586-023-03974-8

ADDITIONAL READING

Healey, B. (2018). *The principles of healthcare leadership*. Health Administration Press.

Hines, A., & Bishop, P. (2006). *Thinking about the future: Guidelines for strategic foresight*. Social Technologies.

Howe, N. (2023). *The fourth turning is here*. Simon & Schuster.

Kouzes, J. M., & Posner, B. Z. (2011). *Credibility: How leaders gain and lose it, why people demand it* (2nd ed.). Jossey-Bass. DOI: 10.1002/9781118983867

Kuhn, T. S. (1962). *The structure of scientific revolutions*. University of Chicago Press.

Loehle, C. (1996). *Thinking strategically: Power tools for Personal and Professional Advancement*. Cambridge University Press. DOI: 10.1017/CBO9780511525308

Pagano, B., & Pagano, E. (2004). *The transparency edge; How credibility can make or break you in business*. McGraw-Hill.

Pine, B. J., & Gilmore, J. H. (2007). *Authenticity: What consumers really want*. Harvard Business Review Press.

Pine, B. J., & Gilmore, J. H. (2020). *The experience economy*. Harvard Business Review Press.

Sanders, T. (1998). *Strategic thinking and the new science: Planning in the midst of chaos, complexity, and change*. The Free Press.

KEY TERMS AND DEFINITIONS

Customer Sacrifice: The gap between what a customer wants exactly and what they settle for; a critical metric for understanding unmet patient needs in healthcare delivery.

Economic Value Progression: The evolution of economic offerings from commodities to goods to services to experiences to transformations, with each stage representing higher value creation.

Environmental Scanning: The process of looking outside of the organization's industry for driving trends that might impact the organization. This process is continual and considers both strong and weak signals.

Healthcare Consolidation: The trend of physicians leaving private practice to join larger organizations such as hospitals, health insurers, and private equity firms, resulting in standardized care delivery.

Mass Customization: The ability to provide individually customized goods or services through flexible processes and organizational structures while maintaining efficiency.

Patient-Centered Care: A healthcare delivery model that prioritizes individual patient needs, preferences, and values, ensuring patient values guide all clinical decisions.

Physician Burnout: A syndrome characterized by emotional exhaustion, depersonalization, and reduced sense of personal accomplishment, particularly prevalent among healthcare providers facing administrative burdens.

STEEPLE Analysis: A strategic planning tool examining Social, Technical, Economic, Environmental, Political, Legal, and Ethical trends that may impact an organization.

Strategic Foresight: The systematic exploration of potential futures through environmental scanning and signal detection to prepare organizations for multiple possible scenarios.

Weak Signals: Early indicators of potential change that are ambiguous and easily overlooked but may herald transformative shifts in the environment.

Worldview: The set of basic assumptions that defines one's reality and provides a framework for decision-making, particularly concerning fundamental questions of purpose, anthropology, and morality.

Chapter 13
Foundations in Practice:
Practical Applications of Strategy Development

Barry A. Doublestein
http://orcid.org/0009-0009-8994-2611
Regent University, USA

Walter T. Lee
http://orcid.org/0000-0002-5487-3603
Duke University School of Medicine, USA

Richard M. Pfohl
Belhaven University, USA

ABSTRACT

This chapter examines how foundational worldview questions and a structured strategy development process translate into practical healthcare transformation. Through three detailed case studies, the chapter demonstrates how identity, purpose, moral vision, vocational understanding, and structural design shape effective strategic outcomes. The analysis highlights behavioral health integration, value-based care innovation, and community centered transformation as examples of strategy grounded in philosophical coherence rather than technical optimization alone. Across diverse organizational contexts, common themes emerge including identity clarity, workforce engagement, balanced measurement systems, and the integration of aspiration with pragmatic implementation. The chapter argues that healthcare strategy must unite analytical rigor with philosophical depth, showing how organizations that align mission, culture, and operational structures are better positioned to achieve sustainable transformation that supports patients, clinicians, and communities.

DOI: 10.4018/979-8-3373-2577-4.ch013

INTRODUCTION

Chapter One established the theoretical foundation for healthcare strategy development grounded in five fundamental worldview questions and a six-stage Strategy Development Process. This chapter transitions from theory to practice, demonstrating how organizations have applied these frameworks to address complex healthcare challenges. Through detailed case studies and practical examples, one will examine how the philosophical foundations translate into actionable strategies that generate meaningful outcomes for patients, clinicians, and communities.

The cases presented here represent diverse contexts within the healthcare landscape: a large integrated delivery system addressing behavioral health access, an innovative health system pioneering value-based care models, and a community hospital navigating organizational transformation. Each example illustrates different aspects of the strategy development framework while highlighting common themes that transcend organizational size, geography, or mission.

These practical applications demonstrate that effective healthcare strategy requires more than analytical rigor or operational excellence. It demands careful attention to the foundational questions of purpose, identity, values, and meaning that shape organizational culture and guide decision-making. When strategy aligns with these deeper elements, organizations create the conditions for sustainable transformation that serves both clinical excellence and human flourishing.

CASE STUDY 1: PROVIDENCE HEALTH & SERVICES—INTEGRATING BEHAVIORAL HEALTH ACROSS THE CARE CONTINUUM

Organizational Context

Providence Health & Services, now Providence St. Joseph Health, is one of the largest not-for-profit healthcare systems in the United States, operating dozens of hospitals and hundreds of clinics across multiple states. Founded in 1856 by the Sisters of Providence, the organization's identity has long been shaped by a moral commitment to serve the poor, the vulnerable, and those pushed to the margins of society. This founding charism was not merely aspirational; it emerged from a theological understanding of healing as an act of mercy, justice, and presence. Over time, this moral narrative became embedded in Providence's institutional memory and public mission statements. However, like many large systems, Providence also faced the pressures of scale, efficiency, and regulatory complexity.

By the early 2010s, Providence confronted a growing contradiction between its stated mission and its lived structures. While the system had developed increasingly sophisticated capabilities for physical health care, patients with behavioral health and substance-use needs were frequently routed into emergency departments as a default point of access. Nationally, emergency departments had become de facto safety nets for mental health crises, a role for which they were poorly designed (Institute of Medicine, 2006). This pattern resulted in prolonged wait times, recurrent crises, and care experiences that often intensified rather than alleviated patient suffering. The system functioned, but it did not heal well.

Internally, clinicians reported moral distress and professional frustration related to this fragmentation. Primary care providers lacked timely access to psychiatric consultation, and frontline caregivers frequently felt ill-equipped to respond to behavioral health needs that presented alongside chronic physical conditions. Caregivers experienced a dissonance between what they believed good care should be and what the system allowed them to provide. Externally, community health needs assessments repeatedly identified behavioral health as one of the most significant unmet needs across Providence service areas. What emerged was not simply an operational deficiency, but a moral contradiction between institutional identity and institutional capability.

I. Application of the Fundamental Questions

The Teleological Question: "What is Healthcare For?"

Providence's behavioral health initiative emerged from a renewed engagement with purpose rather than from purely operational analysis. As a faith-based organization rooted in a long tradition of serving the marginalized, Providence understood healthcare not simply as the delivery of clinical interventions but as participation in whole-person healing. Leadership recognized that the fragmentation of behavioral health services contradicted the organization's historical telos and revealed a misalignment between mission language and institutional practice. Emergency departments functioning as default entry points for mental health crises exposed a system designed for efficiency rather than restoration. By reframing behavioral health integration as a question of purpose, Providence shifted the conversation away from resource scarcity toward moral coherence.

This teleological clarity reshaped strategic decision-making. Leaders acknowledged that integrated behavioral health might not produce immediate financial returns, particularly within reimbursement environments that historically undervalued collaborative care models (Centers for Medicare & Medicaid Services, 2026). Yet the organization concluded that healthcare existed to restore dignity and stability for vulnerable populations, not merely to optimize throughput. Purpose functioned as a governing constraint, limiting acceptable compromises and directing investment toward models aligned with the organization's founding commitments. In this sense, strategy development became an act of fidelity to mission rather than a reactive response to market pressures.

Moreover, the rediscovery of purpose created cultural permission for innovation that might otherwise have appeared financially risky. When purpose precedes planning, difficult decisions can be framed not as departures from tradition but as deeper expressions of it. Providence's leadership framed behavioral health integration as a continuation of its founding charism rather than a modern programmatic addition. This reframing helped align board members, clinicians, and community stakeholders around a shared narrative that healthcare exists to accompany persons in suffering rather than simply to manage disease episodes. Purpose thus served as both ethical compass and strategic catalyst.

The Anthropological Question: "What is a Patient?"

Providence's anthropology challenged reductionist assumptions embedded within traditional healthcare delivery. Patients experiencing behavioral health conditions were frequently treated as disruptions to emergency department flow rather than as persons deserving sustained relational care. Leadership came to recognize that such practices reflected an implicit anthropology inconsistent with the organization's moral commitments. Patients were not defined by diagnoses or utilization patterns but by inherent dignity and complex social realities that required integrated support systems (Blendon & Benson, 2022). This understanding reframed behavioral health not as a specialty silo but as an essential dimension of human wellbeing.

Viewing patients as whole persons reshaped both clinical design and community engagement. Collaborative care models embedded behavioral health specialists within primary care settings, allowing mental health needs to be addressed within trusted relational environments (Archer et al., 2012). Community partnerships extended care beyond hospital walls, acknowledging that healing occurs within social networks rather than isolated clinical encounters. This anthropological shift also addressed stigma, normalizing behavioral health screening and reducing barriers to treatment. By redefining what a patient is, Providence fundamentally altered how care pathways were constructed and how caregivers understood their responsibilities.

Importantly, this anthropological clarity also influenced measurement practices. Rather than focusing exclusively on symptom reduction or utilization metrics, Providence incorporated patient experience and dignity measures into its evaluation framework. Patients were treated as narrators of their own care journeys rather than passive subjects of clinical intervention. Such a perspective reinforced the belief that healing involves relational trust and continuity, elements that cannot be captured fully through quantitative metrics alone.

The Moral Question: "What is the Good We Are Pursuing?"

Providence's leadership articulated a vision of the good that extended beyond traditional measures of efficiency or cost reduction. While reducing emergency department utilization and improving clinical outcomes were important, the organization framed success primarily in terms of dignity, trust, and relational continuity. Behavioral health integration aimed to create care environments where patients felt respected rather than marginalized, challenging prevailing assumptions that value is synonymous with speed or volume (Pine & Gilmore, 2020). The moral good pursued was not merely symptom stabilization but the restoration of human flourishing through compassionate and coordinated care.

Achieving this good required practical wisdom in balancing competing priorities. Investments in workforce training, telehealth infrastructure, and community partnerships demanded significant resources at a time when financial pressures remained high. Leaders recognized that short-term inefficiencies could be morally justified if they contributed to long-term healing outcomes and reduced suffering. By grounding decisions in ethical commitments rather than solely in performance dashboards, Providence demonstrated that healthcare strategy must integrate moral reasoning with operational planning.

The pursuit of the good also required resisting the temptation to define success solely through measurable outputs. Providence leaders acknowledged that certain goods such as restored trust, reduced stigma, and relational continuity are experienced rather than easily quantified. This recognition encouraged a more holistic evaluation of outcomes, reinforcing the idea that healthcare systems must cultivate environments where persons feel seen and accompanied rather than processed.

The Vocational Question: "What Does it Mean to Be a Healer?"

Behavioral health integration forced Providence to reconsider the identity of its caregivers. Historically, clinicians often viewed mental health concerns as outside their scope, contributing to fragmentation and professional frustration. Leadership reframed healing as a shared vocation requiring both technical competence and moral agency. Training initiatives such as trauma-informed care education and Mental Health First Aid sought not only to enhance clinical skill but to cultivate a deeper sense of responsibility for whole-person care (National Council for Mental

Wellbeing, 2021). Formation replaced mere instruction, emphasizing that caregivers participate in a broader mission of accompaniment and restoration.

This vocational framing also addressed widespread burnout and moral distress. Research linking clinician wellbeing to organizational structures underscored the importance of aligning professional identity with institutional expectations (Shanafelt et al., 2016). When caregivers were equipped and supported to address behavioral health needs, they experienced greater coherence between personal calling and daily work. Consultation-liaison psychiatry services and interdisciplinary collaboration reinforced a culture where healing was understood as a collective endeavor rather than an individual burden. The healer became not simply a provider of services but a steward of dignity and relational trust.

The Structural Question: "What Kind of System Best Serves Human Dignity?"

Providence's structural reforms translated philosophical commitments into operational reality. Collaborative care models embedded behavioral health care managers and psychiatric consultants within primary care teams, enabling early intervention and reducing stigma associated with specialty referrals (Archer et al., 2012; Unützer et al., 2013). Tele-behavioral health expanded access across geographically dispersed communities, addressing workforce shortages while preserving continuity of care (Shore et al., 2018; Health Resources and Services Administration, 2025). Electronic health record enhancements supported integrated documentation and communication, reinforcing the relational model of care envisioned by leadership.

Measurement systems further embodied structural alignment with dignity. Providence tracked screening rates, patient experience indicators, caregiver well-being, and clinical outcomes to ensure that integration advanced both operational effectiveness and moral coherence. By designing structures that reinforced justice, prudence, and compassion, the organization demonstrated that systems are not neutral mechanisms but expressions of institutional character. Structure became the durable form of virtue, shaping daily clinical practice in ways consistent with Providence's understanding of healing.

Finally, Providence's structural transformation illustrates that systems shape culture as much as culture shapes systems. When workflows reinforce relational care and interdisciplinary collaboration, caregivers experience alignment between institutional expectations and professional identity. Structural design therefore becomes an ethical act, embedding worldview commitments into daily practice and ensuring that organizational purpose remains visible at the point of care.

II. Results and Key Learnings

Within four years of implementation, Providence achieved significant and measurable improvements across multiple domains (Providence Health & Services, 2022). Depression screening rates in primary care exceeded 85 percent systemwide, reflecting the normalization of behavioral health assessment as part of routine care. More than 20,000 patients were enrolled in collaborative care programs, with approximately 60 percent achieving clinically significant symptom improvement. These outcomes demonstrated that integrated models could deliver both clinical effectiveness and moral coherence.

Emergency department visits for behavioral health conditions decreased by 23 percent in markets with mature implementations, reducing strain on emergency services while improving patient experience (Providence Health & Services, 2022). Importantly, patient experience scores for behavioral health services reached parity with those for general medical care. This parity signaled not only improved access, but reduced stigma and increased dignity in care encounters. The system was no longer routing behavioral health needs to the margins.

Perhaps most significantly, caregiver surveys revealed increased confidence and decreased moral distress related to behavioral health care (Providence Health & Services, 2022). Primary care providers reported feeling supported rather than overwhelmed when caring for patients with mental health and substance-use conditions. This cultural shift represented a fundamental transformation in how the organization understood both care delivery and professional responsibility. Outcomes, in this case, reflected alignment rather than mere optimization.

III. Challenges and Leadership Insights

The transformation was not without significant challenges that required adaptive and sustained leadership responses. Initial resistance emerged from some clinicians who viewed behavioral health as outside their professional scope, reflecting longstanding cultural divisions within medicine. Addressing this resistance required ongoing education, relational engagement, and visible role modeling by physician champions. Leadership learned that cultural change could not be mandated, but had to be cultivated patiently.

Financial pressures during the transition period posed additional challenges. Before alternative payment models matured, Providence faced difficult resource allocation decisions that tested leadership resolve. Behavioral health integration required investment ahead of reimbursement certainty, forcing leaders to prioritize moral commitments over short-term financial predictability. Recruitment and retention of behavioral health professionals also proved more difficult than anticipated, necessitating creative approaches such as tele-behavioral health, loan repayment programs, and partnerships with training institutions (Health Resources and Services Administration, 2023).

Technology implementation introduced further complexity. Integrating behavioral health into electronic health records required significant customization and workflow redesign to avoid creating parallel documentation systems. These challenges yielded important leadership insights. Sustained executive sponsorship proved essential throughout implementation, not merely at initiation, as visible commitment legitimized difficult decisions (Kotter, 2012). Celebrating small wins while maintaining focus on the broader vision helped sustain momentum, and intentional investment in change management and communication infrastructure enabled cultural transformation beyond programmatic success.

V. Reflection on Virtue, Alignment, and Organizational Integrity

Providence's behavioral health integration illustrates how healthcare reform grounded in foundational questions can produce coherent and resilient change. The initiative succeeded not because of technique alone, but because leadership allowed purpose, anthropology, moral goods, and vocation to govern structural decisions. When worldview clarity preceded strategy, alignment followed.

This case underscores a broader lesson for healthcare leaders. When organizations neglect foundational alignment, they compensate with metrics, mandates, and programs that rarely address root causes. When they attend carefully to first principles, strategy becomes an expression of character rather than a substitute for it. Providence's experience demonstrates that virtue is not opposed to strategy, but is its necessary foundation.

Providence's journey does not offer a universal blueprint. It does, however, demonstrate that where purpose is clear, persons are honored, healers are formed, and structures are aligned, healthcare systems are better positioned to serve the dignity and healing of those entrusted to their care.

CASE STUDY 2: GEISINGER HEALTH SYSTEM—CREATING VALUE THROUGH PROVENCARE

Organizational Context

Geisinger Health System, an integrated health services organization serving Pennsylvania and New Jersey, has built a national reputation for clinical innovation and care delivery transformation. Founded in 1915, Geisinger operates 10 hospital campuses, two research centers, and serves approximately 1.5 million patients. The organization integrated structure—combining insurance, hospital, and physician services—positioned it uniquely to experiment with new care and payment models.

In 2005, Geisinger leadership confronted a strategic challenge common across healthcare: variation in clinical quality and outcomes, even for routine surgical procedures. Despite having skilled surgeons and modern facilities, complication rates varied significantly across providers and sites. This variation contradicted Geisinger identity as a quality leader and imposed unnecessary costs and suffering on patients. Leadership recognized an opportunity to fundamentally rethink care delivery in ways that would advance both clinical excellence and financial sustainability.

Applying the Foundational Worldview Questions

The Teleological Question: "What is Healthcare For?"

Geisinger's ProvenCare initiative began with a fundamental reconsideration of healthcare's purpose within an integrated delivery system. Variation in coronary artery bypass graft outcomes revealed that excellence at the individual physician level did not guarantee reliability at the system level. Leadership concluded that healthcare existed not merely to perform technically successful procedures but to provide predictable and trustworthy healing experiences. If the telos of healthcare is the restoration of health through coordinated stewardship of knowledge and resources, then variability represented a failure of organizational purpose rather than simply an operational challenge. ProvenCare therefore emerged as an attempt to align clinical practice with a deeper understanding of healthcare as a system-wide moral responsibility.

This teleological clarity reshaped strategic thinking. Rather than accepting variation as inevitable, Geisinger articulated an aspirational vision of defect-free care grounded in accountability and transparency. Bundled payment guarantees signaled that the organization was willing to assume responsibility for outcomes across the entire episode of care, reinforcing the belief that healthcare exists to reduce preventable harm while strengthening patient confidence. Such an approach reflected a broader shift toward value-based care models emphasizing outcomes over volume (Porter & Lee, 2013). Purpose became the anchor for strategy development, guiding decisions that balanced innovation with prudence.

Importantly, this reframing also altered how success was communicated internally. Healthcare was no longer framed primarily as the exercise of individual expertise but as a shared institutional endeavor aimed at restoring reliability and trust. By grounding the initiative in purpose, leadership created cultural permission for changes that might otherwise have been perceived as administrative intrusion into clinical practice.

The Anthropological Question: "What is a Patient?"

ProvenCare required Geisinger to reconsider its implicit anthropology. Historically, surgical patients were treated as recipients of individualized care shaped by physician preference and experience. While clinical autonomy remained valued, leadership recognized that patients increasingly sought predictable outcomes and transparent care pathways. The organization reframed patients as persons entitled to consistency regardless of provider or facility. This anthropological shift moved the focus from individual performance toward system-level accountability for patient wellbeing.

Viewing patients through this lens also influenced communication and financial design. The bundled pricing model reduced uncertainty surrounding the cost of care, acknowledging that patients experience healthcare emotionally as well as physically. Patients were no longer positioned merely as consumers navigating complex billing structures but as individuals deserving clarity and trust throughout the treatment process. This approach aligned clinical redesign with patient-centered expectations, reinforcing the belief that dignity is upheld through reliability as much as through interpersonal compassion.

Moreover, this anthropological clarity fostered collaboration across disciplines. By understanding patients as participants in a coordinated care journey rather than as isolated surgical cases, Geisinger encouraged multidisciplinary engagement from anesthesiologists, nurses, and care coordinators. The patient became the focal point around which systems were organized, shifting the culture away from siloed expertise toward integrated responsibility.

The Moral Question: "What is the Good We Are Pursuing?"

At the heart of ProvenCare lay a moral commitment to reliability and stewardship. Leadership rejected the assumption that a certain level of complication was unavoidable, framing preventable harm as an ethical failure demanding systemic correction. The pursuit of zero-defect care reflected a vision of the good rooted in accountability and respect for patient vulnerability. Clinical excellence was understood not merely as technical proficiency but as the consistent application of evidence-based practices across the organization.

Financial stewardship also formed part of this moral vision. By introducing bundled payments, Geisinger aligned economic incentives with long-term outcomes rather than procedural volume (Casale et al., 2007). Leaders emphasized that reducing complications served both patients and the broader healthcare ecosystem by lowering costs and preserving resources. The good being pursued therefore integrated clinical, financial, and relational dimensions, demonstrating that ethical responsibility and operational efficiency need not be in tension.

This moral framing helped sustain momentum during periods of resistance. Surgeons and clinical teams were invited to see protocol development not as compliance but as participation in a shared ethical project. By grounding change in a vision of the good rather than in external mandates, leadership fostered deeper engagement and collective ownership of outcomes.

The Vocational Question: "What Does it Mean to Be a Healer?"

ProvenCare challenged traditional notions of professional identity by redefining healers as stewards of evidence and collaborators within a larger system. Initial skepticism among surgeons reflected fears that standardization might undermine professional autonomy or diminish the art of medicine. Geisinger addressed these concerns by positioning physicians as architects of the protocols themselves. Surgeons participated in identifying the forty evidence-based practices that would guide care, reinforcing the idea that professional judgment and standardization could coexist.

This vocational reframing emphasized responsibility rather than restriction. Healers were encouraged to view adherence to shared practices as expressions of professional integrity and commitment to excellence. Transparent outcome reporting further strengthened this identity by enabling clinicians to learn from one another without fear of blame. Leadership development initiatives supported a cultural shift in which healing was understood as a collective vocation grounded in humility, accountability, and scientific rigor.

Over time, this reframing contributed to greater professional satisfaction. When clinicians saw measurable reductions in complications and readmissions, they experienced alignment between their calling to heal and the systems supporting their work. The vocational identity of the healer evolved from independent expert to collaborative steward of patient safety and institutional integrity.

The Structural Question: "What Kind of System Best Serves Human Dignity?"

Structural redesign became the operational embodiment of Geisinger's worldview commitments. Multidisciplinary teams mapped the entire CABG pathway, identifying best practices that would be consistently applied from preoperative evaluation through postoperative recovery. Electronic health record modifications enabled real-time monitoring of compliance, while decision-support tools reinforced adherence without undermining clinical judgment. These structural innovations transformed individual excellence into system-wide reliability.

The bundled payment model further aligned structure with dignity by reducing fragmentation across departments. Financial risk for complications shifted to the organization, incentivizing proactive coordination and continuous improvement. Measurement systems tracked clinical outcomes, patient experience, and workforce engagement, ensuring that success reflected holistic progress rather than isolated metrics. Transparent data sharing cultivated trust and reinforced the belief that systems exist to support, not constrain, the healer's work (Porter & Lee, 2013).

Ultimately, ProvenCare demonstrated that structure is not morally neutral. Workflows, technologies, and payment models shape the conditions under which care occurs. By embedding ethical commitments into operational design, Geisinger created a system capable of delivering consistent, dignified care while maintaining room for innovation and professional growth.

Results and Key Learnings

ProvenCare achieved remarkable results within 18 months of full implementation. Complication rates for CABG surgery decreased by 44%, readmission rates fell by 36%, and length of stay reduced by half a day on average. More strikingly, variation across surgeons and sites essentially disappeared—every patient received consistently excellent care regardless of which surgeon performed the procedure or which facility hosted it. Patient satisfaction scores increased significantly, particularly on dimensions of care coordination and communication (Casale et al., 2007).

Financial results initially appeared counterintuitive. Despite providing care guarantees and absorbing complication costs, Geisinger margins on CABG procedures actually improved. The reduction in complications and readmissions more than offset the warranty costs, and increased market share further enhanced financial performance. Within three years, ProvenCare CABG had generated substantial positive margins while delivering superior clinical outcomes. This demonstrated the value creation possible when quality and efficiency align rather than trade off.

Perhaps most significantly, ProvenCare established organizational capabilities and culture that enabled replication across other conditions. Geisinger successfully extended the model to other surgical procedures, chronic disease management, and eventually preventive care. The methodology became embedded in how the organization approached quality improvement, creating lasting transformation beyond any single program.

Challenges and Leadership Insights

Success required navigating substantial challenges. Initial physician skepticism was high, with many surgeons questioning whether standardization would compromise their clinical judgment or limit appropriate individualization. Building trust required transparent data sharing, involving physicians directly in protocol development, and clearly distinguishing between evidence-based requirements and areas of legitimate professional judgment. Early wins in complication reduction helped convert skeptics into champions.

Information technology limitations created significant implementation hurdles. Electronic health records were not initially designed to support the level of real-time process monitoring and decision support required. Substantial custom development was necessary, requiring ongoing negotiation of IT priorities and investment. Workflow integration proved more complex than anticipated, necessitating multiple iterative adjustments based on user feedback.

Financial risk management required sophisticated capabilities that many organizations lack. Geisinger needed accurate cost accounting, risk stratification methodologies, and actuarial modeling to set appropriate bundled prices. Early iterations underestimated certain costs, requiring price adjustments and refined approaches to risk assessment. The organization integrated structure and analytic capabilities enabled this learning, but implementation would be more challenging for less integrated providers.

Key leadership insights emerged from the implementation journey. First, starting with a well-defined clinical domain where evidence was clear and outcomes measurable provided important early wins that built credibility and momentum. Second, maintaining physician leadership of the initiative was non-negotiable—administrative drive alone could not overcome professional culture barriers. Third, transparent data sharing and collaborative problem-solving created psychological safety for identifying and addressing problems without blame. Finally, celebrating progress while maintaining focus on continuous improvement sustained motivation and prevented complacency.

Reflection on Foundational Alignment

Geisinger ProvenCare exemplifies how organizational identity and structural characteristics shape strategic possibilities. The initiative succeeded because it aligned with Geisinger identity as an innovator and quality leader, giving the organization permission to attempt something genuinely novel. The integrated structure created economic conditions that enabled risk-taking impossible in fragmented delivery systems. Strategy did not emerge despite organizational context but rather leveraged that context as a strategic asset.

The case also demonstrates the interplay between aspirational vision and pragmatic implementation. The zero-defect goal was deliberately aspirational, designed to stretch thinking beyond incremental improvement. However, implementation was intensely pragmatic, starting with one well-defined condition and building capabilities systematically. This combination of bold vision and disciplined execution characterizes effective strategic change.

Finally, ProvenCare illustrates how measurement creates accountability while shaping culture. Geisinger commitment to transparent outcome reporting, both internally and publicly, reinforced the cultural message that quality was the institutional priority. This transparency created positive peer pressure while providing data for continuous improvement. The organization recognized that what gets measured and shared signals what matters, and designed measurement systems accordingly.

The case ultimately demonstrates that value creation in healthcare requires rethinking fundamental assumptions about quality, efficiency, and professional practice. When organizations ground strategy in clear identity and values while systematically addressing implementation barriers, transformation becomes possible even in areas where conventional wisdom suggests change is too difficult.

CASE STUDY 3: REGIONAL COMMUNITY HOSPITAL—NAVIGATING ORGANIZATIONAL TRANSFORMATION

Organizational Context

This case examines a 250-bed community hospital in the Midwest serving a mixed urban-rural population of approximately 200,000. The hospital has deep community roots spanning 75 years, with generations of families having received care there. Like many community hospitals, it faces significant strategic pressures: declining inpatient volumes, increasing competition from specialized centers and academic medical centers in nearby cities, narrow operating margins, and workforce recruitment challenges.

In 2018, the board and executive leadership confronted a critical strategic decision. A larger regional health system offered acquisition terms that would provide capital investment and reduce administrative burden. However, the offer also threatened community identity and local governance autonomy. The alternative—remaining independent—required significant transformation to ensure financial sustainability and competitive viability. The decision represented more than a business transaction;

it touched fundamental questions of organizational identity, community commitment, and long-term viability.

Applying the Foundational Worldview Questions

The Teleological Question: "What is Healthcare For?"

For the regional community hospital, the question of purpose emerged as the most decisive factor shaping its transformation. Facing declining inpatient volumes, mounting financial pressures, and the possibility of acquisition by a larger health system, leadership recognized that strategic decisions could not be made solely on economic grounds. The hospital's seventy-five-year history of serving its surrounding communities raised deeper questions about what healthcare existed to accomplish within that context. Rather than defining success exclusively through expansion or competitive positioning, leaders reframed healthcare as a vocation of presence and accessibility for local populations whose needs extended beyond acute clinical interventions.

This teleological clarity shifted the strategic conversation away from imitation of academic medical centers toward a renewed commitment to community-centered care. Healthcare was understood as a means of sustaining relational continuity, supporting preventive and chronic disease management, and preserving local trust in an increasingly consolidated industry. The hospital's decision to remain independent reflected a conviction that healthcare exists not only to deliver services efficiently but to cultivate stability and belonging within the communities it serves. Purpose became the lens through which difficult choices were evaluated, allowing leadership to interpret transformation not as abandonment of tradition but as fidelity to its deepest calling.

Furthermore, teleological reflection enabled stakeholders to navigate competing visions of the hospital's future. Some advocated aggressive service expansion, while others emphasized financial survival. By returning to foundational questions about what healthcare is ultimately for, leadership established a shared narrative that balanced aspiration with realism. Healthcare was not defined merely by institutional growth but by its capacity to promote wellbeing and human flourishing within the community. This reframing provided coherence during a period of uncertainty and created a foundation for subsequent strategic decisions.

The Anthropological Question: "What is a Patient?"

The hospital's transformation required a reexamination of its understanding of patients within a changing healthcare landscape. Historically, patients were viewed primarily as recipients of inpatient services, reflecting the hospital-centric model that shaped its early decades. However, shifting demographics and chronic disease patterns revealed that patients increasingly required longitudinal relationships rather than episodic encounters. Leadership came to recognize that patients were members of interconnected communities whose health outcomes were influenced by social determinants, access barriers, and relational trust.

This anthropological shift encouraged the hospital to invest in expanded primary care access, care coordination programs, and community partnerships designed to address health needs beyond traditional hospital walls. Patients were understood not simply as clinical cases but as persons navigating complex life circumstances. The chronic disease management initiative exemplified this perspective by integrating nurse care managers, social workers, and community health workers into care teams. By recognizing patients as relational beings rather than isolated individuals, the hospital reoriented its services toward continuity and prevention.

Moreover, this understanding influenced how the organization approached patient experience and communication. Surveys revealed that community members valued familiarity, compassion, and accessibility as much as technological sophistication. The hospital's strategic response emphasized these relational strengths, positioning itself as a trusted community health partner rather than a competitor to large tertiary centers. Anthropology thus shaped not only clinical design but also institutional identity, reinforcing the belief that healthcare must honor the lived experiences and dignity of those it serves (Blendon & Benson, 2022).

The Moral Question: "What is the Good We Are Pursuing?"

In the midst of transformation, leadership grappled with competing visions of what constituted good healthcare. Financial sustainability was necessary, yet defining success solely through margin improvement risked undermining the hospital's community mission. The organization articulated a moral vision that integrated clinical excellence, accessibility, and stewardship of resources. Good care was defined as care that preserved local access while maintaining quality and trust, even when that required difficult decisions such as closing underutilized service lines.

These decisions illustrated the tension between short-term loss and long-term good. Eliminating certain programs provoked emotional responses from staff and community members, yet leadership framed these actions as necessary to sustain the hospital's broader mission. The pursuit of the good involved balancing prudence with compassion, recognizing that maintaining every historical service could ultimately threaten the organization's survival. By grounding decisions in ethical reflection rather than purely financial logic, the hospital-maintained credibility during a period of significant change.

The moral vision also emphasized workforce wellbeing and professional integrity. Leaders acknowledged that sustainable transformation required environments where clinicians could practice meaningful care without excessive burnout. Integrating workforce engagement into the strategic vision reflected a commitment to the quadruple aim, recognizing that the good pursued includes both patient outcomes and caregiver flourishing (Bodenheimer & Sinsky, 2014; West et al., 2019). Moral clarity thus guided the hospital's efforts to balance operational efficiency with relational care.

The Vocational Question: "What Does it Mean to Be a Healer?"

As the hospital transitioned from an inpatient-focused model to a community-centered health partner, the identity of its caregivers evolved. Physicians, nurses, and allied health professionals were invited to see themselves not merely as providers of episodic treatment but as partners in long-term health journeys. Leadership invested in physician engagement initiatives, interdisciplinary collaboration, and leadership development programs that reinforced a sense of shared responsibility for community wellbeing. The healer was understood as both clinician and advocate, participating in a broader effort to sustain local access to care.

This vocational reframing helped address skepticism among some clinicians who initially resisted changes to service lines or workflow redesign. By connecting transformation to professional purpose rather than administrative mandate, leadership fostered a culture of ownership and creativity. Caregivers were encouraged to contribute to strategic discussions, reinforcing the belief that healing involves collaborative problem-solving rather than top-down directives. Over time, this approach strengthened alignment between individual calling and institutional mission.

The vocational dimension also supported resilience during periods of uncertainty. Workforce challenges, including recruitment difficulties and operational pressures, required caregivers to adapt to new roles and expectations. Framing these changes within a shared sense of vocation helped sustain morale and reinforced the belief that transformation was an expression of commitment to patients rather than a departure from professional values.

The Structural Question: "What Kind of System Best Serves Human Dignity?"

Structural redesign represented the tangible expression of the hospital's worldview commitments. Service line restructuring aligned resources with community needs, while partnerships with regional centers ensured access to specialized care without compromising local identity. Infrastructure modernization improved patient flow and supported virtual care options, enabling more flexible and accessible service delivery. These structural changes reflected a commitment to dignity by prioritizing accessibility, coordination, and sustainability over institutional prestige.

The balanced scorecard approach embodied this structural philosophy. By measuring financial performance alongside clinical quality, community impact, and workforce engagement, leadership created accountability for holistic success rather than narrow optimization. Transparent reporting fostered trust among stakeholders and reinforced the belief that systems exist to serve persons rather than metrics alone. Measurement became a form of moral architecture, guiding decisions in ways consistent with the hospital's purpose.

Ultimately, the hospital's structural transformation illustrated that systems shape culture as much as culture shapes systems. When workflows reinforce collaboration and community connection, caregivers experience alignment between institutional expectations and professional identity. Structure became the mechanism through which teleological and anthropological commitments were translated into daily practice, ensuring that the organization's transformation remained grounded in dignity and relational care.

Progress and Key Learnings

Three years into transformation, the hospital demonstrated substantial progress across most strategic objectives. Operating margins improved to 3.2%, with positive trends continuing. The chronic disease management program enrolled over 1,200 patients, reducing hospital readmissions by 28% for program participants and achieving strong quality metrics. Patient experience scores improved significantly, moving from below national average to above average across most domains. Physician and staff satisfaction surveys showed marked improvement, though some areas required continued attention.

Strategic repositioning was generating results. Primary care access expanded with two new clinics opening in underserved communities. Partnership arrangements for specialized services functioned well, maintaining local access for routine needs while appropriately referring complex cases. The hospital gained recognition as a community health leader, strengthening brand position even while reducing bed capacity and certain clinical services.

Perhaps most significantly, community support intensified. A recent capital campaign for facility modernization exceeded its goal by 30%, demonstrating community confidence in the hospital direction. Patient satisfaction comments frequently mentioned care team compassion and coordination, suggesting culture was evolving as intended. Board and leadership reported renewed energy and clarity of purpose.

However, challenges persisted. Workforce recruitment remained difficult despite improvements, particularly for nursing and specialized clinical roles. Some physicians remained skeptical about population health strategy, preferring traditional acute care focus. Technology implementations delivered some benefits but also created workflow disruptions requiring ongoing adjustment. Financial performance, while improved, remained vulnerable to payor rate pressures and volume fluctuations.

The transformation remained incomplete and ongoing. Leadership recognized that sustainable change required continued commitment beyond the initial three-year timeline. Nevertheless, the hospital had fundamentally altered its trajectory, moving from decline toward vitality.

Challenges and Leadership Insights

Several challenges required adaptive leadership and creative problem-solving. Emotionally, closing services with deep community history proved wrenching despite strategic necessity. Leadership learned the importance of extensive community dialogue, transparent rationale sharing, and demonstrating how service restructuring actually strengthened the hospital ability to serve community needs. Honoring the past while building the future required careful communication and genuine empathy for losses even as the organization moved forward.

Maintaining transformation momentum through inevitable setbacks tested organizational resilience. When certain initiatives showed slower progress than hoped, some stakeholders questioned the entire strategy. Leadership responded by distinguishing between course corrections expected and healthy and fundamental strategy failures requiring reassessment. This required transparent communication about challenges while maintaining confidence in core direction. Celebrating meaningful progress while acknowledging persistent difficulties helped sustain momentum and psychological safety.

Managing multiple simultaneous change initiatives created real risks of change fatigue and organizational overload. Not everything could happen at once, yet transformation required comprehensive change across domains. Leadership learned to sequence initiatives carefully, create integration mechanisms preventing siloed efforts, and build explicit rest periods into change plans allowing consolidation and recovery. This pacing discipline proved essential to sustainable change rather than burnout-inducing heroics.

Key leadership insights emerged from navigating transformation:

First, identity clarity proved foundational to all subsequent decisions. When leadership had genuine clarity about who the organization was and aspired to be, difficult decisions became more navigable. Strategic choices could reference core identity rather than relying solely on financial analysis or competitive positioning. This identity anchor provided stability during turbulent change.

Second, honest assessment of current reality—including both strengths and challenges—enabled realistic strategy. Denying financial pressures or competitive threats would have been comforting but ultimately destructive. Conversely, fixating solely on problems without recognizing strengths would have undermined confidence and missed strategic assets. Balanced assessment created foundation for transformation rather than either complacency or despair.

Third, meaningful stakeholder engagement throughout the process-built trust and generated better strategies. Early involvement of physicians, staff, board members, and community representatives not only improved strategy quality through diverse perspectives but also created psychological ownership supporting implementation. This engagement required significant time investment but paid dividends in reduced resistance and enhanced collective problem-solving.

Fourth, balancing multiple performance dimensions through the balanced scorecard prevented the single-minded optimization that often undermines sustainability. When leaders were accountable for simultaneous progress on financial, clinical, community, and workforce dimensions, they necessarily sought integrated solutions rather than narrow fixes. This aligned daily decisions with comprehensive strategic vision.

Finally, leadership learned that transformation is fundamentally about meaning as much as mechanics. Helping people understand why the hospital was transforming, how their work connected to larger purpose, and what success would mean for their professional lives proved as important as technical implementation plans. When transformation connected to people sense of calling and professional identity, energy and creativity followed.

Reflection on Foundational Alignment

This case illuminates how the foundational worldview questions guide strategic decision-making in contexts of genuine uncertainty and competing pressures. Unlike the previous cases featuring larger, better-resourced organizations, this community hospital faced existential strategic choices with limited margin for error. The worldview questions framework provided structure for navigating this complexity without offering false certainty or simplistic answers.

The identity question proved particularly powerful because it had no predetermined answer. Different stakeholders held different views, and the question prompted genuine inquiry rather than confirmation of existing beliefs. This inquiry surfaced both deep community roots and professional excellence aspirations as core identity elements, leading to a strategy balancing these values rather than forcing artificial choice between them.

The situational assessment demonstrated the importance of honest environmental understanding. Financial pressures were real and ignoring them would have been irresponsible. However, the assessment also identified genuine strengths and community assets that provided strategic foundation. Strategy emerged from understanding both constraints and capabilities, neither denying difficulties nor succumbing to them.

The vision question required reconciling aspiration with realism. Pure aspiration disconnected from financial reality would have led to bankruptcy. Pure pragmatism focused solely on financial survival would have lost mission and community support. The articulated vision integrated both dimensions, describing an inspiring future that was ambitious yet achievable given disciplined execution.

Implementation strategy demonstrated that knowing the destination is insufficient without realistic pathways. The hospital developed concrete initiatives across multiple domains, sequenced for maximum impact with available resources, and adapted based on implementation learning. This pragmatic approach honored the vision while remaining grounded in operational reality.

Finally, the measurement question showed how balanced accountability shapes organizational behavior. By measuring financial, clinical, community, and workforce dimensions equally, the hospital created accountability for integrated success rather than narrow optimization. This measurement approach reinforced the strategy and made progress visible, sustaining commitment through difficult periods.

The case ultimately demonstrates that the worldview questions framework serves organizations of any size and resource level. While specific answers vary dramatically based on organizational context, the questions themselves provide universal structure for strategic thinking that aligns purpose, identity, capabilities, and aspirations into coherent direction.

SYNTHESIS: PATTERNS ACROSS PRACTICE CONTEXTS

Common Themes Across Diverse Contexts

While the three case studies represent dramatically different organizational contexts—a large integrated delivery system, an innovative regional health system, and an independent community hospital—several common themes emerge that transcend organizational size, structure, or resources. These themes illuminate fundamental principles of effective healthcare strategy regardless of specific circumstances.

Identity as Strategic Foundation

All three organizations discovered that clarity about organizational identity provided essential foundation for strategic decision-making. For Providence, identity as a mission-driven organization serving vulnerable populations created both permission and expectation for ambitious behavioral health integration. For Geisinger, identity as a quality innovator and integrated system enabled experimentation with care delivery and payment models. For the community hospital, achieving identity clarity about community roots and appropriate clinical scope guided difficult service line decisions and transformation direction.

In each case, identity served not as constraint but as liberation—providing clear criteria for difficult choices and creating focus amid competing demands. When leaders understood their organization authentic identity, strategy became less about responding to every external pressure and more about selectively engaging opportunities aligned with core purpose and capabilities. Identity clarity also provided the foundation for cultural coherence and meaningful work, as staff could understand how their daily efforts connected to larger organizational purpose.

Importantly, identity was not static or monolithic. Organizations clarified and sometimes redefined identity through the strategy development process itself. Identity emerged through dialogue, reflection, and honest examination of history, current reality, and aspirations. This iterative identity clarification process was strategic work, not merely precursor to strategy.

Strategic Tension Between Aspiration and Pragmatism

Each case demonstrated the productive tension between aspirational vision and pragmatic implementation. Providence envisioned behavioral health integration while pragmatically building infrastructure and capabilities over years. Geisinger articulated zero-defect care while methodically developing standardized processes and monitoring systems. The community hospital aspired to population health leadership while realistically sequencing initiatives and managing financial constraints.

This tension was not a problem to be resolved but rather a dynamic to be managed. Purely aspirational strategy disconnected from operational reality becomes empty rhetoric. Purely pragmatic strategy focused solely on immediate constraints loses the inspirational power necessary for sustained commitment and innovation. Effective strategy maintains both poles in tension—aspirational vision that stretches thinking while pragmatic pathways that enable progress.

Leadership role in managing this tension involved constant translation between vision and execution, helping people understand how daily work contributes to aspirational goals while ensuring vision remains grounded enough to guide practical decisions. This translation work required both strategic patience recognizing transformation takes time and operational urgency maintaining momentum through tangible progress.

Measurement as Cultural Reinforcement

All three organizations recognized that measurement systems shape organizational culture and behavior. Providence measured patient dignity alongside clinical outcomes, signaling that behavioral health integration was fundamentally about respect and whole-person care, not just efficient service delivery. Geisinger public reporting of quality metrics reinforced a culture of transparency and continuous improvement. The community hospital balanced scorecard prevented financial optimization at the expense of mission or workforce wellbeing.

In each case, measurement served multiple functions simultaneously: accountability for results, early warning system for emerging problems, basis for celebration and recognition, and cultural communication about organizational priorities. What organizations choose to measure and report signals what matters, often more powerfully than explicit statements. Effective measurement aligned with strategy and values, creating positive feedback loops reinforcing desired behaviors and outcomes.

Critically, measurement avoided becoming reductionist or mechanistic. Organizations tracked quantitative metrics while also attending to qualitative indicators of cultural health, meaning, and purpose. They recognized that not everything important is easily measurable, and that over-reliance on measurable metrics can distort priorities toward what is quantifiable rather than what is meaningful. Balanced measurement approached strategy as both art and science, combining rigorous data analysis with qualitative judgment (Porter & Lee, 2013).

Workforce Engagement as Strategic Imperative

Each organization discovered that workforce engagement was not a soft human resources concern but rather a hard strategic imperative. Providence could not achieve behavioral health integration without caregiver buy-in and capability development. Geisinger ProvenCare required physician leadership and front-line clinician engagement in process design. The community hospital transformation depended on staff and medical staff commitment through difficult change.

This workforce centrality reflected healthcare fundamental reality: quality, experience, and efficiency all depend on the knowledge, skill, judgment, and engagement of clinical and support staff. Unlike manufacturing where processes can be automated, healthcare improvement ultimately requires human behavioral change and professional development. Strategy that treats workforce as cost to be minimized rather than asset to be developed inevitably undermines its own objectives.

Organizations approached workforce engagement through multiple levers: meaningful involvement in strategy development and implementation, transparent communication about challenges and progress, professional development opportunities, reduction of administrative burdens interfering with meaningful work, and recognition of contributions to strategic goals. They also measured and addressed burnout and satisfaction, recognizing that unsustainable work environments undermine both human wellbeing and strategic success (Bodenheimer & Sinsky, 2014; West et al., 2018).

Stakeholder Engagement Throughout Strategic Process

All three cases demonstrated the value of genuine stakeholder engagement throughout strategic planning and implementation rather than simply at the beginning or end. Providence involved community partners, patients, and front-line staff in designing behavioral health programs. Geisinger engaged physicians in ProvenCare protocol development and iteration. The community hospital conducted extensive dialogue with board, physicians, staff, and community during strategy formulation.

This engagement served multiple purposes. It improved strategy quality by incorporating diverse perspectives and practical knowledge. It built psychological ownership supporting implementation by giving stakeholders voice in shaping direction. It enhanced legitimacy by demonstrating respect for stakeholder concerns and ideas. It created feedback loops enabling course correction based on implementation learning.

Importantly, engagement was authentic rather than performative. Organizations genuinely incorporated stakeholder input and adapted strategies based on what they learned. When engagement is merely going through the motions, stakeholders recognize the manipulation and trust erodes. When engagement genuinely shapes decisions, stakeholders become strategic partners rather than resistant obstacles.

Environmental Understanding Without Environmental Determinism

Each organization demonstrated sophisticated understanding of its competitive, regulatory, and community environment while avoiding environmental determinism. They recognized external pressures and constraints without allowing those forces to completely dictate strategy. Providence understood payment system limitations while still pursuing mission-aligned behavioral health integration. Geisinger worked within existing quality measurement frameworks while pioneering more comprehensive approaches. The community hospital faced market pressures without simply capitulating to them.

This balance required distinguishing between constraints that must be accommodated such as regulatory requirements, financial realities, and competitive dynamics and constraints that could be challenged or changed through innovation. Organizations asked not just what does the environment require of us but also how might we shape the environment to better enable our mission. This agentic stance toward environment prevented passive reactivity while maintaining realistic understanding of boundaries and pressures.

Strategy emerged from dialogue between environmental reality and organizational aspiration. Organizations neither ignored market forces nor allowed markets to override mission and values. They found creative ways to advance purpose within constraints, sometimes even leveraging constraints as catalysts for innovation. This sophisticated environmental engagement characterized strategic leadership rather than simply environmental adaptation.

Meaning and Purpose as Strategic Assets

Perhaps most fundamentally, all three cases demonstrated that meaning and purpose are not soft concerns peripheral to strategic success but rather strategic assets central to achievement. Providence behavioral health initiative succeeded partly because it connected to caregivers' sense of calling to serve vulnerable populations. Geisinger quality transformation resonated with physicians' professional identity and commitment to excellence. The community hospital transformation maintained support partly because people understood the meaningful connection between change and community service.

When strategy connects to sources of meaning—whether organizational mission, professional identity, community commitment, or patient service—it generates energy, creativity, and resilience that cannot be manufactured through extrinsic incentives alone. People endure difficulty and uncertainty when they believe their work matters and contributes to purposes beyond themselves. Conversely, when strategy is purely instrumental or financial, commitment remains fragile and motivation superficial.

This is not to suggest that meaning alone suffices. Organizations must also attend to financial sustainability, operational efficiency, and competitive viability. However, the cases suggest that meaning and purpose are necessary if not sufficient conditions for strategic success. They provide the motivational foundation on which operational excellence and financial performance can build. Strategy disconnected from meaning may achieve short-term results but rarely sustains transformation or builds cultures of excellence.

IMPLICATIONS FOR HEALTHCARE STRATEGY DEVELOPMENT PRACTICE

These common themes across diverse contexts suggest several implications for healthcare strategy development practice:

First, strategy development should begin with foundational questions about identity, purpose, and values before proceeding to environmental analysis and strategic options. These questions are not mere preliminaries but rather core strategic work that shapes everything that follows. Organizations that skip quickly to SWOT analysis or strategic option evaluation without foundational clarity often produce technically sophisticated plans disconnected from organizational DNA and incapable of generating sustained commitment.

Second, strategy development should be genuinely participatory, involving diverse stakeholders throughout the process rather than only at selected moments. This participation requires time investment and tolerating messy dialogue, but produces better strategies and stronger implementation commitment. The alternative—executive-driven plans presented for stakeholder endorsement—rarely generates the ownership necessary for difficult organizational change.

Third, measurement systems should be designed as cultural tools reinforcing strategic priorities, not merely as accountability mechanisms. What gets measured signals what matters, and comprehensive measurement across multiple dimensions prevents narrow optimization undermining broader goals. Organizations should measure mission achievement, not just financial performance, and should attend to workforce wellbeing alongside productivity.

Fourth, strategy implementation requires sustained leadership attention and adaptive management, not simply execution of predetermined plans. The cases showed that initial strategies required iteration and adjustment based on implementation learning. Leaders who treated strategy as fixed and implementation as mechanical failed to adapt effectively. Those who maintained strategic intent while flexibly adjusting tactics based on emerging information navigated complexity more successfully.

Fifth, effective healthcare strategy balances aspiration and pragmatism, maintaining productive tension between them rather than collapsing into either pure idealism or pure incrementalism. Aspiration without pragmatism becomes rhetoric; pragmatism without aspiration becomes incrementalism. Strategic leadership holds both dimensions in creative tension, using aspiration to stretch thinking while employing pragmatism to enable progress.

Finally, meaning and purpose should be recognized as strategic assets to be cultivated rather than peripheral concerns. When organizations connect strategy to sources of meaning, they generate commitment, creativity, and resilience beyond what instrumental incentives alone can achieve. This requires explicit attention to how strategic choices relate to professional identity, organizational mission, and human flourishing. Strategy that ignores meaning may optimize metrics but often fails to inspire the human excellence required for healthcare transformation.

FUTURE DIRECTIONS

Part 3 will extend these practical insights by examining common strategy development pitfalls and how to avoid them, exploring additional industry examples across different healthcare segments, and providing practical tools and templates for implementing the strategy development framework in other organizational settings. The goal remains translating philosophical principles into practical application that serves patients, supports clinicians, and strengthens communities.

CONCLUSION: FROM PRINCIPLES TO PRACTICE

The cases presented in this chapter demonstrate how the foundational worldview questions and strategy development framework translate from theoretical principles into practical organizational transformation. Whether addressing behavioral health integration, pioneering value-based care delivery, or navigating community hospital transformation, effective strategy begins with clarity about identity and purpose, proceeds through honest environmental assessment, articulates aspirational yet achievable vision, develops pragmatic implementation pathways, and creates measurement systems enabling accountability and learning.

These practical applications reveal that healthcare strategy development is fundamentally both analytical and philosophical work. It requires rigorous data analysis, competitive assessment, and operational planning. But it also requires careful attention to questions of meaning, purpose, identity, and values that cannot be reduced to spreadsheets or strategic matrices. The most effective healthcare strategies integrate both dimensions, combining analytical sophistication with philosophical depth.

The diversity of contexts represented in these cases—from large integrated delivery systems to independent community hospitals—demonstrates that the strategic planning framework applies across organizational types and circumstances. While specific strategies necessarily vary based on organizational resources, market position, and community needs, the underlying process and foundational questions remain remarkably consistent. This suggests that effective strategy development reflects universal principles adapted to particular contexts rather than context-specific tactics without broader application.

Looking forward, healthcare organizations face unprecedented complexity and uncertainty. Payment models continue evolving toward value-based arrangements. Technology creates both opportunities and disruptions. Workforce challenges persist and evolve. Patient expectations shift. Environmental pressures intensify. In this context, strategy grounded in foundational clarity about identity and purpose provides stability amid turbulence. When organizations know who they are and why they exist, they can navigate uncertainty with greater confidence and consistency.

REFERENCES

Archer, J., Bower, P., Gilbody, S., Lovell, K., Richards, D., Gask, L., Dickens, C., & Coventry, P. (2012). Collaborative care for depression and anxiety problems. *Cochrane Database of Systematic Reviews*, *10*(10), CD006525. Advance online publication. DOI: 10.1002/14651858.CD006525.pub2 PMID: 23076925

Blendon, R. J., & Benson, J. M. (2022). Trust in medicine, the health system & public health. *Daedalus*, *151*(4), 67–82. DOI: 10.1162/daed_a_01944

Bodenheimer, T., & Sinsky, C. (2014). From triple to quadruple aim: Care of the patient requires care of the provider. *Annals of Family Medicine*, *12*(6), 573–576. DOI: 10.1370/afm.1713 PMID: 25384822

Casale, A., Paulus, R., Selna, M., Doll, M., Bothe, A., McKinley, K., Berry, S., Davis, D., Gilfillan, R., Hamory, B., & Steele, G. (2007). "ProvenCareSM": A Provider-Driven Pay-for-Performance Program for Acute Episodic Cardiac Surgical Care. *Annals of Surgery*, *246*(4), 613–621. DOI: 10.1097/SLA.0b013e318155a996 PMID: 17893498

Centers for Medicare & Medicaid Services. (2016). *Behavioral health integration services*. https://www.cms.gov/files/document/mln909432-behavioral-health-integration-services.pdf

Health Resources and Services Administration. (2025). *Behavioral health workforce projections*. U.S. Department of Health and Human Services. https://data.hrsa.gov/topics/health-workforce/nchwa/workforce-projections

Institute of Medicine (US) Committee on Crossing the Quality Chasm. Adaptation to Mental Health and Addictive Disorders. (2006). *Improving the Quality of Health Care for Mental and Substance-Use Conditions: Quality Chasm Series*. National Academies Press (US). DOI: 10.17226/11470

Kotter, J. P. (2012). *Leading change*. Harvard Business Review Press.

National Council for Mental Wellbeing. (2021). Mental Health First Aid USA. https://www.mentalhealthfirstaid.org

Pine, B. J., & Gilmore, J. H. (2020). *The experience economy* (Updated ed.). Harvard Business Review Press.

Porter, M. E., & Lee, T. H. (2013). The strategy that will fix health care. *Harvard Business Review*, *91*(10), 50–70.

Providence, St. Joseph Health. (2023). *About us*. https://www.providence.org/about

Providence Health & Services. (2022). *Behavioral health integration outcomes report*. Providence St. Joseph Health.

Providence Health & Services. (2022, June 1). Providence program builds bridge to behavioral health care, recovery. *Catholic Health World*. https://www.chausa.org/news-and-publications/publications/catholic-health-world/archives/june-1-2022/providence-program-builds-bridge-to-behavioral-health-care-recovery

Shanafelt, T. D., Hasan, O., Dyrbye, L. N., Sinsky, C., Satele, D., Sloan, J., & West, C. P. (2016). Changes in burnout and satisfaction with work–life balance in physicians and the general U.S. working population between 2011 and 2014. *Mayo Clinic Proceedings*, *90*(12), 1600–1613. DOI: 10.1016/j.mayocp.2015.08.023 PMID: 26653297

Shore, J. H., Yellowlees, P., Caudill, R., Johnston, B., Turvey, C., Mishkind, M., Krupinski, E., Myers, K., Shore, P., Kaftarian, E., & Hilty, D. (2018). Best Practices in Videoconferencing-Based Telemental Health April 2018. *Telemedicine journal and e-health: the official journal of the American Telemedicine Association*, 24(11), 827–832. DOI: 10.1089/tmj.2018.0237

The Beryl Institute. (2024). *Consumer perspectives on patient experience in the U.S.* Retrieved from https://theberylinstitute.org/wp-content/uploads/woocommerce_uploads/2024/10/Consumer-Perspectives-on-Patient-Experience-2024-1-mqh0nm.pdf

Unützer, J., Katon, W. J., Fan, M. Y., Schoenbaum, M. C., Lin, E. H., Della Penna, R. D., & Powers, D. (2013). Long-term cost effects of collaborative care for late-life depression. *The American Journal of Managed Care*, *14*(2), 95–100. PMID: 18269305

West, C. P., Dyrbye, L. N., & Shanafelt, T. D. (2018). Physician burnout: Contributors, consequences and solutions. *Journal of Internal Medicine*, *283*(6), 516–529. DOI: 10.1111/joim.12752 PMID: 29505159

ADDITIONAL READING

Healey, B. (2018). *The principles of healthcare leadership*. Health Administration Press.

Hines, A., & Bishop, P. (2006). *Thinking about the future: Guidelines for strategic foresight*. Social Technologies.

Howe, N. (2023). *The fourth turning is here*. Simon & Schuster.

Kouzes, J. M., & Posner, B. Z. (2011). *Credibility: How leaders gain and lose it, why people demand it* (2nd ed.). Jossey-Bass. DOI: 10.1002/9781118983867

Kuhn, T. S. (1962). *The structure of scientific revolutions*. University of Chicago Press.

Loehle, C. (1996). *Thinking strategically: Power tools for Personal and Professional Advancement*. Cambridge University Press. DOI: 10.1017/CBO9780511525308

Pagano, B., & Pagano, E. (2004). *The transparency edge; How credibility can make or break you in business*. McGraw-Hill.

Pine, B. J., & Gilmore, J. H. (2007). *Authenticity: What consumers really want*. Harvard Business Review Press.

Pine, B. J., & Gilmore, J. H. (2020). *The experience economy*. Harvard Business Review Press.

Sanders, T. (1998). *Strategic thinking and the new science: Planning in the midst of chaos, complexity, and change*. The Free Press.

KEY TERMS AND DEFINITIONS

Anthropological Question: An examination of how organizations understand patients and human dignity, influencing care design and relational practices.

Behavioral Health Integration: The embedding of mental health services within primary or coordinated care models to improve access, continuity, and outcomes.

Community Centered Transformation: Strategic change focused on preserving local access, relational continuity, and population health within community-based healthcare organizations.

Fundamental Worldview Questions: Five guiding inquiries concerning purpose, anthropology, moral vision, vocation, and structure that shape organizational identity and decision making.

Moral Question: The evaluation of what constitutes the good being pursued, including ethical commitments related to healing, trust, and stewardship.

Organizational Identity: The collective understanding of mission, values, and historical purpose that shapes strategic direction and cultural coherence.

ProvenCare Model: A value-based care initiative emphasizing standardized evidence-based protocols, bundled payments, and system wide accountability for outcomes.

Strategy Development Process: A structured framework guiding organizations from foundational worldview questions through implementation and measurement to achieve aligned strategic outcomes.

Structural Question: The analysis of organizational systems, workflows, and governance structures that embody institutional values.

Teleological Question: The exploration of organizational purpose and the ultimate ends healthcare seeks to achieve beyond operational efficiency.

Value Based Care: A healthcare delivery approach prioritizing patient outcomes and long-term value rather than procedural volume.

Vocational Question: A reflection on the identity and calling of caregivers and leaders within healthcare systems.

Compilation of References

AAMC (2024). *The complexities of physician supply and demand: Projections from 2021 to 2036*. Retrieved from The Complexities of Physician Supply and Demand: Projections From 2021 to 2036.

Abdel-Razig, S., & Stoller, J. (2024). Addressing physician shortage in the United States with novel legislation to bypass traditional training pathways: The fine print. [Retrieved from Addressing Physician Shortages in the United States With Novel Legislation to Bypass Traditional Training Pathways: The Fine Print - PMC]. *Journal of Graduate Medical Education, 17*(1), 16–19.

Abramson, B., Boerma, J., & Tsyvinski, A. (2024). Macroeconomics of Mental Health, NBER Working Paper 32354, DOI: 10.3386/w32354

Accelerant Research. (2025, September 2). *Branding backlash: What Cracker Barrel, Target, and Bud Lite can teach us about the power of market research*. https://www.accelerantresearch.com/articles/branding-backlash-what-cracker-barrel-target-and-bud-light-can-teach-us-about-the-power-of-market-research

Accreditation Council for Graduate Medical Education (ACGME). (2025). *Common program requirements*. Retrieved from Common Program Requirements.

Adashi, E., O'Mahony, D., & Cohen, G. (2024). The national physician statement: The imperative of Congressional action. The National Physician Shortage: The Imperative of Congressional Action. [The National Physician Shortage: The Imperative of Congressional Action - The American Journal of Medicine]. *The American Journal of Medicine, 137*(11), 1030–1031. DOI: 10.1016/j.amjmed.2024.05.032 PMID: 38876332

Adeniyi, A. O., Arowoogun, J. O., Chidi, R., Okolo, C. A., & Babawarun, O. (2024). The impact of electronic health records on patient care and outcomes: A comprehensive review. *World Journal of Advanced Research and Reviews, 21*(2), 1446–1455. DOI: 10.30574/wjarr.2024.21.2.0592

Adler-Milstein, J., & Jha, A. K. (2017). HITECH Act drove large gains in hospital electronic health record adoption. *Health Affairs*, *36*(8), 1416–1422. DOI: 10.1377/hlthaff.2016.1651 PMID: 28784734

Advanced Medical Reviews (AMR). (2022). Telemedicine: A solution to the predicted physician shortage? Retrieved from Telemedicine: a Solution to the Predicted Physician Shortage?

Advanced Medical Reviews (AMR). (2022). Telemedicine: A solution to the predicted physician shortage? Retrieved from Telemedicine: a Solution to the Predicted Physician Shortage? AMA, (2021). *2021 Telehealth Survey Report*. Retrieved from 2021 Telehealth Survey Report | AMA

Advisory Board. (2025). *One Big Beautiful Bill Act: Understanding the healthcare impacts*. Retrieved from One Big Beautiful Bill Act: Understanding the healthcare impacts

Ahmed, N. (2005). 23 years of the discovery of *Helicobacter pylori*: Is the debate over? *Annals of Clinical Microbiology and Antimicrobials*, *4*(1), 17. Advance online publication. DOI: 10.1186/1476-0711-4-17 PMID: 16262889

Ali, I., Ahmad, W., Ullah, A. R., Khan, F., Ijaz, M., Khan, S., & Khan, T. M. (2021). Knowledge, attitude, and barriers toward ADRs reporting among health-care professionals at tertiary care health settings in Peshawar, Pakistan: A web based study. *Hospital Pharmacy*, *56*(4), 384–391. DOI: 10.1177/0018578720910401 PMID: 34381279

Alkhamis, Z. (2025). *The Implementation of Telehealth and AI in Pediatrics: Smarter Solutions for the Modern World*. Independently published.

America Next. (2014). *The freedom and empowerment plan: The prescription for conservative consumer-focused health reform*. America Next.

American Association of Medical Colleges. (2024). New AAMC report shows continuing projected physician shortage. https://www.aamc.org/news/press-releases/new-aamc-report-shows-continuing-projected-physician-shortage

American College of Healthcare Executives. (2024). *Hospital leadership crisis 2025: CEO action plan*. https://www.thehealthcareexecutive.net/blog/blog-hospital-leadership-crisis-2025

American Hospital Association (AHA). (2026). *Improvements in safety culture linked to better patient and staff outcomes*. Retrieved from Improvement in Safety Culture Linked to Better Patient and Staff Outcomes | AHA

American Hospital Association. (2025) Fast facts on U.S. hospitals, 2025, https://www.aha.org/statistics/fast-facts-us-hospitals. Retrieved May 30, 2025.

American Hospital Association. (2025, July). *Fact sheet: Extending the hospital-at-home program.* https://www.aha.org/fact-sheets/2024-08-06-fact-sheet-extending-hospital-home-program

American Medical Association. (2023). 2 in 3 physicians are using health AI—up 78% from 2023. https://www.ama-assn.org/practice-management/digital-health/2-3-physicians-are-using-health-ai-78-2023

Anderson, K. K., Fuhrer, R., Schmitz, N., & Malla, A. K. (2013). Determinants of negative pathways to care and their impact on service disengagement in first-episode psychosis. *Social Psychiatry and Psychiatric Epidemiology, 48*(1), 125–136. DOI: 10.1007/s00127-012-0571-0 PMID: 22976337

Angus, L. (2025). *Healthcare executive coaching - MEDI Leadership.* MEDI Leadership. Retrieved from https://medileadership.org/beyond-role-clarity-unlocking-excellence-in-healthcare-dyad-and-triad-leadership-teams/

AnilKumar. A. (2026). Reimagining rural healthcare ecosystems in the age of AI and other enabling technologies. In R. Selladurai, C.Hobson, R. Selladurai, & T. Spaulding. (Eds.). (2026). *New perspectives on post-2020 healthcare reform: Opportunities and challenges.* Hershey, PA: IGI Global, Inc.

Annas, G. J. (2003). HIPAA regulations—A new era of medical-record privacy? *The New England Journal of Medicine, 348*(15), 1486–1490. DOI: 10.1056/NEJMlim035027 PMID: 12686707

Ansoff, H. I. (1975). Managing strategic surprise by response to weak signals. *California Management Review, 18*(2), 21–33. DOI: 10.2307/41164635

Archer, J., Bower, P., Gilbody, S., Lovell, K., Richards, D., Gask, L., Dickens, C., & Coventry, P. (2012). Collaborative care for depression and anxiety problems. *Cochrane Database of Systematic Reviews, 10*(10), CD006525. Advance online publication. DOI: 10.1002/14651858.CD006525.pub2 PMID: 23076925

Ardekani, A. M., Vahdat, S., Hojati, A., Moradi, H., Tousi, A. Z., Ebrahimzadeh, F., & Farhangi, M. A. (2023). Evaluating the association between the Mediterranean-DASH Intervention for Neurodegenerative Delay (MIND) diet, mental health, and cardio-metabolic risk factors among individuals with obesity. *BMC Endocrine Disorders, 23*(1), 29. DOI: 10.1186/s12902-023-01284-8 PMID: 36726099

Arrieta, A. B., Díaz-Rodríguez, N., Del Ser, J., Bennetot, A., Tabik, S., Barbado, A., & Herrera, F. (2020). Explainable Artificial Intelligence (XAI): Concepts, taxonomies, opportunities and challenges toward responsible AI. *Information Fusion*, *58*, 82–115. DOI: 10.1016/j.inffus.2019.12.012

Association of American Medical Colleges (AAMC). (2025). *Tomorrow's doctors, tomorrow's cures.* Retrieved from Tomorrow's Doctors, Tomorrow's Cures | AAMC

Association of American Medical Colleges AAMC (2024). *The complexities of physician supply and demand: Projections from 2021 to 2036*. Retrieved from The Complexities of Physician Supply and Demand: Projections From 2021 to 2036.

Astral Codex Ten. (n.d.). Best of Moltbook. https://www.astralcodexten.com/p/best-of-moltbook

August, J. (2024) Healthcare insights: How medical debt is crushing 100 million Americans. Cornell ILR Scheinman Institute, Oct. 21, 2024. https://www.ilr.cornell.edu/scheinman-institute/blog/john-august-healthcare/healthcare-insights-how-medical-debt-crushing-100-million-americans

Aviello, G., Cristiano, C., Luckman, S. M., & D'Agostino, G. (2021). Brain control of appetite during sickness. *British Journal of Pharmacology*, *178*(10), 2096–2110. DOI: 10.1111/bph.15189 PMID: 32627171

Aylward, B. S., Abbas, H., Taraman, S., Salomon, C., Gal-Szabo, D., Kraft, C., Ehwerhemuepha, L., Chang, A., & Wall, D. P. (2022). An Introduction to Artificial Intelligence in Developmental and Behavioral Pediatrics. *Journal of Behavioral Pediatrics*, *44*(2), e126–e134. DOI: 0.1097/DBP.0000000000001149 PMID: 36730317

Azalea Health. (n.d.). The importance of rural health: Building a strong local network. https://www.azaleahealth.com/blog/importance-of-rural-health-strong-local-networks/

Bailey-Hughes, B. (2021). A communication audit exercise to enhance virtual team and individual communication skills. *Management Teaching Review*, *6*(4), 298–308. DOI: 10.1177/23792981211001527

Baker, D. P., Horvath, L., Campion, M. A., Offermann, L., & Salas, E. (2005). The ALL Teamwork Framework. In Murray, T. S., Clermont, Y., & Binkley, M. (Eds.), *International Adult Literacy Survey, Measuring Adult Literacy and Life Skills: New Frameworks for Assessment*. Ministry of Industry.

Bales, R. F. (1950). A set of categories for the analysis of small group interaction. *American Sociological Review*, *15*(2), 257–263. DOI: 10.2307/2086790

Bambra, J. (n.d.). When 250 files can compromise an AI model: What the latest research tells us about LLM security. LinkedIn. https://www.linkedin.com/pulse/when-250-files-can-compromise-ai-model-what-latest-research-bambra-3bvhe/

Barbuto J., & Wheeler, D. (2006). Scale development and construct clarification of servant leadership. *Group Organization Management,* 31(3):300–326. Retrieved from Scale Development and Construct Clarification of Servant Leadership - John E. Barbuto, Daniel W. Wheeler, 2006.

Bardosh, K., De Figueiredo, A., Gur-Arie, R., Jamrozik, E., Doidge, J., Lemmens, T., Keshavjee, S., Graham, J. E., & Baral, S. (2022). The unintended consequences of COVID-19 vaccine policy: Why mandates, passports and restrictions may cause more harm than good. *BMJ Global Health, 7*(5), e008684. Advance online publication. DOI: 10.1136/bmjgh-2022-008684 PMID: 35618306

Bates, D. W., Saria, S., Ohno-Machado, L., Shah, A., & Escobar, G. (2018). Big data in health care: Using analytics to identify and manage high-risk and high-cost patients. *Health Affairs, 33*(7), 1123–1131. DOI: 10.1377/hlthaff.2014.0041 PMID: 25006137

Beauchamp, T. L., & Childress, J. F. (2019). *Principles of Biomedical Ethics* (8th ed.). Oxford University Press.

Bebinger, M. (2025). *Can artificial intelligence help with a primary care provider shortage?* Rerieved from Can artificial intelligence help with a primary care provider shortage?: NPR

Bednarczyk, L., Reichenpfader, D., Gaudet-Blavignac, C., Ette, A. K., Zaghir, J., Zheng, Y., Bensahla, A , Bjelogrlic, M., & Lovis, C. (2025). Scientific evidence for clinical text summarization using large language models: Scoping review. *Journal of Medical Internet Research, 27*, e68998. DOI: 10.2196/68998 PMID: 40371947

Beigzadeh, A., Adibi, P., Bahaadinbeigy, K., & Yamani, N. (2019). Strategies for teaching in clinical rounds: A systematic review of the literature. *Journal of Research in Medical Sciences : the Official Journal of Isfahan University of Medical Sciences, 24*(1), 33.

Benbassat, J. (2014). Role modeling in medical education: The importance of a reflective imitation. *Academic Medicine, 89*(4), 550–554.

Berghea, E. C., Ionescu, M. D., Gheorghiu, R. M., Tincu, J. F., Cobilinschi, C. O., Craiu, M., Bălgrădean, M., & Berghea, F. (2024). Integrating Artificial Intelligence in Pediatric Healthcare: Parental Perceptions and Ethical Implications. *Children (Basel, Switzerland), 11*(2), 240–252. DOI: 10.3390/children11020240 PMID: 38397353

Bern University of Applied Sciences. (2011). Tiny turbine in human artery harvests energy from blood flow. Phys.org. https://phys.org/news/2011-05-tiny-turbine-human-artery-harvests.html

Betancourt, J. (2025). *Looking to 2025: Changing healthcare, and the need for courage.* Retrieved from Looking to 2025: Changing Health Care, and the Need for Courage – Commonwealth Fund | healthcarereimagined

Bhargava, H., Salomon, C., Suresh, S., Chang, A., Kilian, R., van Stijn, D., Orio, A., Low, D., Knebel, A., & Taraman, S. (2024). Promises, Pitfalls, and Clinical Applications of Artificial Intelligence in Pediatrics. *Journal of Medical Internet Research*, *26*, e49022. DOI: 10.2196/49022 PMID: 38421690

Binkley, C., & Loftus, T. (2024). *Encoding Bioethics: AI in Clinical Decision-Making*. University of California Press.

Blake, R. R., & Mouton, J. J. (1964). *The managerial grid.* Gulf Publishers.

Blendon, R. J., & Benson, J. M. (2022). Trust in medicine, the health system & public health. *Daedalus*, *151*(4), 67–82. DOI: 10.1162/daed_a_01944

Board on Health Care Services, & the Board Institute of Medicine. (2012). *The Role of Telehealth in an Evolving Health Care Environment: Workshop Summary.* Washington (DC): National Academies Press (US). Available from: https://www.ncbi.nlm.nih.gov/books/NBK207146)

Boch, S., Sezgin, E., & Linwood, S. L. (2022). Ethical Artificial Intelligence in Paediatrics. *The Lancet. Child & Adolescent Health*, *6*(12), 833–835. DOI: 10.1016/S2352-4642(22)00243-7 PMID: 36084667

Bodenheimer, T., & Sinsky, C. (2014). From triple to quadruple aim: Care of the patient requires care of the provider. *Annals of Family Medicine*, *12*(6), 573–576. DOI: 10.1370/afm.1713 PMID: 25384822

Bodenreider, O., Cornet, R., & Vreeman, D. J. (2018). Recent developments in clinical terminologies—SNOMED CT, LOINC, and RxNorm. *Yearbook of Medical Informatics*, *27*(01), 129–139. DOI: 10.1055/s-0038-1667077 PMID: 30157516

Bonnabry, P., & François, O. (2020). Return on investment: A practical calculation tool to convince your institution. *European Journal of Hospital Pharmacy. Science and Practice*, *27*(2), 111–113. DOI: 10.1136/ejhpharm-2018-001733 PMID: 32133138

Brereton, T. A., Malik, M. M., Rost, L. M., Ohde, J. W., Zheng, L., Jose, K. A., . . . Overgaard, S. M. (2024). AImedReport: A Prototype Tool to Facilitate Research Reporting and Translation of AI Technologies in Healthcare. medRxiv, 2024-01. DOI: 10.1101/2024.01.16.24301358

Bretthauer, M., Gerke, S., Hassan, C., Ahmad, O. F., & Mori, Y. (2023). The new European medical device regulation: Balancing innovation and patient safety. *Annals of Internal Medicine*, *176*(6), 844–848. DOI: 10.7326/M23-0454 PMID: 37068279

Brock, D. C. (2018). Learning from artificial intelligence's previous awakenings: The history of expert systems. *AI Magazine*, *39*(3), 3–15. DOI: 10.1609/aimag.v39i3.2809

Budach, L., Feuerpfeil, M., Ihde, N., Nathansen, A., Noack, N., Patzlaff, H., . . . Harmouch, H. (2022). The effects of data quality on machine learning performance. arXiv preprint arXiv:2207.14529.

Budd, J. (2023). Burnout related to electronic health record use in primary care. *Journal of Primary Care & Community Health*, *14*, 21501319231166921. DOI: 10.1177/21501319231166921 PMID: 37073905

Buell, J. (2017). The Dyad Leadership Model: Four case studies. Retrieved from PRMT-Mod3-CreateChange-CaseStudies_1_.pdf

Buoli, M., Dell'osso, B., Zaytseva, Y., Gurovich, I. Y., Movina, L., Dorodnova, A., Shmuckler, A., & Altamura, A. C. (2013). Duration of untreated illness (DUI) and schizophrenia sub-types: A collaborative study between the universities of Milan and Moscow. *The International Journal of Social Psychiatry*, *59*(8), 765–770. DOI: 10.1177/0020764012456807 PMID: 23034286

Burde, H. (2011). The HITECH act: An overview. *AMA Journal of Ethics*, *13*(3), 172–175. DOI: 10.1001/virtualmentor.2011.13.3.hlaw1-1103 PMID: 23127320

Burke, C. S., Stagl, K. C., Klein, C., Goodwin, G. F., Salas, E., & Halpin, S. M. (2006). What type of leadership behaviors are functional in teams? A meta-analysis. *The Leadership Quarterly*, *17*(3), 288–307. DOI: 10.1016/j.leaqua.2006.02.007

Business Continuity Institute. (2025). Business continuity and risk management. https://www.thebci.org

Cabo, R., & Mattson, M. P. (2019). Effects of intermittent fasting on health, aging, and disease. *The New England Journal of Medicine*, *381*(26), 2541–2551. DOI: 10.1056/NEJMra1905136 PMID: 31881139

California Institute of Technology. (n.d.). Electronic skin fully powered by sweat can monitor health, serve as human-machine interface. https://www.caltech.edu/about/news/electronic-skin-fully-powered-sweat-can-monitor-health-serve-human-machine-interface

Cannon-Bowers, J. A., Tannenbaum, S. I., Salas, E., & Volpe, C. E. (1995). Defining competencies and establishing team training requirements. In Guzzo, R., & Salas, E. (Eds.), *Team effectiveness and decision making in organizations* (pp. 333–380). Jossey-Bass.

Caron, J. P., Kreher, M. A., Mickle, A. M., Wu, S., Przkora, R., Estores, I. M., & Sibille, K. T. (2022). Intermittent fasting: Potential utility in the treatment of chronic pain across the clinical spectrum. *Nutrients, 14*(12), 2536. DOI: 10.3390/nu14122536 PMID: 35745266

Casale, A., Paulus, R., Selna, M., Doll, M., Bothe, A., McKinley, K., Berry, S., Davis, D., Gilfillan, R., Hamory, B., & Steele, G. (2007). "ProvenCareSM": A Provider-Driven Pay-for-Performance Program for Acute Episodic Cardiac Surgical Care. *Annals of Surgery, 246*(4), 613–621. DOI: 10.1097/SLA.0b013e318155a996 PMID: 17893498

Cassie, B. (2025, September 4). *Big Pharma's worst nightmare? FDA now exposes drug harms in real time.* https://www.newstarget.com/2025-09-04-big-pharma-nightmare-fda-drug-harms.html

Castro Martínez, J. C., & Santamaría-García, H. (2023). Understanding mental health through computers: An introduction to computational psychiatry. *Frontiers in Psychiatry, 14*, 1092471. DOI: 10.3389/fpsyt.2023.1092471 PMID: 36824671

Center on Budget and Policy Priorities. (2025) Policy basics: Where do our federal tax dollars go? https://www.chpp.org/research/federal-budget/where-do-our-federal-tax-dollars-go. Retrieved February 22, 2025.

Centers for Medicare & Medicaid Services. (2016). *Behavioral health integration services.* https://www.cms.gov/files/document/mln909432-behavioral-health-integration-services.pdf

Centers for Medicare and Medicaid Service – CMS. (2025) National health expenditures (NHE) fact sheet. https://www.cms.gov/data-research/statistics-trents-and-reports/national-health-expenditures-data/nhe-fact-sheet. Retrieved January 20, 2025.

Centers for Medicare and Medicaid Services (CMS). (2025). *CMS announces $50 billion in awards to strengthen rural health in all 50 states.* CMS Announces $50 Billion in Awards to Strengthen Rural Health in All 50 States | CMS

Chen, G., Donahue, L. M., & Klimoski, R. J. (2004). Training undergraduates to work in organizational teams. *Academy of Management Learning & Education, 3*(1), 27–40. DOI: 10.5465/amle.2004.12436817

Chen, Y., Wang, P., & Li, Z. (2025). Exploring genetic and epigenetic markers for predicting or monitoring response to cognitive-behavioral therapy in obsessive-compulsive disorder: A systematic review. *Neuroscience and Biobehavioral Reviews, 174*, 106192. DOI: 10.1016/j.neubiorev.2025.106192 PMID: 40324706

Chishtie, J., Sapiro, N., Wiebe, N., Rabatach, L., Lorenzetti, D., Leung, A. A., Rabi, D., Quan, H., & Eastwood, C. A. (2023). Use of epic electronic health record system for health care research: Scoping review. *Journal of Medical Internet Research, 25*, e51003. DOI: 10.2196/51003 PMID: 38100185

Chng, S. Y., Tern, M. J. W., Lee, Y. S., Cheng, L. T., Kapur, J., Eriksson, J. G., Chong, Y. S., & Savulescu, J. (2025). Ethical Considerations in AI for Child Health and Recommendations for Child-Centered Medical AI. *NPJ Digital Medicine, 8*(1), 152. DOI: 10.1038/s41746-025-01541-1 PMID: 40065130

Christensen, C. M. (2003). *The innovator's dilemma*. HarperBusiness Essentials.

Cloud, G. (n.d.). Federated learning: What it is and how it works. Retrieved from https://cloud.google.com/blog/products/ai-machine-learning/federated-learning-what-it-is-and-how-it-works

CMS. (2020). *CMS announces comprehensive strategy to enhance hospital capacity amid COVID-19 surge*. Retrieved from CMS Announces Comprehensive Strategy to Enhance Hospital Capacity Amid COVID-19 Surge | CMS

Cohen, S., Doyle, W.J., Alper, C.M., Janicki-Deverts, D. & Turner, R.B. (2009). Sleep habits and susceptibility to the common cold. Archives of Internal Medicine, Jan, 169 (1), 62-67. DOI: 10.1001/archinternmed.2008.505

Cohen, G., & Slottje, A. (2024). Artificial Intelligence and the Law of Informed Consent. In Solaiman, B., & Cohen, G. (Eds.), *Research Handbook on Health, AI and the Law* (pp. 167–182). Edward Elgar Publishing. DOI: 10.4337/9781802205657.ch10

Cohen, I. G., & Mello, M. M. (2018). HIPAA and protecting health information in the 21st century. *Journal of the American Medical Association, 320*(3), 231–232. DOI: 10.1001/jama.2018.5630 PMID: 29800120

Congress.gov. (2025). *H.R. 6703 Lower health care premiums for all Americans Act*. Retrieved from H.R.6703 - 119th Congress (2025-2026): Lower Health Care Premiums for All Americans Act | Congress.gov | Library of Congress

Congress.gov. (2025). H.R.2433 - *Reducing Medically Unnecessary Delays in Care Act of 2025.* Retrieved from H.R.2433 - 119th Congress (2025-2026): Reducing Medically Unnecessary Delays in Care Act of 2025 | Congress.gov | Library of Congress

Congress.gov. (2025). *H.R.4731 - 119th Congress (2025-2026): Resident Physician Shortage Reduction Act of 2025.* Retrieved from H.R.4731 - 119th Congress (2025-2026): Resident Physician Shortage Reduction Act of 2025 | Congress.gov | Library of Congress

Congress.gov. (2025). *Text – H. R. 1 – 119th Congress (2025-2026): An act to provide for reconciliation pursuant to title II of H. Con. Res. 14.* Retrieved from Text - H.R.1 - 119th Congress (2025-2026): An act to provide for reconciliation pursuant to title II of H. Con. Res. 14. | Congress.gov | Library of Congress

Congressional Budget Office (CBO). (2025). *CBO's Review of the Reconciliation Recommendations of the House Committee on Energy and Commerce.* Retrieved from CBO's Review of the Reconciliation Recommendations of the House Committee on Energy and Commerce | Congressional Budget Office

Congressional Budget Office (CBO). (2025). *Estimated budgetary effects of public law 119-21, to provide for reconciliation pursuant to Title II of H. Con. Res. 14, Relative to CBO's January 2025 baseline.* Retrieved from Estimated Budgetary Effects of Public Law 119-21, to Provide for Reconciliation Pursuant to Title II of H. Con. Res. 14, Relative to CBO's January 2025 Baseline | Congressional Budget Office

Congressional Budget Office (CBO). (2025). *Estimated effects on the number of uninsured people in 2034 resulting from policies incorporated within CBO's baseline projections and H.R. 1, the One Big Beautiful Bill Act.* Retrieved from Estimated Effects on the Number of Uninsured People in 2034 Resulting From Policies Incorporated Within CBO's Baseline Projections and H.R. 1, the One Big Beautiful Bill Act | Congressional Budget Office

Congressional Budget Office (CBO). (2025). *H.R. 1, One Big Beautiful Bill Act (Dynamic Estimate).* Retrieved from H.R. 1, One Big Beautiful Bill Act (Dynamic Estimate) | Congressional Budget Office

Coombs, N. C., Meriwether, W. E., Caringi, J., & Newcomer, S. R. (2021). Barriers to healthcare access among US adults with mental health challenges: A population-based study. *SSM - Population Health, 15*, 100847. DOI: 10.1016/j.ssmph.2021.100847 PMID: 34179332

Cooper, A. (2025). *How Many Individuals Are Content With Health Insurance?* Retrieved from How Many People Satisfied With Health Insurance.

Cornell University. (2024). AI tools reveal complexity of mental health measurement. https://news.cornell.edu/stories/2024/07/ai-tools-reveal-complexity-mental-health-measurement

Corrigan, P. W., Larson, J. E., & Rüsch, N. (2009). Self-stigma and the "why try" effect: Impact on life goals and evidence-based practices. *World Psychiatry; Official Journal of the World Psychiatric Association (WPA)*, *8*(2), 75–81. DOI: 10.1002/j.2051-5545.2009.tb00218.x PMID: 19516923

Cottier, B., Rahman, R., Fattorini, L., Maslej, N., Besiroglu, T., & Owen, D. (2024). The rising costs of training frontier AI models. arXiv preprint arXiv:2405.21015.

Crichton, M. (2003, January 17). *Aliens cause global warming* [Caltech Michelin Lecture]. https://stephenschneider.stanford.edu/Publications/PDF_Papers/Crichton2003.pdf

Cruz, M. F., Cavalcante, C. A. M. T., & Sá Barretto, S. T. (2018). Using OPC and HL7 standards to incorporate an industrial Big Data historian in a health IT environment. *Journal of Medical Systems*, *42*(7), 122. DOI: 10.1007/s10916-018-0979-5 PMID: 29846812

Dal, N., & Bilici, S. (2024). An Overview of the Potential Role of Nutrition in Mental Disorders in the Light of Advances in Nutripsychiatry. *Current Nutrition Reports*, *13*(2), 69–81. DOI: 10.1007/s13668-024-00520-4 PMID: 38329691

Davis, M. (2024). How many doctors commit suicide every year? *Advance Study.org*. Retrieved from How Many Doctors Commit Suicide Every Year? - Advance Study

Davis, M., & Fang, A. (2025). Emancipated Minor. *StatPearls*. StatPearls Publishing. https://www.ncbi.nlm.nih.gov/books/NBK554594

Day, G. S., & Schoemaker, P. J. H. (2005). *Peripheral vision: Detecting the weak signals that will make or break your company*. Harvard Business Review Press.

Diamandis, P. H., & Kraft, D. (2025). *Exponential medicine* [Conference]. https://danielkraftmd.net/exponential-medicine

Duggan, M. J., Gervase, J., Schoenbaum, A., Hanson, W., Howell, J. T. III, Sheinberg, M., & Johnson, K. B. (2025). Clinician experiences with ambient scribe technology to assist with documentation burden and efficiency. *JAMA Network Open*, *8*(2), e2460637–e2460637. DOI: 10.1001/jamanetworkopen.2024.60637 PMID: 39969880

ECRI. (2026). Challenges facing rural healthcare in the current policy landscape. https://home.ecri.org/blogs/ecri-blog/safety-challenges-facing-rural-healthcare

Education Workforce (2022). *Five reasons Obamacare is a failure.* Retrieved from Five Reasons Obamacare is a Failure | Committee on Education & the Workforce

Ehsan, U., Liao, Q. V., Muller, M., Riedl, M. O., & Weisz, J. D. (2021, May). Expanding explainability: Towards social transparency in ai systems. In *Proceedings of the 2021 CHI conference on human factors in computing systems* (pp. 1-19). DOI: 10.1145/3411764.3445188

Eldin, M. M., Huynh, C., Eldin, R. A., Khan, S., Nguyen, B., & Kim, G. (2024). 8 The current state of nutrition education in medical schools in the United States: An analysis of curriculum, faculty perspectives, and resources. *BMJ Nutrition, Prevention & Health*, *7*, A4.1–A4. Advance online publication. DOI: 10.1136/bmjnph-2024-nnedprosummit2023.8

Elhaddad, M., & Hamam, S. (2024). AI-driven clinical decision support systems: An ongoing pursuit of potential. *Cureus*, *16*(4). Advance online publication. DOI: 10.7759/cureus.57728 PMID: 38711724

Evans, R. S. (2016). Electronic health records: then, now, and in the future. Yearbook of medical informatics, 25(S 01), S48-S61.

Faridimehr, S., Venkatachalam, S., & Chinnam, R. B. (2021). Managing access to primary care clinics using scheduling templates. *Health Care Management Science*, *24*(3), 482–498. DOI: 10.1007/s10729-020-09535-z PMID: 33400050

FDA M15 General Principles for Model-Informed Drug Development. (2024). https://www.fda.gov/regulatory-information-search-fda-guidance-documents/m15-general-prinicples-model-informed-drug-development

Federal Housing Finance Agency. (n.d.). Helping restore the American dream for all Americans. https://www.fhfa.gov/

Ferres, J. M. L. (2024). Artificial Intelligence: Its Applications andLlimitations. In Ferres, J. M. L., & Weeks, W. B. (Eds.), *AI for Good: Applications in Sustainability, Humanitarian Action, and Health* (pp. 9–32). Wiley.

Flint, A. (2024, October 22). *Avoiding discussion of vaccine side effects isn't pro-vaccine. It's anti-science.* https://harvardpublichealth.org/policy-practice/vaccine-side-effects-are-real-we-should-talk-about-them/

Fortin, E., Baca-Motes, K., Steinhubl, S., & Topol, E. (2019). Characteristics of the modern-day physician house call. [Baltimore]. *Medicine*, *98*(8), 14671. DOI: 10.1097/MD.0000000000014671 PMID: 30813215

Fradkov, A. L. (2020). Early history of machine learning. *IFAC-PapersOnLine, 53*(2), 1385–1390. DOI: 10.1016/j.ifacol.2020.12.1888

Fuhrman, J. (1995). *Fasting and eating for health: A Medical doctor's program for conquering disease*. St. Martin's Griffin.

Gabay, M. (2017). 21st century cures act. *Hospital Pharmacy, 52*(4), 264–265. DOI: 10.1310/hpx5204-264 PMID: 28515504

Gallup. (2025a). *2025 confidence in institutions poll*. https://news.gallup.com/poll/1597/confidence-institutions.aspx

Gallup. (2025b). *2025 healthcare system poll*. https://news.gallup.com/poll/4708/healthcare-system.aspx

Gardner, R. L., Cooper, E., Haskell, J., Harris, D. A., Poplau, S., Kroth, P. J., & Linzer, M. (2019). Physician stress and burnout: The impact of health information technology. *Journal of the American Medical Informatics Association : JAMIA, 26*(2), 106–114. DOI: 10.1093/jamia/ocy145 PMID: 30517663

Gartner. (2024). Gartner Announces Ranking of the Gartner Healthcare Supply Chain Top 25 for 2024. https://www.gartner.com/en/newsroom/press-releases/2024-11-13-gartner-announces-ranking-of-the-gartner-healthcare-supply-chain-top-25-for-2024

George, P., Jones, N., Goldman, H., & Rosenblatt, A. (2023). Cycles of reform in the history of psychosis treatment in the United States. *SSM. Mental Health, 3*, 100205. DOI: 10.1016/j.ssmmh.2023.100205 PMID: 37388405

Gillum, R. F. (2013). From papyrus to the electronic tablet: A brief history of the clinical medical record with lessons for the digital age. *The American Journal of Medicine, 126*(10), 853–857. DOI: 10.1016/j.amjmed.2013.03.024 PMID: 24054954

Grandview Research (2025). *U.S. concierge medicine market size*. Retrieved from U.S. Concierge Medicine Market Size | Industry Report, 2030

Grandview Research. (2024) U.S. hospital services market size and outlooks, https://www.grandviewresearch.com/horizon/outlook/hosptial-servicesmarket. Retrieved May 30, 2025.

Greenhalgh, T., Wherton, J., Papoutsi, C., Lynch, J., Hughes, G., A'Court, C., Hinder, S., Fahy, N., Procter, R., & Shaw, S. (2020). Beyond adoption: A new framework for theorizing and evaluating nonadoption, abandonment, and challenges to the scale-up, spread, and sustainability of health and care technologies. *Journal of Medical Internet Research, 19*(11), e367. DOI: 10.2196/jmir.8775 PMID: 29092808

Greer, A., Selladurai, R. I., Pfeifle, A., Selladurai, R., & Hobson, C. (2020). Effective teamwork and healthcare delivery outcomes. In Selladurai, R., Hobson, C., Selladurai, R. I., & Greer, A. (Eds.), *Evaluating challenges and opportunities for healthcare reform*. IGI Global, Inc. DOI: 10.4018/978-1-7998-2949-2.ch004

Grundler, F., Mesnage, R., Ruppert, P. M. M., Kouretas, D., & Toledo, F. W. (2024). Long-term fasting-induced ketosis in 1610 subjects: Metabolic regulation and safety. *Nutrients*, *16*(12), 1849. DOI: 10.3390/nu16121849 PMID: 38931204

Gupt, A., Naudiyal, S., Rani, A., & Kumar, S. (2024). Mental Health and the Microbiome: A Review of Psychological Impacts of Gut Microflora. *Current Pharmacology Reports*, *10*(4), 223–236. DOI: 10.1007/s40495-024-00357-z

Haakman, M., Cruz, L., Huijgens, H., & Van Deursen, A. (2021). AI lifecycle models need to be revised: An exploratory study in Fintech. *Empirical Software Engineering*, *26*(5), 95. DOI: 10.1007/s10664-021-09993-1

Habka, D., Hsu, W. C., & Antoun, J. (2025). Economic evaluation of fasting mimicking diet versus standard care in diabetic patients on dual or triple medications at baseline in the United States: A cost-utility analysis. *Value in Health*, *28*(1), 51–59. DOI: 10.1016/j.jval.2024.08.003 PMID: 39343090

Hackman, R., & Oldham, G. (1980). Job Characteristics Model in *Work Redesign*. Retrieved from Work Redesign - J. Richard Hackman, Greg R. Oldham - Google Books

Haenlein, M., & Kaplan, A. (2019). A brief history of artificial intelligence: On the past, present, and future of artificial intelligence. *California Management Review*, *61*(4), 5–14. DOI: 10.1177/0008125619864925

Haga, S. B., & LaPointe, N. M. (2013). The potential impact of pharmacogenetic testing on medication adherence. *The Pharmacogenomics Journal*, *13*(6), 481–483. DOI: 10.1038/tpj.2013.33 PMID: 23999596

Hargreaves, D. S., Sizmur, S., Pitchforth, J., Tallett, A., Toomey, S., Toomey, S. L., Hopwood, B., Schuster, M. A., & Viner, R. M. (2018). Children and Young People's Versus Parents' Responses in an English National Inpatient Survey. *Archives of Disease in Childhood*, *103*(5), 486–491. DOI: 10.1136/archdischild-2017-313801 PMID: 29434020

Harrer, S., Shah, P., Antony, B., & Hu, J. (2019). Artificial intelligence for clinical trial design. *Trends in Pharmacological Sciences*, *40*(8), 577–591. DOI: 10.1016/j.tips.2019.05.005 PMID: 31326235

Harvard Business Review. (2021). A simpler way to modernize your supply chain. Harvard Business Review. https://hbr.org/2021/09/a-simpler-way-to-modernize-your-supply-chain

Harvard Health Publishing. (2025). *Telehealth: The advantages and disadvantages.* Retrieved from Telehealth: The advantages and disadvantages - Harvard Health

Hasan, M. M., Li, H., Fallahzadeh, E., Rajbahadur, G. K., Adams, B., & Hassan, A. E. (2025). Model context protocol (mcp) at first glance: Studying the security and maintainability of mcp servers. arXiv preprint arXiv:2506.13538.

Hatzenbuehler, M. L., & Link, B. G. (2014). Introduction to the special issue on structural stigma and health. *Social Science & Medicine*, *103*, 1–6. DOI: 10.1016/j.socscimed.2013.12.017 PMID: 24445152

Haugstetter, M., Hines, S., Sousane, Z., & Mossburg, S. (2024). *Revising TeamSTEPPS: The evolution ofpatient safety teamwork training*. Retrieved from Revising TeamSTEPPS: The Evolution of Patient Safety Teamwork Training | PSNet

Haupt, A. (2025, May 12). 5 questions you should always ask at doctor's appointments. *Time*, •••, 8.

Health Resources and Services Administration. (2025). *Behavioral health workforce projections*. U.S. Department of Health and Human Services. https://data.hrsa.gov/topics/health-workforce/nchwa/workforce-projections

Hendricks, S. (2022) The oldest cure in the world: Adventures in the art and science of fasting. New York: Abrams Press Johns Hopkins Medicine (2025) Intermittent fasting: What is it, and how does it work? https://www.hopkinsmedicine.org/health/wellness-and-prevention/intermittent-fasting-what-is-it-and-how-does-it-work. Retrieved January 20, 2025.

HHS.gov. (2025). *Telehealth research recap: Quality of care*. Retrieved from Telehealth.HHS.gov: Learn how to access or provide telehealth care

Hiatt, G. (2021). *A phenomenological study of rotational leadership experiences' potential influence on promotability within organizations*. Retrieved from A Phenomenological Study of Rotational Leadership - ProQuest.

Hiltunen, E. (2008). The future sign and its three dimensions. *Futures*, *40*(3), 247–260. DOI: 10.1016/j.futures.2007.08.021

Himes, J. R. (2011). The UN Convention on the Rights of the Child: More Than a New Utopia? In C. Rutgers (Ed.). *Creating a World Fit for Children: Understanding the UN Convention on the Rights of the Child,* (pp 37-44). International Debate Educational Association.

Hirani, R., Noruzi, K., Khuram, H., Hussaini, A. S., Aifuwa, E. I., Ely, K. E., Lewis, J. M., Gabr, A. E., Smiley, A., Tiwari, R. K., & Etienne, M. (2024). Artificial intelligence and healthcare: A journey through history, present innovations, and future possibilities. *Life (Chicago, Ill.), 14*(5), 557. DOI: 10.3390/life14050557 PMID: 38792579

Hobson, C. J., Strupeck, D., Griffin, A., Szostek, J., & Rominger, A. S. (2014). Teaching MBA students teamwork and team leadership skills: An empirical evaluation of a classroom educational program. *American Journal of Business Education, 7*(3), 191–212. DOI: 10.19030/ajbe.v7i3.8629

Hobson, C. J., Strupeck, D., Griffin, A., Szostek, J., Selladurai, R., & Rominger, A. (2013). Facilitating and documenting behavioral improvements in business student teamwork skills. *Business Education Innovation Journal, 5*(1), 83–95.

Holt, C. A., & Roth, A. E. (2004). The Nash equilibrium: A perspective. *Proceedings of the National Academy of Sciences of the United States of America, 101*(12), 3999–4002. DOI: 10.1073/pnas.0308738101 PMID: 15024100

Hospital Consumer Assessment of Healthcare Providers and Systems (HCAHPS). *CAHPS Hospital Survey*. Retrieved from https://hcahpsonline.org/en/summary-analyses/

Howe, N. (2023). *The fourth turning is here*. Simon & Schuster.

HRSA Health Workforce (2024). *Physician Workforce: Projections, 2022-2037*. Retrieved from Physician Workforce: Projections, 2022-2037

Hubley, S., Lynch, S., Schneck, C., Thomas, M., & Shore. (2016). *Review of key telepsychiatry outcomes*. Retrieved from Review of key telepsychiatry outcomes - PMC

Indrio, F., Pettoello-Mantovani, M., Giardino, I., & Masciari, E. (2024). The Role of Artificial Intelligence in Pediatrics From Treating Illnesses to Managing Children's Overall Well-Being. *The Journal of Pediatrics, 275*, 11429. DOI: 10.1016/j.jpeds.2024.114291 PMID: 39242077

Inglis, S. (2015). *Structured telephone support or non-invasive telemonitoring for patients with heart failure*. Retrieved from Structured telephone support or non-invasive telemonitoring for patients with heart failure - PMC

Insel, T. R. (2014). Mental disorders in childhood: Shifting the focus from behavioral symptoms to neurodevelopmental trajectories. *Journal of the American Medical Association, 311*(17), 1727–1728. DOI: 10.1001/jama.2014.1193 PMID: 24794359

Institute of Medicine (US) Committee on Crossing the Quality Chasm. Adaptation to Mental Health and Addictive Disorders. (2006). *Improving the Quality of Health Care for Mental and Substance-Use Conditions: Quality Chasm Series*. National Academies Press (US). DOI: 10.17226/11470

Ivanova, J. (2025). *Digital equity in Telehealth: Ensuring access for all*. Retrieved from Digital Equity in Telehealth: Ensuring Access for All | Telehealth.org

Jacka, F. N., O'Neil, A., Opie, R., Itsiopoulos, C., Cotton, S., Mohebbi, M., Castle, D., Dash, S., Mihalopoulos, C., Chatterton, M. L., Brazionis, L., Dean, O. M., Hodge, A. M., & Berk, M. (2017). A randomised controlled trial of dietary improvement for adults with major depression (the 'SMILES' trial). *BMC Medicine, 15*(1), 23. DOI: 10.1186/s12916-017-0791-y PMID: 28137247

Jagarapu, J., & Savani, R. (2021). *A brief history of telemedicine and the evolution of teleneonatology*. Retrieved from A brief history of telemedicine and the evolution of teleneonatology - ScienceDirect

James, T. (2021). *Teamwork as a core value in health care*. Retrieved from Teamwork as a Core Value in Health Care | Harvard Medical School Professional, Corporate, and Continuing Education

Javed, A. (2025). Bridging the health care gap in rural populations: Challenges, innovations, and solutions. *The American Journal of Medicine, 138*(5), 761–762. DOI: 10.1016/j.amjmed.2025.01.008 PMID: 39848392

Jeevanandam, N. (2024). Making AI smarter: Why machines need to unlearn to learn, *Emeritus,* https://emeritusorg/in/non-montonic-reasoning-in-ai.

Jiang, F., Jiang, Y., Zhi, H., Dong, Y., Li, H., Ma, S., Wang, Y., Dong, Q., Shen, H., & Wang, Y. (2017). Artificial intelligence in healthcare: Past, present and future. *Stroke and Vascular Neurology, 2*(4), 230–243. DOI: 10.1136/svn-2017-000101 PMID: 29507784

Jones, K. S. (1994). Natural language processing: a historical review. Current issues in computational linguistics: in honour of Don Walker, 3-16.

Jost, T. J., & Pollock, H. (2016). Making Healthcare Truly Affordable after Healthcare Reform. *The Journal of Law, Medicine & Ethics, 44*(4), 546–554. DOI: 10.1177/1073110516684785 PMID: 28661251

Judson, T. J., Odisho, A. Y., Neinstein, A. B., Chao, J., Williams, A., Miller, C., Moriarty, T., Gleason, N., Intinarelli, G., & Gonzales, R. (2020). Rapid design and implementation of an integrated patient self-triage and self-scheduling tool for COVID-19. *Journal of the American Medical Informatics Association : JAMIA*, *27*(6), 860–866. DOI: 10.1093/jamia/ocaa051 PMID: 32267928

Jutley, G. S., Pucci, M., Ferner, R. E., & Coleman, J. J. (2024). Adverse drug reactions and interactions. *Medicine*, *52*(1), 15–22. DOI: 10.1016/j.mpmed.2023.10.006 PMID: 38221612

Kamel Boulos, M. N., & Zhang, P. (2021). Digital twins: From personalised medicine to precision public health. *Journal of Personalized Medicine*, *11*(8), 745. DOI: 10.3390/jpm11080745 PMID: 34442389

Kao, H., Conant, R., Soriano, T., & McCormick, W. (2009). The past, present, and future of house calls. *Clinics in Geriatric Medicine*, *25*(1), 19–34. DOI: 10.1016/j.cger.2008.10.005 PMID: 19217490

Kapadia, K., Ruwali, S., Malav, T., Seshadri, S., Seidmann, A., Press, D. Z., & Kolachalama, V. B. (2024). Enhancing efficiency with an AI-augmented clinician in neurology. *Aging and Disease*, *16*(5), 2498. DOI: 10.14336/AD.2024.1249 PMID: 39500349

Kaur, G., Aggarwal, H., & Goel, N. (2025). Artificial intelligence driven neuropsychiatry: A systematic review of electroencephalography-based computational techniques for major depressive disorder prediction. *Neuroscience*, *581*, 179–207. DOI: 10.1016/j.neuroscience.2025.07.010 PMID: 40639536

Kaye, J., Curren, L., Anderson, N., Edwards, K., Fullerton, S. M., Kanellopoulou, N., Lund, D., MacArthur, D. G., Mascalzoni, D., Shepherd, J., Taylor, P. L., Terry, S. F., & Winter, S. F. (2012). From Patients to Partners: Participant-Centric Initiatives in Biomedical Research. *Nature Reviews. Genetics*, *13*(5), 371–376. DOI: 10.1038/nrg3218 PMID: 22473380

Kaye, J., Whitley, E. A., Lund, D., Morrison, M., Teare, H., & Melham, K. (2015). Dynamic Consent: A Patient Interface for Twenty-First Century Research Networks. *European Journal of Human Genetics : EJHG*, *23*(2), 141–146. DOI: 10.1038/ejhg.2014.71 PMID: 24801761

Kayser, A. (2025). *World's best hospitals 2025 – United State of America*. Retrieved from World's Best Hospitals 2025 - United States of America.

Kayser, A. (2025). *World's best hospitals 2025 – United States of America*. Retrieved from World's Best Hospitals 2025 - United States of America

Keeley, P., Wolf, Z., Regul, L., & Jadwin, A. (2015). Effectiveness of standard of care protocol on patient satisfaction and perceived staff caring. *Clinical Journal of Oncology Nursing, 19*(3), 352–360. DOI: 10.1188/15.CJON.352-360 PMID: 26000585

Keenan, T. (2025). *Rural adults wait longer and travel farther for medical appointments. AARP.org*. Retrieved from Medical Appointment Waiting and Travel Time.

Kelly, A., & Tangalakis-Lippert, K. (2025). *The longest government shutdown in US history is over after 43 days.* Retrieved from The Longest Government Shutdown in US History Is Over After 43 Days - Business Insider

Kelly, R., & Lavelle, A. (2024). *Teamwork matters: team situation awareness to build high-performing healthcare teams.* Retrieved from Teamwork matters: team situation awareness to build high-performing healthcare teams.

KFF. (2025). International comparison of health systems. https://www.kff.org/health-policy-101/

Khan, B., Talha, K., & Ul, W.. (2025). Reshaping the healthcare world by AI-integrated wearable sensors following COVID-19. [Retrieved from Google Scholar]. *Chemical Engineering Journal, 505*, 159478. DOI: 10.1016/j.cej.2025.159478

Kilkelly, U. (2016). The Best Interests of the Child: A Gateway to Children's Rights? In Sutherland, E. E., & Macfarlane, L. B. (Eds.), *Implementing Article 3 of the United Nations Convention on the Rights of the Child: Best Interests, Welfare and Well-being* (pp. 51–66). Cambridge University Press. DOI: 10.1017/9781316662977.004

Kim, T., & Zuckerman, J. (2019). Realizing the potential of telemedicine in global health. Retrieved from Realizing the potential of telemedicine in global health - PMC

Kim, J. S., Vivas, A., Arvind, V., Lombardi, J., Reidler, J., Zuckerman, S. L., Lee, N. J., Vulapalli, M., Geng, E. A., Cho, B. H., Morizane, K., Cho, S. K., Lehman, R. A., Lenke, L. G., & Riew, K. D. (2023). Can natural language processing and artificial intelligence automate the generation of billing codes from operative note dictations? *Global Spine Journal, 13*(7), 1946–1955. DOI: 10.1177/21925682211062831 PMID: 35225694

KiranKumar, Y. (2023). *Role of management in healthcare.* Retrieved from Role of Management in Healthcare

Kiss, J. (2023). *6 types of concierge medicine fees.* Retrieved from *6 Types of Concierge Medicine Fees*

Koch, E., Pardiñas, A. F., O'Connell, K. S., Selvaggi, P., Collados, J. C., Babic, A., Marshall, S. E., Eycken, E. V., Angulo, C., Lu, Y., Sullivan, P. F., Dale, A. M., Molden, E., Posthuma, D., White, N., Schubert, A., Djurovic, S., Heimer, H., Stefánsson, H., & Andreassen, O. A. (2024). How Real-World Data Can Facilitate the Development of Precision Medicine Treatment in Psychiatry. *Biological Psychiatry*, *96*(7), 543–551. DOI: 10.1016/j.biopsych.2024.01.001 PMID: 38185234

Kocher, R., Emanuel, E. J., & DeParle, N. A. M. (2010). The Affordable Care Act and the future of clinical medicine: The opportunities and challenges. *Annals of Internal Medicine*, *153*(8), 536–539. DOI: 10.7326/0003-4819-153-8-201010190-00274 PMID: 20733178

Kononenko, I. (2001). Machine learning for medical diagnosis: History, state of the art and perspective. *Artificial Intelligence in Medicine*, *23*(1), 89–109. DOI: 10.1016/S0933-3657(01)00077-X PMID: 11470218

Koonin L., Hoots, B., Tsang C., Leroy Z., Farris K., Jolly B., Antall, P., McCabe B., Zelis, C., Tong, I., Harris, A. (2020). *Trends in telehealth use during the emergence of the COVID-19 pandemic*. Retrieved from Trends in the Use of Telehealth D... preview & related info | Mendeley

Koppold, D. A., Breinlinger, C., Hanslian, E., Kessler, C., Cramer, H., Rajput Khokhar, A., Peterson, C. M., Tinsley, G., Vernieri, C., Bloomer, R., Boschmann, M., Bragazzi, N., Brandhorst, S., Gabel, K., Goldhamer, A. C., Grajower, M., Harvie, M., Heilbronn, L., Home, B., & Michalsen, A. (2024). International consensus on fasting terminology. *Cell Metabolism*, *36*(8), 1779–1794. DOI: 10.1016/j.cmet.2024.06.013 PMID: 39059384

Kotter, J. P. (2012). *Leading change*. Harvard Business Review Press.

Kouzes, J. M., & Posner, B. Z. (2011). *Credibility: How leaders gain and lose it, why people demand it* (2nd ed.). Jossey-Bass. DOI: 10.1002/9781118983867

Kruse, K. (2022). *How Mayo Clinic develops leaders who drive engagement and reduce burnout*. Retrieved from How Mayo Clinic Develops Leaders Who Drive Engagement And Reduce Burnout.

Kuhn, T. S. (1962). *The structure of scientific revolutions*. University of Chicago Press.

Kushnick, H. L. (2015) Medicine and the market AMA Journal of Ethics, From the Editor, August 2015, https://journalofethics.ama-assn.org/article/medicine-and-market/2015-08

Kwon, M., Jolin, J., & Shachar, C. (2024). Telehealth after the Federal COVID-19 Public Health Emergency: Implications and Future Directions. *The Journal of Law, Medicine & Ethics*, *52*(2), 412–418. DOI: 10.1017/jme.2024.118 PMID: 39435920

Labkoff, S., Oladimeji, B., Kannry, J., Solomonides, A., Leftwich, R., Koski, E., Joseph, A. L., Lopez-Gonzalez, M., Fleisher, L. A., Nolen, K., Dutta, S., Levy, D. R., Price, A., Barr, P. J., Hron, J. D., Lin, B., Srivastava, G., Pastor, N., Luque, U. S., & Quintana, Y. (2024). Toward a responsible future: Recommendations for AI-enabled clinical decision support. *Journal of the American Medical Informatics Association : JAMIA*, *31*(11), 2730–2739. DOI: 10.1093/jamia/ocae209 PMID: 39325508

Lamb, H. R., & Bachrach, L. L. (2001). Some Perspectives on Deinstitutionalization. *Psychiatric Services (Washington, D.C.)*, *52*(8), 999–1118. DOI: 10.1176/appi.ps.52.8.1039 PMID: 11474048

Laubenbacher, R., Mehrad, B., Shmulevich, I., & Trayanova, N. (2024). Digital twins in medicine. *Nature Computational Science*, *4*(3), 184–191. DOI: 10.1038/s43588-024-00607-6 PMID: 38532133

Liang, W., Tadesse, G. A., Ho, D., Fei-Fei, L., Zaharia, M., Zhang, C., & Zou, J. (2022). Advances, challenges and opportunities in creating data for trustworthy AI. *Nature Machine Intelligence*, *4*(8), 669–677. DOI: 10.1038/s42256-022-00516-1

Liden, R., Wayne, S., Zhao, H., & Henderson, D. (2008, April). Servant leadership: Development of a multidimensional measure and multi-level assessment. [Retrieved from Servant leadership: Development of a multidimensional measure and multi-level assessment - ScienceDirect]. *The Leadership Quarterly*, *19*(2), 161–177. DOI: 10.1016/j.leaqua.2008.01.006

Likert, R. (1961). *New patterns of management*. McGraw-Hill.

Lincoff, N. (2015). *The future of healthcare could be in concierge medicine*. Retrieved from https://www.healthline.com/health-news/the-future-of-healthcare-could-be-in-concierge-medicine-063015

Lira-Junior, R., Aogain, M. M., Crncalo, E., Ekberg, N. R., Chotirmall, S. H., Pettersson, S., Gustafsson, A., Brismar, K., & Bostanci, N. (2024). Effects of intermittent fasting on periodontal inflammation and subgingival microbiota. *Journal of Periodontology*, *95*(7), 640–649. DOI: 10.1002/JPER.23-0676 PMID: 38655661

Luengo-Fernandez, R., Walli-Attaei, M., Gray, A., Torbica, A., Maggioni, A. P., Huculeci, R., Bairami, F., Aboyans, V., Timmis, A. D., Vardas, P., & Leal, J. (2023). Economic burden of cardiovascular diseases in the European Union: A population-based cost study. *European Heart Journal, 44*(45), 4752–4767. DOI: 10.1093/eurheartj/ehad583 PMID: 37632363

Mahdavi, S., Fekri, M., Mohammadi-Sarab, S., Mehmandoost, M., & Zarei, E. (2025). *The use of telemedicine in family medicine: A scoping review*. Retrieved from The use of telemedicine in family medicine: A scoping review | BMC Health Services Research | Springer Nature Link

Makiwa, T. (2025). *The job characteristics model: everything you need to know*. Retrieved from The job characteristic model: everything you need to know | The Human Capital Hub

Mandel, J. C., Kreda, D. A., Mandl, K. D., Kohane, I. S., & Ramoni, R. B. (2016). SMART on FHIR: A standards-based, interoperable apps platform for electronic health records. *Journal of the American Medical Informatics Association : JAMIA, 23*(5), 899–908. DOI: 10.1093/jamia/ocv189 PMID: 26911829

Maraniss, D. (2000). *When pride still mattered: A life of Vince Lombardi*. Simon & Schuster.

Marshall, B. J., & Warren, J. R. (2005). *Helicobacter pylori and peptic ulcer disease* [Nobel Prize in Physiology or Medicine]. https://www.nobelprize.org/prizes/medicine/2005/marshall/facts/

Massachusetts Institute of Technology. (2019). Robotic thread is designed to slip through the brain's blood vessels. https://meche.mit.edu/news-media/robotic-thread-designed-slip-through-brain%E2%80%99s-blood-vessels

Massachusetts Institute of Technology. (2022). Handheld surgical robot can help stem fatal blood loss. https://news.mit.edu/2022/handheld-surgical-robot-can-help-stem-fatal-blood-loss-0317

Massachusetts Institute of Technology. (2025). Wearable device tracks individual cells in the bloodstream in real time. https://news.mit.edu/2025/circtrek-wearable-device-tracks-individual-cells-bloodstream-real-time-0423

Matar, M., Massaad, C., Itani, A., Kreidly, S., Chedid, G., Salameh, P., & Nakib, H. (2025). Attitudes and practices toward medical literature: A cross-sectional study at LAU Medical Center-Rizk. *Future Science OA, 11*(1), 2526314. DOI: 10.1080/20565623.2025.2526314 PMID: 40588374

Maternal Mental Health Leadership Alliance (MMHLA). (2025). *The One Big Beautiful Bill Act (OBBBA) and its Impact on Maternal Mental Health*. The One Big Beautiful Bill Act (OBBBA) and its Impact on Maternal Mental Health — Maternal Mental Health Leadership Alliance: MMHLA

Mayer, K. (2024) Employers project 8% - 9% rise in health care costs for 2025. Society for Human Resource Management, https://www.shrm.org/topics-tool/news/benefits-compensation/employers-project-8-9-rise-in-health-care-costs-for-2025. Retrieved May 26, 2025.

Mayo Clinic Finance. (2025). Mayo Clinic Financial Operating Budget. [Unpublished].

Mayo Clinic Supply Chain. (2025a). Mayo Clinic 2025 Operating Budget. [Unpublished].

Mayo Clinic Supply Chain. (2025b). Mayo Clinic Five Step CQVA Process. [Unpublished].

Mayo Clinic Supply Chain. (2025c). Mayo Clinic Supply Chain Automation Assessment. [Unpublished].

Mayo Clinic Supply Chain. (2025d). Mayo Clinic Supply Chain Strategic Plan. [Unpublished}. Nadeau, K. L. (2019). Value-based care: The role and impact of healthcare supply chains. https://www.ghx.com/the-healthcare-hub/role-supply-chain-management-healthcare/

Mayo Clinic. (2025). "*The Mayo Effect*:" *Ten things you may not know about Mayo*. Retrieved from https://share.google/ZqnWlKFoTzFDKXSk2

Mayo Clinic. (2025). *How Mayo Clinic measures patient experience*. Retrieved from Patient Experience - Mayo Clinic.

Mayo Clinic. (2025). *Why Mayo Clinic*? Retrieved from https://executiveeducation.mayo.edu/catalog?pagename=why-mayo-clinic

Mayo Clinic. (2026). *Mission and values*. Rerieved from Mission and values - Mayo Clinic

McCall, B. (2018). What does the GDPR mean for the medical community? *Lancet, 391*(10127), 1249–1250. DOI: 10.1016/S0140-6736(18)30739-6 PMID: 29619949

McCarthy, J. (2018, December 7). Most Americans rate still rate their healthcare quality quite positively. *Well-Being*. Retrieved from https://news.gallup.com/poll/245195/americans-rate-healthcare-quite-positively.aspx

McCarthy, J. (1956). https://www.formal.stanford.edu/jmc/index.html

McCarthy, J. (1959, December). Programs with Common Sense. *Proceedings of the Teddington Conference on the Mechanization of Thought Processes.*

McClain, C. R. (2025). Trade secrets and transparency in medical research. *Journal of Healthcare Ethics*, *14*(2), 112–128.

McDermottt+ Consulting (2025). *Health-related provisions in the One Big Beautiful Bill Act.* Retrieved from Health-related provisions in the One Big Beautiful Bill Act - McDermott+

Medbridge (2026). *Why the Quadruple Aim matters for healthcare systems today.* Retrieved from Quadruple Aim in Healthcare: 4 Key Goals | Medbridge

Mehta, N., & Devarakonda, M. V. (2018). Machine learning, natural language programming, and electronic health records: The next step in the artificial intelligence journey? *The Journal of Allergy and Clinical Immunology*, *141*(6), 2019–2021. DOI: 10.1016/j.jaci.2018.02.025 PMID: 29518424

Mello, M. M., & Guha, N. (2024). Understanding liability risk from using health care artificial intelligence tools. *The New England Journal of Medicine*, *390*(3), 271–278. DOI: 10.1056/NEJMhle2308901 PMID: 38231630

Meskó, B., Kristóf, T., Dhunnoo, P., Árvai, N., & Katonai, G. (2024). Exploring the need for medical futures studies: Insights from a scoping review of health care foresight. *Journal of Medical Internet Research*, *26*, e57148. DOI: 10.2196/57148 PMID: 39383528

Meurers, D. (2012). Natural language processing and language learning. Encyclopedia of applied linguistics, 4193-4205. DOI: 10.1002/9781405198431.wbeal0858

Meyer, H. (2026). AI in 2026: Combatting the healthcare staffing shortage. [Combatting the Healthcare Staffing Shortage - Providertech]. *AI*, •••, 2026.

Miller, A. H., Berk, M., Bloch, G., Briquet-Laugier, V., Brouillon, C., Cuthbert, B. N., Dantzer, R., Davis, M. C., De Picker, L. J., Drevets, W. C., Eyre, H. A., Hack, L. M., Harrison, N. A., Krystal, A. D., Lombardo, G., Mondelli, V., Pariante, C. M., Pulvirenti, L., Salvadore, G., & Leboyer, M. (2025). Advancing precision psychiatry and targeted treatments: Insights from immunopsychiatry. *Brain, Behavior, and Immunity*, *125*, 319–329. DOI: 10.1016/j.bbi.2025.01.002 PMID: 39828008

Miller, J. E., Wilenzick, M., Ritcey, N., Ross, J. S., & Mello, M. M. (2017). Measuring clinical trial transparency: An empirical analysis of newly approved drugs and large pharmaceutical companies. *BMJ Open*, *7*(12), e017917. Advance online publication. DOI: 10.1136/bmjopen-2017-017917 PMID: 29208616

Minh, D., Wang, H. X., Li, Y. F., & Nguyen, T. N. (2022). Explainable artificial intelligence: A comprehensive review. *Artificial Intelligence Review*, *55*(5), 3503–3568. DOI: 10.1007/s10462-021-10088-y

Miranda, L., Paul, R., Pütz, B., Koutsouleris, N., & Müller-Myhsok, B. (2021). Systematic Review of Functional MRI Applications for Psychiatric Disease Subtyping. *Frontiers in Psychiatry*, *12*, 665536. DOI: 10.3389/fpsyt.2021.665536 PMID: 34744805

Mittermaier, M., Raza, M. M., & Kvedar, J. C. (2023). Bias in AI-based models for medical applications: Challenges and mitigation strategies. *NPJ Digital Medicine*, *6*(1), 113. DOI: 10.1038/s41746-023-00858-z PMID: 37311802

Mojtabai, R. (2021). US. Health Care Reform and Enduring Barriers to Mental Health Care Among Low-Income Adults With Psychological Distress. *Psychiatric Services (Washington, D.C.)*, *72*(3), 338–342. DOI: 10.1176/appi.ps.202000194 PMID: 33467868

Mokwena, K. E. (2021). Neglecting Maternal Depression Compromises Child Health and Development Outcomes, and Violates Children's Rights in South Africa. *Children (Basel, Switzerland)*, *8*(7), 609. DOI: 10.3390/children8070609 PMID: 34356588

Mukkamala, B. (2025). *The physician shortage will worsen – unless Congress acts now*. Retrieved from The physician shortage will worsen—unless Congress acts now | American Medical Association

Murad, M. H., Vaa Stelling, B. E., West, C. P., Hasan, B., Simha, S., Saadi, S., Firwana, M., Viola, K. E., Prokop, L. J., Nayfeh, T., & Wang, Z. (2024). Measuring documentation burden in healthcare. *Journal of General Internal Medicine*, *39*(14), 2837–2848. DOI: 10.1007/s11606-024-08956-8 PMID: 39073484

Naddaf, M. (2025, September 23). Journals infiltrated with 'copycat' papers that can be written by AI. *Nature*. https://www.nature.com/articles/d41586-025-03046-z

National Council for Mental Wellbeing. (2021). Mental Health First Aid USA. https://www.mentalhealthfirstaid.org

Nazer, L. H., Zatarah, R., Waldrip, S., Ke, J. X. C., Moukheiber, M., Khanna, A. K., Hicklen, R. S., Moukheiber, L., Moukheiber, D., Ma, H., & Mathur, P. (2023). Bias in artificial intelligence algorithms and recommendations for mitigation. *PLOS Digital Health*, *2*(6), e0000278. DOI: 10.1371/journal.pdig.0000278 PMID: 37347721

Neuner, I., Veselinović, T., Ramkiran, S., Rajkumar, R., Schnellbaecher, G. J., & Shah, N. J. (2022). 7T ultra-high-field neuroimaging for mental health: An emerging tool for precision psychiatry? *Translational Psychiatry*, *12*(1), 36. DOI: 10.1038/s41398-022-01787-3 PMID: 35082273

Nevada State University. (2025). Rural healthcare: How is it unique? https://nevadastate.edu/son/rn-bsn/rural-healthcare-how-is-it-unique/

Newitt, P. (2025). *The biggest threat to physicians in 2026*. The biggest threat to physicians in 2026 - Becker's Physician Leadership

Niekerk, G., Loos, B., Nell, T., & Engelbrecht, A.M. Autophagy-A free meal in sickness-associated anorexia, Autophagy, 12 (4), 727-734, .DOI: 10.1080/15548627.2016.1147672

NTCA–The Rural Broadband Association. (2025). Broadband/internet availability survey report 2025. https://www.ntca.org/sites/default/files/documents/2025-12/2025BroadbandInternetAvailabilityReport.pdf

Nyarko, E. N., Santa, S., & Diaba-Nuhoho, P. (2025). AI and digital health for childhood cancer care in Ghana. *Communications Medicine*, *5*(1), 344. DOI: 10.1038/s43856-025-01047-7 PMID: 40781166

Nye, K., Cherrin, C., & Meires, J. (2024). Intermittent fasting: Exploring approaches, benefits, and implications for health and weight management. *The Journal for Nurse Practitioners*, *20*(3), 104893. DOI: 10.1016/j.nurpra.2023.104893

O'Brien, J. (2024). *Category Management in Purchasing*. Kogan Page.

Obermeyer, Z., Powers, B., Vogeli, C., & Mullainathan, S. (2019). Dissecting racial bias in an algorithm used to manage the health of populations. *Science*, *366*(6464), 447–453. DOI: 10.1126/science.aax2342 PMID: 31649194

Obuchowicz, R., Piórkowski, A., Nurzyńska, K., Obuchowicz, B., Strzelecki, M., & Bielecka, M. (2026). Will AI Replace Physicians in the Near Future? AI Adoption Barriers in Medicine. *Diagnostics (Basel)*, *16*(3), 396. DOI: 10.3390/diagnostics16030396 PMID: 41681714

Olawade, D. B., Wada, O. J., David-Olawade, A. C., Kunonga, E., Abaire, O., & Ling, J. (2023). Using artificial intelligence to improve public health: A narrative review. *Frontiers in Public Health*, *11*, 1196397. DOI: 10.3389/fpubh.2023.1196397 PMID: 37954052

Osheroff, J. A., Teich, J., Levick, D., Saldana, L., Velasco, F., Sittig, D., & Jenders, R. (2012). *Improving outcomes with clinical decision support: an implementer's guide*. Himss Publishing. DOI: 10.4324/9781498757461

Parletta, N., Zarnowiecki, D., Cho, J., Wilson, A., Bogomolova, S., Villani, A., Itsiopoulos, C., Niyonsenga, T., Blunden, S., Meyer, B., Segal, L., Baune, B. T., & O'Dea, K. (2017). A Mediterranean-style dietary intervention supplemented with fish oil improves diet quality and mental health in people with depression: A randomized controlled trial (HELFIMED). *Nutritional Neuroscience*, *22*(7), 474–487. DOI: 10.1080/1028415X.2017.1411320 PMID: 29215971

Patel, J. (2019). Bridging data silos using big data integration. International Journal of Database Management Systems, 11(3), 01-06.

Permanente, K. (n.d.). Housing security: Programs and partnerships. https://about.kaiserpermanente.org/expertise-and-impact/healthy-communities/our-programs-and-partnerships/housing-security

Pescosolido, B. A. (2013). The public stigma of mental illness: What do we think; what do we know; what can we prove? *Journal of Health and Social Behavior*, *54*(1), 1–21. DOI: 10.1177/0022146512471197 PMID: 23325423

Petersen, C., Smith, J., Freimuth, R. R., Goodman, K. W., Jackson, G. P., Kannry, J., Liu, H., Madhavan, S., Sittig, D. F., & Wright, A. (2021). Recommendations for the Safe, Effective Use of Adaptive CDS in the U.S. Healthcare System: An AMIA Position Paper. *Journal of the American Medical Informatics Association : JAMIA*, *28*(4), 677–684. DOI: 10.1093/jamia/ocaa319 PMID: 33447854

Peters, Z., Lendon, J., Caffrey, C., Myrick, K., Mahar, M., & DeFrances, C. (2024, September). Telemedicine use during the COVID-19 pandemic by office-based physicians and long-term care providers. *Retrieved from CDC National Health Statistics Reports*, (210), 18. PMID: 39471289

Pew Research Center. (2025). *How Americans view AI and its impact on people and society*. https://www.pewresearch.org/wp-content/uploads/sites/20/2025/09/PS_2025.9.15_AI-and-its-impact_report.pdf

Physician Advisory Institute (2024). *Over 77% of physicians are employed. Here's how that's shaping healthcare.* Retrieved from Over 77% of physicians are employed. Here's how that's shaping healthcare.

Physicians Practice. (2024, April 23). *What over 2 million patients say about their healthcare experiences*. https://www.physicianspractice.com/view/what-over-2-million-patients-say-about-their-healthcare-experiences

Pine, B. J., & Gilmore, J. H. (2020). *The experience economy* (Updated ed.). Harvard Business Review Press.

Pine, B. J., & Gilmore, J. H. (2007). *Authenticity: What consumers really want*. Harvard Business Review Press.

Pine, B. J., & Gilmore, J. H. (2020). *The experience economy*. Harvard Business Review Press.

Porterfield, C. (2021, December 21). Dr. Fauci on GOP criticism: 'Attacks on me, quite frankly, are attacks on science.' *Forbes*. https://www.forbes.com/sites/carlieporterfield/2021/06/09/fauci-on-gop-criticism-attacks-on-me-quite-frankly-are-attacks-on-science/

Porter, M. E., & Lee, T. H. (2013). The strategy that will fix health care. *Harvard Business Review*, *91*(10), 50–70.

Powles, J., & Hodson, H. (2017). Google DeepMind and healthcare in an age of algorithms. *Health and Technology*, *7*(4), 351–357. DOI: 10.1007/s12553-017-0179-1 PMID: 29308344

Pratt, M. (2025). *How AI is changing telemedicine in 2025*. Retrieved from How AI is Changing Telemedicine in 2025 | Informa TechTarget

Prins, S. J. (2011). Does Transinstitutionalization Explain the Overrepresentation of People with Serious Mental Illnesses in the Criminal Justice System? *Community Mental Health Journal*, *47*(6), 716–722. DOI: 10.1007/s10597-011-9420-y PMID: 21655941

Probul, N., Huang, Z., Saak, C. C., Baumbach, J., & List, M. (2024). AI in microbiome-related healthcare. *Microbial Biotechnology*, *17*(11), e70027. DOI: 10.1111/1751-7915.70027 PMID: 39487766

Prosci. (2025). ADKAR model. https://www.prosci.com

Protection, P., & Act, A. C. (2010). affordable Care Act. Public law, (111-148), 124.

Providence Health & Services. (2022). *Behavioral health integration outcomes report*. Providence St. Joseph Health.

Providence Health & Services. (2022, June 1). Providence program builds bridge to behavioral health care, recovery. *Catholic Health World*. https://www.chausa.org/news-and-publications/publications/catholic-health-world/archives/june-1-2022/providence-program-builds-bridge-to-behavioral-health-care-recovery

Providence, St. Joseph Health. (2023). *About us*. https://www.providence.org/about

PwC. (2025, May 29). *Healthcare execs rethink strategy amid market and policy volatility*. Fierce Healthcare. https://www.fiercehealthcare.com/providers/healthcare-leaders-rethinking-short-term-strategy-amid-market-policy-volatility-pwc

Rahman, S., Jiang, L. Y., Gabriel, S., Aphinyanaphongs, Y., Oermann, E. K., & Chunara, R. (2024). Generalization in healthcare ai: Evaluation of a clinical large language model. arXiv preprint arXiv:2402.10965.

Rajaraman, V. (2014). John McCarthy: Father of Artificial Intelligence. *Resonance, 19*(3), 198–207. DOI: 10.1007/s12045-014-0027-9

Ramgopal, S., Sanchez-Pinto, L. N., Horvat, C. M., Carroll, M. S., Luo, Y., & Florin, T. A. (2023). Artificial intelligence-based clinical decision support in pediatrics. *Pediatric Research, 93*(2), 334–341. DOI: 10.1038/s41390-022-02226-1 PMID: 35906317

Reichert, A., & Jacobs, R. (2018). The impact of waiting time on patient outcomes: Evidence from early intervention in psychosis services in England. *Health Economics, 27*(11), 1772–1787. DOI: 10.1002/hec.3800 PMID: 30014544

Reinhard, S. C., Caldera, S., Houser, A., & Choula, R. B. (2023). Valuing the Invaluable 2023 Update: Strengthening Supports for Family Caregivers. Washington, DC: AARP Public Policy Institute. March 8, 2023. DOI: 10.26419/ppi.00082.006

Rittel, H. W. J., & Webber, M. M. (1973). Dilemmas in a general theory of planning. *Policy Sciences, 4*(2), 155–169. DOI: 10.1007/BF01405730

Robinson, S. (2011). Children's Rights: Historic Developments. In C. Rutgers (Ed.). *Creating a World Fit for Children: Understanding the UN Convention on the rights of the Child,* (pp. 16-25). International Debate Education Association.

Rodriguez, J. A., Clark, C. R., & Bates, D. W. (2020). Digital health equity as a necessity in the 21st century cures act era. *Journal of the American Medical Association, 323*(23), 2381–2382. DOI: 10.1001/jama.2020.7858 PMID: 32463421

Rossi, M., & Rehman, S. (2025). *Integrating Artificial Intelligence into telemedicine: Evidence, challenges, and future directions*. Retrieved from Integrating Artificial Intelligence Into Telemedicine: Evidence, Challenges, and Future Directions - PMC

Roth A. (2018). Insane: America's Criminal Treatment of Mental Illness

Rucker, P., Miller, M., & Armstrong, D. (2023, March 25). How Cigna saves millions by having its doctors reject claims without reading them. *ProPublica*. https://www.propublica.org/article/cigna-pxdx-medical-health-insurance-rejection-claims

Runge, M. (2025). *The great healthcare disruption: big tech, bold policy, and the future of american medicine*. Forbes Books.

Saad, L (2023). *Gallup: Historically low faith in U.S. institutions continues*. Retrieved from Historically Low Faith in U.S. Institutions Continues

Saberi, M. A., Mcheick, H., & Adda, M. (2025). From data silos to health records without borders: A systematic survey on patient-centered data interoperability. *Information (Basel)*, *16*(2), 106. DOI: 10.3390/info16020106

Saharkhiz, M., Rao, T., Parker-Lue, S., Borelli, S., Johnson, K., & Cataife, G. (2024). Telehealth expansion and Medicare beneficiaries' care quality and access. *JAMA Network Open*, *7*(5), e2411006. DOI: 10.1001/jamanetworkopen.2024.11006 PMID: 38739388

Salari-Moghaddam, A., Keshteli, A. H., Mousavi, S. M., Afshar, H., Esmaillzadeh, A., & Adibi, P. (2019). Adherence to the MIND diet and prevalence of psychological disorders in adults. *Journal of Affective Disorders*, *256*, 96–102. DOI: 10.1016/j.jad.2019.05.056 PMID: 31170621

Salas, E., Sims, D. E., & Burke, C. S. (2005). Is there a "Big Five" in teamwork? *Small Group Research*, *36*(5), 555–599. DOI: 10.1177/1046496405277134

Salter, E. K., Hester, D. M., Vinarcsik, L., Antommaria, A. H. M., Bester, J., Blustein, J., Clayton, E. W., Diekema, D. S., Itlis, A. S., Kopelman, L., Malone, J. R., Mercurio, M. R., Navin, M. C., Paquette, E. T., Pope, T. M., Rhodes, R., & Ross, L. F. (2024). Pediatric Decision Making: Consensus Recommendations. *Pediatrics*, *152*(3), e2023061832. DOI: 10.1542/peds.2023-061832 PMID: 37555276

Sambasivan, N., ... ""Everyone wants to do the model work, not the data work": Data Cascades in High-Stakes AI." proceedings of the 2021 CHI Conference on Human Factors in Computing Systems. 2021. DOI: 10.1145/3411764.3445518

Sánchez-Salmerón, R., Gómez-Urquiza, J. L., Albendín-García, L., Correa-Rodríguez, M., Martos-Cabrera, M. B., Velando-Soriano, A., & Suleiman-Martos, N. (2022). Machine learning methods applied to triage in emergency services: A systematic review. *International Emergency Nursing*, *60*, 101109. DOI: 10.1016/j.ienj.2021.101109 PMID: 34952482

Sarpong, D., Maclean, M., & Davies, C. (2013). A matter of foresight: How practices enable (or impede) organizational foresightfulness. *European Management Journal*, *31*(6), 613–625. DOI: 10.1016/j.emj.2013.03.004

Schildbach, S., & Schildbach, C. (2018). Criminalization Through Transinstitutionalization: A Critical Review of the Penrose Hypothesis in the Context of Compensation Imprisonment. *Frontiers in Psychiatry*, *9*, 534. DOI: 10.3389/fpsyt.2018.00534 PMID: 30410452

Schmutz, J., Meier, L., & Manser, T. (2019). *How effective is teamwork really? The relationship between teamwork and performance in healthcare teams: A systematic review and meta-analysis*. Retrieved from Schmutz: How effective is teamwork really? The relationsh... - Google Scholar

Science Direct. (2013). Product Variety Management. https://www.sciencedirect.com/science/article/pii/S0007850613001972

Scott, B. (2024). *Inaugural address at the 2024 AMA annual meeting*. Retrieved from There is a perfect storm coming, with increased demand for prior authorizations from the insurance company by Bruce Scott, MD - Search Videos

Scott, R. (2025). *Sen. Rick Scott introduces bill to fix Obamacare and drive down health care costs*. Retrieved from Sen. Rick Scott Introduces Bill to Fix Obamacare and Drive Down Health Care Costs.

Selladurai, R., & Carraher, S. (2014). Lead like the greatest leader! Case Study. In Selladurai, R., & Carraher, S. (Eds.), *Servant leadership: Research and Practice* (pp. 350–355). IGI Global. DOI: 10.4018/978-1-4666-5840-0.ch026

Selladurai, R., Hobson, C., Selladurai, R. I., & Greer, A. (2020). *Evaluating challenges and opportunities for healthcare reform. IGI Global, Inc.*

Sepluveda, J. L., & Young, D. S. (2013). The ideal laboratory information system. *Archives of Pathology & Laboratory Medicine*, *137*(8), 1129–1140. DOI: 10.5858/arpa.2012-0362-RA PMID: 23216205

Seymour, T., Frantsvog, D., & Graeber, T. (2012). Electronic health records (EHR). *American Journal of Health Sciences*, *3*(3), 201–210. DOI: 10.19030/ajhs.v3i3.7139

Shanafelt, T. D., Hasan, O., Dyrbye, L. N., Sinsky, C., Satele, D., Sloan, J., & West, C. P. (2016). Changes in burnout and satisfaction with work–life balance in physicians and the general U.S. working population between 2011 and 2014. *Mayo Clinic Proceedings*, *90*(12), 1600–1613. DOI: 10.1016/j.mayocp.2015.08.023 PMID: 26653297

Shanafelt, T. D., West, C. P., Dyrbye, L. N., Trockel, M., Tutty, M., Wang, H., Carlasare, L. E., & Sinsky, C. (2022). Changes in burnout and satisfaction with work-life integration in physicians during the first 2 years of the COVID-19 pandemic. *Mayo Clinic Proceedings*, *97*(12), 2248–2258. DOI: 10.1016/j.mayocp.2022.09.002 PMID: 36229269

Shandafelt, T., Dyrbe, L., West, C., Wang, H., Carlasare, L., & Sinsky, C. (2023). Career Plans of U.S. Physicians After the First 2 Years of the COVID-19 Pandemic. *Mayo Clinic Proceedings*, p. 1629-1640. Retrieved from Career Plans of U.S. Physicians After the First 2 Years of the COVID-19 Pandemic - Mayo Clinic Proceedings

Shi, Q., Luzuriaga, K., Allison, J. J., Oztekin, A., Faro, J. M., Lee, J. L., Hafter, N., McManus, M., & Zai, A. H. (2025). Transforming Informed Consent Generation Using Large Language Models: Mixed Methods Study. *JMIR Medical Informatics*, *13*, e368139. DOI: 10.2196/68139 PMID: 39946400

Shore, J. H., Yellowlees, P., Caudill, R., Johnston, B., Turvey, C., Mishkind, M., Krupinski, E., Myers, K., Shore, P., Kaftarian, E., & Hilty, D. (2018). Best Practices in Videoconferencing-Based Telemental Health April 2018. *Telemedicine journal and e-health: the official journal of the American Telemedicine Association*, 24(11), 827–832. DOI: 10.1089/tmj.2018.0237

Shortliffe, E. H., & Sepúlveda, M. J. (2018). Clinical decision support in the era of artificial intelligence. *Journal of the American Medical Association*, *320*(21), 2199–2200. DOI: 10.1001/jama.2018.17163 PMID: 30398550

Shoubridge, A. P., Choo, J. M., Martin, A. M., Keating, D. J., Wong, M.-L., Licinio, J., & Rogers, G. B. (2022). The gut microbiome and mental health: Advances in research and emerging priorities. *Molecular Psychiatry*, *27*(4), 1908–1919. DOI: 10.1038/s41380-022-01479-w PMID: 35236957

Singh, J., Sillerud, B., & Singh, A. (2023). Artificial intelligence, chatbots and ChatGPT in healthcare—Narrative review of historical evolution, current application, and change management approach to increase adoption. *Journal of Medical Artificial Intelligence*, *6*, 6. DOI: 10.21037/jmai-23-92

Sisk, B. A., Antes, A. L., & DuBois, J. M. (2020). Parental Attitudes Toward Artificial Intelligence-Driven Precision Medicine Technologies in Pediatric Healthcare. *Children (Basel, Switzerland)*, *7*(9), 145. DOI: 10.3390/children7090145 PMID: 32962204

Skulmowski, A. (2025). Informed Consent in Educational AI Research Needs to Be Transparent, Flexible and Dynamic. *Mind, Brain and Education : the Official Journal of the International Mind, Brain, and Education Society*, *19*(1), 32–36. DOI: 10.1111/mbe.12435

Slater, B., & Schur, M. (2023). *The future of healthcare as an integrated ecosystem of health and care.* Retrieved from https://www.gensler.com/blog/future-of-healthcare-as-integrated-ecosystem

Slater, B., & Schur, M. (2023, August 23). The future of healthcare as an integrated ecosystem of health and care. Gensler. https://www.gensler.com/blog/future-of-healthcare-as-integrated-ecosystem

Sloss, E. A., Abdul, S., Aboagyewah, M. A., Beebe, A., Kendle, K., Marshall, K., Rosenbloom, S. T., Rossetti, S., Grigg, A., Smith, K. D., & Mishuris, R. G. (2024). Toward alleviating clinician documentation burden: A scoping review of burden reduction efforts. *Applied Clinical Informatics*, *15*(03), 446–455. DOI: 10.1055/s-0044-1787007 PMID: 38839063

Smith, K. A., Blease, C., Faurholt-Jepsen, M., Firth, J., Van Daele, T., Moreno, C., Carlbring, P., Ebner-Priemer, U. W., Koutsouleris, N., Riper, H., Mouchabac, S., Torous, J., & Cipriani, A. (2023). Digital mental health: Challenges and next steps. *BMJ Mental Health*, *26*(1), e300670. DOI: 10.1136/bmjment-2023-300670 PMID: 37197797

Softheon. (2025, September). *Strategy in action healthcare executive survey: 4 key insights for health plans.* https://www.softheon.com/blog/strategy-in-action-healthcare-executive-survey-4-key-insights-for-health-plans

Sonka Medical. (n.d.). https://www.sonkamedical.com/

Spaans, I., Verbree, A. R., de Kleijn, R., & Dilaver, G. (2026). Role models in medicine and beyond: A survey study exploring the relationship between role models, academic performance and sense of belonging. *BMC Medical Education*, *26*(1), 5.

Spears, L. C. (2004). Practicing servant leadership. *Leader to Leader*, *34*(34), 7–11. DOI: 10.1002/ltl.94

Spies, C., & Ranzani, O. (2025). *Telemedicine in critical care.* Telemedicine in critical care | Intensive Care Medicine | Springer Nature Link

Spredemann, A. (2025, November 9). How AI is supercharging scientific fraud. *The Epoch Times*. https://www.theepochtimes.com/article/how-ai-is-supercharging-scientific-fraud-5937211

St. Mary' University. (2026). *Exploring effective leadership and team management in healthcare*. Retrieved from Exploring effective leadership and team management in healthcare - Blog

Statifacts (2025) U.S. pharmaceutical market – Industry report. https://www.statifacts.com/outlook/us-pharmaceutical-market. Retrieved May 29, 2025.

Statista (2025) OTC pharmaceuticals – United States – market forecast. https://www.statista.com/outlook/hmo/otc-pharmaceuticals/united-states. Retrieved May 29, 2025.

Stevens, M. J., & Campion, M. A. (1994). The knowledge, skill, and ability requirements for teamwork: Implications for human resource management. *Journal of Management*, *20*(2), 503–530. DOI: 10.1177/014920639402000210

Stevens, R. (1998). *American Medicine and the Public Interest*. University of California Press.

Stobierski, T. (2021, March 23). What is health care economics? Harvard Business School Online. https://online.hbs.edu/blog/post/what-is-healthcare-economics

Stogdill, R. M., & Coons, A. E. (1957). *Leader behavior: Its description and measurement*. Ohio State University, Bureau of Business Research.

Substance Abuse and Mental Health Services Administration. (2021). Key substance use and mental health indicators in the United States: Results from the 2020 National Survey on Drug Use and Health (HHS Publication No.PEP21-07-01-003, NSDUH Series H-56). Rockville, MD: Center for Behavioral Health Statistics and Quality, Substance Abuse and Mental Health Services Administration. Retrieved from https://www.samhsa.gov/data/

Sun, M. L., Yao, W., Wang, X. Y., Gao, S., Varady, K. A., Forslund, S. K., Zhang, M. Z. Y., Cao, F., Zou, B. J., Sun, M. H., Liu, K. X., Bao, Q., Xu, J., Qin, X., Xiao, Q., Wu, L., Zhao, Y. H., Zhang, D. Y., Wu, Q. J., & Gong, T. T. (2024, April). Intermittent fasting and health outcomes: An umbrella review of systematic reviews and meta-analyses of randomized controlled trials. *EClinicalMedicine*, *70*, 102519. DOI: 10.1016/j.eclinm.2024.102519 PMID: 38500840

Sun, Y., Sheng, D., Zhou, Z., & Wu, Y. (2024). AI hallucination: Towards a comprehensive classification of distorted information in artificial intelligence-generated content. *Humanities & Social Sciences Communications*, *11*(1), 1278. DOI: 10.1057/s41599-024-03811-x

Sya'ban, S., Wazir, A., & Horneffer, P. (2024). *Active learning in medical education*. Retrieved from Active Learning in Medical Education | Lecturio

Syamsir, S., Saputra, N., & Mulia, R. (2025). Leadership agility in a VUCA world: A systematic review, conceptual insights, and research directions. *Cogent Business & Management, 12*(1), 2482022. Advance online publication. DOI: 10.1080/23311975.2025.2482022

Szabo, C. (2025). *Unreliable: Bias, fraud, and the reproducibility crisis in biomedical research.* Columbia University Press. DOI: 10.7312/szab21623

Tan, H. (2017, September). A brief history and technical review of the expert system research. [). IOP Publishing.]. *IOP Conference Series. Materials Science and Engineering, 242*(1), 012111. DOI: 10.1088/1757-899X/242/1/012111

Telehealth.HHS.gov. (2025). *Learn how to access or provide telehealth care.* Retrieved from Telehealth.HHS.gov: Learn how to access or provide telehealth care

Telehealth.HHS.gov. (2026). *Telehealth policy updates.* Retrieved from Telehealth policy updates | Telehealth.HHS.gov

Teo, Z. L., Jin, L., Liu, N., Li, S., Miao, D., Zhang, X., Ng, W. Y., Tan, T. F., Lee, D. M., Chua, K. J., Heng, J., Liu, Y., Goh, R. S. M., & Ting, D. S. W. (2024). Federated machine learning in healthcare: A systematic review on clinical applications and technical architecture. *Cell Reports Medicine, 5*(2), 101419. DOI: 10.1016/j.xcrm.2024.101419 PMID: 38340728

The Beryl Institute. (2023, January). *Consumer perspectives on patient experience in the U.S. PX Pulse.* https://theberylinstitute.org/wp-content/uploads/woocommerce_uploads/2023/02/PXPulse_Q1_Jan2023-nc4w5c.pdf

The Beryl Institute. (2024). *Consumer perspectives on patient experience in the U.S.* Retrieved from https://theberylinstitute.org/wp-content/uploads/woocommerce_uploads/2024/10/Consumer-Perspectives-on-Patient-Experience-2024-1-mqh0nm.pdf

The Physicians Foundation. (2018). *2018 survey of America's physicians: Practice patterns and perspectives.* https://physiciansfoundation.org/wp-content/uploads/2018/09/physicians-survey-results-final-2018.pdf

The White House Executive Order. (2025, May 12). *Delivering most-favored-nation prescription drug pricing to American patients.* Retrieved from Delivering Most-Favored-Nation Prescription Drug Pricing to American Patients – The White House

The White House. (2025, July 4). *The One Big Beautiful Bill.* Retrieved from The One Big Beautiful Bill – The White House

The White House. (2026). *President Trump unveils the Great Healthcare Plan to Lower Costs and Deliver Money Directly to the People*. Retrieved from President Trump Unveils The Great Healthcare Plan to Lower Costs and Deliver Money Directly to the People – The White House.

Thornicroft, G., Sunkel, C., Alikhon Aliev, A., Baker, S., Brohan, E., El Chammay, R., Davies, K., Demissie, M., Duncan, J., Fekadu, W., Gronholm, P. C., Guerrero, Z., Gurung, D., Habtamu, K., Hanlon, C., Heim, E., Henderson, C., Hijazi, Z., Hoffman, C., & Winkler, P. (2022). The Lancet Commission on ending stigma and discrimination in mental health. *Lancet*, *400*(10361), 1438–1480. DOI: 10.1016/S0140-6736(22)01470-2 PMID: 36223799

Tierney, A. A., Gayre, G., Hoberman, B., Mattern, B., Ballesca, M., Kipnis, P., Liu, V., & Lee, K. (2024). Ambient artificial intelligence scribes to alleviate the burden of clinical documentation. *NEJM Catalyst Innovations in Care Delivery*, *5*(3), CAT-23. DOI: 10.1056/CAT.23.0404

Topol, E. (2019). *Deep Medicine: How Artificial Intelligence Can Make Healthcare Human Again*. Basic Books.

Toynbee, M. (2015). The Penrose hypothesis in the 21st century: Revisiting the asylum. *Evidence-Based Mental Health*, *18*(3), 76. DOI: 10.1136/eb-2015-102115 PMID: 26116302

Tozzi, L., Zhang, X., Pines, A., Olmsted, A. M., Zhai, E. S., Anene, E. T., Chesnut, M., Holt-Gosselin, B., Chang, S., Stetz, P. C., Ramirez, C. A., Hack, L. M., Korgaonkar, M. S., Wintermark, M., Gotlib, I. H., Ma, J., & Williams, L. M. (2024). Personalized brain circuit scores identify clinically distinct biotypes in depression and anxiety. *Nature Medicine*, *30*(7), 2076–2087. DOI: 10.1038/s41591-024-03057-9 PMID: 38886626

Trastek, V. F., Hamilton, N. W., & Niles, E. E. (2014). Leadership models in healthcare – A case for servant leadership. *Mayo Clinic Proceedings*, *89*(3), 374–381. DOI: 10.1016/j.mayocp.2013.10.012 PMID: 24486078

U.S. Bureau of Labor Statistics. (2024). Physicians and Surgeons: Occupational Outlook Handbook. Retrieved from Physicians and Surgeons: Occupational Outlook Handbook: U.S. Bureau of Labor Statistics

U.S. Government Accountability Office. (2025, September 25). *Healthcare is becoming more consolidated—including physicians. What effect is it having?* https://www.gao.gov/blog/health-care-becoming-more-consolidated-including-physicians.-what-effect-it-having

Ulrich, A. (2025, July 8). *8 best AI medical documentation tools for healthcare in 2025*. https://austinulrich.com/best-ai-medical-documentation-tools-for-healthcare

UNESCO. (2006, June). Universal declaration on bioethics and human rights. Paris. https://unesdoc.unesco.org/images/0014/001461/146180E.pdf

United Nations Convention on the Rights of the Child, Nov. 20, 1989, 1577 U.N.T.S. 3.

University of Hawaiʻi. (2023). Breakthrough for sweat: Health monitoring device from UH researchers. https://www.hawaii.edu/news/2023/05/03/sweatainer-health-device/

Unützer, J., Katon, W. J., Fan, M. Y., Schoenbaum, M. C., Lin, E. H., Della Penna, R. D., & Powers, D. (2013). Long-term cost effects of collaborative care for late-life depression. *The American Journal of Managed Care, 14*(2), 95–100. PMID: 18269305

US Department of Health and Human Services (2025). *HHS Secretary Kennedy and CMC Administrator Oz secure industry pledge to fix the broken prior authorization system*. Retrieved from HHS Secretary Kennedy, CMS Administrator Oz Secure Industry Pledge to Fix Broken Prior Authorization System | HHS.gov

US House Committee on Ways & Means. (2025, December 30). *Ways & Means Committee delivered historic tax relief for families in 2025.* Retrieved from Ways & Means Committee Delivered Historic Tax Relief for Working Families in 2025 - Ways and Means

US House Committee on Ways & Means. (2025, November 13). *Republicans Deliver Lower Health Costs, More Choice, and Greater Control for Working Families.* Retrieved from Republicans Deliver Lower Health Costs, More Choice, and Greater Control for Working Families - Ways and Means

US News. (2026). America's Best Hospitals: 2025-2026 Honor Roll and Overview. America's Best Hospitals: The 2025-2026 Honor Roll and Overview | U.S. News

van Dellen, E. (2024). Precision psychiatry: Predicting predictability. *Psychological Medicine, 54*(8), 1500–1509. DOI: 10.1017/S0033291724000370 PMID: 38497091

Van Noorden, R. (2023, December 12). More than 10,000 research papers were retracted in 2023—a new record. *Nature*. https://www.nature.com/articles/d41586-023-03974-8

van Westrhenen, R., Young, A. H., Heilbronner, U., Juruena, M., Ingelman-Sundberg, M., Jukic, M., Kaprio, J., Kas, M. J. H., Moldovan, R., Nöthen, M. M., Philipsen, A., Shomron, N., Van der Eycken, E., Vieta, E., & Schulze, T. G. (2025). PSY-PGx: A new intervention for the implementation of pharmacogenetics in psychiatry. *World Psychiatry; Official Journal of the World Psychiatric Association (WPA)*, *24*(1), 141–142. DOI: 10.1002/wps.21289 PMID: 39810666

Varadan, S. (2020). Article 5: The Role of Parents in the Proxy Informed Consent Process in Medical Research Involving Children. *International Journal of Children's Rights*, *28*(3), 521–546. DOI: 10.1163/15718182-02803009

Vertex, A. I. (n.d.). Google Cloud. https://cloud.google.com/vertex-ai?hl=en

Visram, S., Leyden, D., Annesley, O., Bappa, D., & Sebire, N. J. (2023). Engaging Children and Young People on the Potential Role of Artificial Intelligence in Medicine. *Pediatric Research*, *93*(2), 440–444. DOI: 10.1038/s41390-022-02053-4 PMID: 35393524

Viswanadham, N. (2021). Ecosystem model for healthcare platform. *Sadhana*, *46*(4), 188. DOI: 10.1007/s12046-021-01708-y

Wade, S.B. (2023). *Transforming Healthcare: AI in Healthcare Leads to Greater Accuracy and Precision, Minimizing Discrepancies and Improving Patient Outcomes*. Independently published.

Wang, F., & Beecy, A. (2025). Implementing AI models in clinical workflows: A roadmap. *BMJ Evidence-Based Medicine*, *30*(5), 285–287. PMID: 38914450

Wang, P. S., Berglund, P. A., Olfson, M., & Kessler, R. C. (2004). Delays in initial treatment contact after the first onset of a mental disorder. *Health Services Research*, *39*(2), 393–415. DOI: 10.1111/j.1475-6773.2004.00234.x PMID: 15032961

Wang, Y., & Ma, Z. (2023). Ethical and Legal Examples of Medical AI on Informed Consent: China as an Example. *Developing World Bioethics*, *25*(1), 46–54. DOI: 10.1111/dewb.12442 PMID: 38240080

Wang, Z., Chu, Z., Doan, T. V., Ni, S., Yang, M., & Zhang, W. (2025). History, development, and principles of large language models: An introductory survey. *AI and Ethics*, *5*(3), 1955–1971. DOI: 10.1007/s43681-024-00583-7

Wanzer, R., Booth-Butterfield, M., & Grueber, K. (2014). Perceptions of health-care providers' communication: Relationships between patient-centered communication and satisfaction. *Health Communication*, *16*(3), 363–383. DOI: 10.1207/S15327027HC1603_6 PMID: 15265756

Wasylewicz, A. T., & Scheepers-Hoeks, A. M. J. W. (2018). Clinical decision support systems. Fundamentals of clinical data science, 153-169.

Webster, C., Coomber, T., Liu, S., Allen, K., & Jowsey, T. (2023). *Interprofessional learning in multidisciplinary healthcare teams is associated with reduced patient mortality: A quantitative systematic review and meta-analysis*. Retrieved from Webster: Interprofessional learning in multidisciplinary... - Google Scholar

Weineke, K., Berkland, B., Kruse, G., Priestly, M., Teal, D., & West, C. (2025). *Charting a New Path Forward in Addressing Employee Well-being in Health Care.* Retrieved from Charting a New Path Forward in Addressing Employee Well-being in Health Care -. *Mayo Clinic Proceedings*, *100*(3), 501–513. DOI: 10.1016/j.mayocp.2024.11.018

Weller, J., Mahajan, R., Fahey-Williams, K., & Wesbster, C. (2024). "*Teamwork matters: team situation awareness to build high-performing healthcare teams, a narrative review.*" Retrieved from Teamwork matters: team situation awareness to build high-performing healthcare teams, a narrative review - ScienceDirect

West, C. P., Dyrbye, L. N., & Shanafelt, T. D. (2018). Physician burnout: Contributors, consequences and solutions. *Journal of Internal Medicine*, *283*(6), 516–529. DOI: 10.1111/joim.12752 PMID: 29505159

Whereby. (2025). *5 predictions for the future of telehealth.* Retrieved from https://whereby.com/blog/5-predictions-for-the-future-of-telehealth/

Wilhelm, C., Surendar, J., & Karagiannis, F. (2021) Enemy or ally? Fasting as an essential regulator of immune responses. Trends in Immunology, May, 42 (5), 389-400. .DOI: 10.1016/j.it.2021.03.007

Wong, A., Otles, E., Donnelly, J. P., Krumm, A., McCullough, J., DeTroyer-Cooley, O., Pestrue, J., Phillips, M., Konye, J., Penoza, C., Ghous, M., & Singh, K. (2021). External validation of a widely implemented proprietary sepsis prediction model in hospitalized patients. *JAMA Internal Medicine*, *181*(8), 1065–1070. DOI: 10.1001/jamainternmed.2021.2626 PMID: 34152373

World Economic Forum. (2025). Ways AI is transforming healthcare. https://www.weforum.org/stories/2025/08/ai-transforming-global-health/

World Health Organization & International Telecommunication Union. (2025). Mapping the application of artificial intelligence in traditional medicine: Technical brief.

World Health Organization. (2025). India first country to launch a Traditional Knowledge Digital Library. https://economictimes.indiatimes.com/news/india/india-first-country-to-launch-a-traditional-knowledge-digital-library-who/articleshow/122403845.cms

World Medical Association. (2024). Declaration of Helsinki ethical principles for medical research involving human subjects. https://www.wma.net/what-we-do/medical-ethics/declaration-of-helsinki

Xu, F., Uszkoreit, H., Du, Y., Fan, W., Zhao, D., & Zhu, J. (2019, September). Explainable AI: A brief survey on history, research areas, approaches and challenges. In *CCF international conference on natural language processing and Chinese computing* (pp. 563–574). Springer International Publishing. DOI: 10.1007/978-3-030-32236-6_51

Yang, Q., Liu, Y., Chen, T., & Tong, Y. (2019). Federated machine learning: Concept and applications. [TIST]. *ACM Transactions on Intelligent Systems and Technology*, *10*(2), 1–19. DOI: 10.1145/3298981

Youth Mental Health and Substance Use Task Force. (2025). Redesigning the health care delivery system to better meet the needs of youth. Bipartisan Policy Center. https://bipartisanpolicy.org/report/health-care-redesign-youth/

Yu, J., Zhang, J., & Sengoku, S. (2023). Innovation process and industrial system of US Food and Drug Administration–approved software as a medical device: Review and content analysis. *Journal of Medical Internet Research*, *25*, e47505. DOI: 10.2196/47505 PMID: 37999948

Zach, G. (2024). *The AI Advantage in Healthcare: Unlocking the Power of Artificial Intelligence to Enhance Precision, Elevate Diagnostics, and Streamline Patient Care*. GZ Publishing.

Zajac, S., Woods, A., Tannenbaum, S., Salas, E., & Holladay, C. (2021). "*Overcoming Challenges to Teamwork in Healthcare: A Team Effectiveness Framework and Evidence-Based Guidance,*" Retrieved from Frontiers | Overcoming Challenges to Teamwork in Healthcare: A Team Effectiveness Framework and Evidence-Based Guidance

Zayas-Cabán, T., Okubo, T. H., & Posnack, S. (2023). Priorities to accelerate workflow automation in health care. *Journal of the American Medical Informatics Association : JAMIA*, *30*(1), 195–201. DOI: 10.1093/jamia/ocac197 PMID: 36259967

Zhou, C., Li, Q., Li, C., Yu, J., Liu, Y., Wang, G., Zhang, K., Ji, C., Yan, Q., He, L., Feng, H., Li, J., Wu, J., Liu, Z., Xie, P., Xiong, C., Pei, J., Yu, P. S., & Sun, L. (2025). A comprehensive survey on pretrained foundation models: A history from bert to chatgpt. *International Journal of Machine Learning and Cybernetics*, *16*(12), 9851–9915. DOI: 10.1007/s13042-024-02443-6

Zhu, J., Zeveney, A., Read, S., & Crowley, R. (2024). Physician perspectives on private equity investment in healthcare. [Retrieved from Physician Perspectives on Private Equity Investment in Health Care | Health Care Economics, Insurance, Payment | JAMA Internal Medicine | JAMA Network]. *JAMA Internal Medicine*, *184*(5), 579–580. DOI: 10.1001/jamainternmed.2024.0062 PMID: 38466275

Zucker, H. (2025). Where have all the physicians gone? AARP.org/Bulletin. Retrieved from America Is Facing a Shortage of Doctors

About the Contributors

Raj Selladurai is an Associate Professor of Management in the School of Business and Economics at Indiana University Northwest. He also serves as Small Business Institute (SBI) Director for the School of Business and Economics. In addition, he has owned and managed a consulting business in the energy industry and other related areas. His research interests focus on servant leadership, business-healthcare collaboration, leadership effectiveness, operations/supply chain management, and high-speed rail/supply chain management. Recently, he led a project team as the Lead Project Director and completed a book project, "Challenges and Opportunities for Healthcare Reform." The team consisted of two business professors (Dr. Raj Selladurai and Dr. Charlie Hobson (Professors, Indiana University Northwest), and two physicians (Dr. Roshini Selladurai, MD, In His Image, OK, and Dr. Adam Greer (MD, St John, Ascension Healthcare, OK)) who worked collaboratively on the healthcare project. They completed it in 2019, and IGI Global published it in February 2020. In addition, Raj Selladurai was invited to participate in Harvard University's "What's next for US healthcare reform? Seminar at Harvard University School of Public Health in Boston, MA. Healthcare Reform in the US is an ongoing, significant national initiative with strategic policy implications, which would affect several millions of stakeholders in the US, especially in the coming election. Incidentally, some of the significant healthcare reform-related issues that we in the US are facing and managing today and will be in the future have been addressed and discussed in our book, completed in 2019! Dr. Selladurai has published several papers, chapters, and case studies in various management and operations management-related business publications and journals, including co-editing (with Shawn Carraher) a book on "Servant Leadership: Research and Practice." He also co-edited with Peggy Daniels Lee and George VandeWerken his other recent book, "Emerging Challenges and Opportunities of High-Speed Rail on Business and Society," which was published by IGI Global, Inc. All his innovative books are being actively promoted on social media like Twitter, with impressive results of around 33,000+ impressions per month and growing! He has over 30 years of academic and professional business experience, including completing a Professional Certificate in "Servant Leadership: Path to High Performance" Executive Education Seminar at the prestigious Darden School of Business, University of Virginia. He also completed another Certificate in Organizational Behavior at Harvard Business School, Harvard University. He has also taught business management courses as Visiting Professor at universities in Austria and Switzerland. He has diverse leadership and administrative experiences in various organizations, including serving as a Lead Elder, finance deacon, and Group Leader at Bethel Church, Crown Point, Indiana, as a Group Leader at Bible Study Fellowship (BSF), and in other roles at the university, community, business, and other professional service organizations. Raj also serves as a Board member of the Agape Asia nonprofit organization that provides holistic services to children worldwide. Dr. Selladurai's current project is to continue integrating SAP (Systems, Applications, Products), the world-renowned Enterprise Resource Planning (ERP) software, in the Operations Management courses and the IU Online programs to help benefit students gain a competitive edge in their jobs and careers.

Charles J. Hobson Charlie has a Ph.D. in Industrial/Organizational Psychology from Purdue and is currently a Professor of Management in the AACSB-accredited School of Business and Economics at Indiana University Northwest, where he has taught MBA and undergraduate classes in Human Resource Management, Leadership, Teamwork, Organizational Behavior, and Entrepreneurship since 1981. In addition, Charlie has 189 professional publications/presentations, 4 books, and 1 book chapter on HR-related topics, has provided training/consultation services to 205 organizations (Fortune 100 to new start-ups), and functioned as an expert witness in 41 cases involving workplace and educational discrimination.

Roshini Selladurai, M.D., is a board certified Family Medicine physician at Mayo Clinic with additional board certification in Obesity Medicine. She is also an Assistant Professor in Family Medicine at Mayo Clinic School of Medicine. Dr. Selladurai attended medical school at Indiana University. She trained in Family Medicine with an emphasis on whole person care, global health, and medical missions at In His Image Family Medicine residency in Tulsa, OK. She received her board certification in Obesity Medicine in 2021. Dr. Selladurai's clinical practice focuses on whole person care, education, preventative medicine, and obesity medicine. She aims to provide compassionate, holistic care and education so patients feel heard and experience hope. Her research interests include physician burnout, research writing, teamwork in healthcare, and lifestyle medicine. She and her husband enjoy spending time with family, friends, church community, and exploring the outdoors with their golden retriever.

Tony Spaulding joined Mayo Clinic as Quality Improvement Advisor in August of 2008. Since then, Tony has held roles as Senior Health Systems Engineering Analyst and Operations Manager within General Internal Medicine. In 2015, Tony joined Provider Relations as an Operations Administrator working with the Mayo Clinic Care Network. Tony has also served as an instructor with the Mayo Clinic Quality Academy, helping to develop and deliver a broad-based quality management curriculum for Mayo Clinic staff. In 2021 Tony joined the Midwest Department of Family Medicine as an Operations Administrator that oversees 50+ clinics throughout the midwest. Tony has Bachelor of Science Degree in Business from Saint Mary's University and a Master's Degree in Business Management from Saint Mary's. Tony also holds a Certification in Lean Principles from the University of Michigan. Tony holds academic ranks as an Assistant Professor in Health Care System Engineering and as an Assistant Professor of Health Care Administration with the Mayo Clinic School of Health Sciences. Prior to his employment at Mayo Clinic, Tony spent fifteen years as an Engineer and Lean Engineer for a large manufacturer of heavy construction equipment. Tony is a Minnesota native. He and his wife, Kelly, have four children.

***

Barry Doublestein is Adjunct Associate Professor in the School of Business & Leadership at Regent University. He currently teaches strategy development in the Masters in Organizational Leadership Program, leadership theory & communications, healthcare leadership, and chair of numerous doctoral project committees in the Doctor of Strategic Leadership Program. He is also Senior Director of Leadership Solutions (a leadership consulting practice) and Chairman of the Board of Peace Mountain Enterprises (a Georgia Not-for Profit institution whose purpose is to advance training on developing leaders of virtuous character). He has spent the entirety of his vocational career in pre-and post-graduate medical education leadership roles and advocacy for physician policy initiatives at the state and national level. Dr. Doublestein earned his BA in Psychology from Albion College, his MA in Educational Administration from Truman State University, and his DSL (Doctor of Strategic Leadership) from the Regent University School of Business & Leadership. He is an author of numerous articles and book chapters on the role of professionalism in medicine and is an international speaker on leadership development in healthcare.

Joe Dudas is responsible for providing oversight and coordination of Mayo's Supply Chain Strategic Initiatives. Additionally, Joe is the Inspirity Systems and Operations EVP as well as Board Member. The Mayo Clinic Supply Chain manages Purchasing, Distribution, and Inventory Management functions across Mayo Clinic. Over the past 15+ years, Mayo's Supply Chain has been on a transformative journey to move a decentralized and autonomous function to that of a highly integrated and, in part, commercial shared service. The results to-date total over $1B in value to Mayo Clinic.

James Francis is the Chief Supply Chain Officer for Mayo Clinic based in Rochester, MN. He has worked at Mayo Clinic for 26 years managing an enterprise-wide supply chain of $7.4B annually. Prior to joining Mayo Clinic he was the Vice President of Supply Chain at BJC Health in St. Louis, MO. Mr. Francis holds a Masters degree in Health Administration from the Washington University School of Medicine in St. Louis. He participates in numerous community and professional organizations. He is an Assistant Professor in Mayo's College of Medicine and Science.

Jason Greenwood holds an MS in Electrical Engineering from the University of Wisconsin–Madison. He has experience with engineering start-ups as well as larger companies such as IBM and has contributed to both software and hardware development. He earned his MD from the University of North Dakota, completed his Family Medicine residency at Mayo Clinic in Rochester, MN, and pursued fellowship training in Clinical Informatics at Mayo Clinic in Rochester, MN. Currently, he serves as Assistant Professor and Director of Artificial Intelligence and Clinical Informatics in the Department of Family Medicine at Mayo Clinic Rochester, MN. He carries a full panel of patients, lectures at the Mayo Clinic Alix School of Medicine, and has been an invited speaker at multiple board review courses. He publishes on a diverse range of topics in primary care and informatics.

Abburi Kumar obtained his Ph.D. in Physics from the Indian Institute of Science, Bangalore. After working on a variety of research projects on device modeling and communication theory aspects, he focused on what he recognized as proper preparation in STEM disciplines at the middle and high school levels. imperative for better college level performance. He worked with multiple school districts on state and national standards, relevance of science in the global economy and expanding opportunities for students, teachers and faculty in STEM disciplines. For the over five years he directed Project XLR8 (ACCELERATE), a high school redesign project, funded by the Thurgood Marshall College Fund, with support from the Bill and Melinda Gates Foundation. He is currently working on a monograph on redesigning education. For his work in public education and his achievements in research, he was one of five faculty members in the TAMU System to have received the Distinguished Achievement Award from the Board of Regents, a recipient of the Thurgood Marshall College Fund's Outstanding Achievement Award for School Reform and the Harmony Public Schools Public Servant Award. His current interests include modeling of cancer metastasis and learning in the age of reengineered humanity.

Lawrence Lee, MD, received a medical degree from the Medical College of Wisconsin, completed Family Medicine residency training at In His Image Family Medicine Residency program, and completed a Hospital Medicine fellowship at the University of Alabama. Currently serving as a hospitalist and adjunct faculty member with the In His Image Family Medicine Residency, Lee has over sixteen years of experience in clinical practice and medical education. Primary areas of focus include clinical reasoning, evidence-based decision-making, and the cultivation of growth and resilience mindsets among resident physicians. Additional interests include mentoring in professional and spiritual development, as well as real estate investing, playing the piano, home renovation, and time with family and friends.

Walter Lee is Professor in the Duke Departments of Head and Neck Surgery & Communication Sciences and Radiation Oncology. He currently serves as the Department Chief of Staff and Co-Director of the Head and Neck Program in the Duke Cancer Institute. He is also an affiliate faculty member at the Duke Global Health Institute and holds joint appointment with Duke-National University of Singapore. His research interests are focused on two areas. The first is the development of taking "first world" technology to improve the diagnosis and treatment of head and neck cancers in patients living in low resource settings. This has included device development and nanotechnology for early cancer detection. He holds several NIH funded grants that currently work with collaborators in Vietnam, Singapore, and Laos. The second is a focus on professional formation and leadership development. He was co-creator of a curriculum that is based on a virtue-based approach to leadership and professional development. He has been awarded the Mentor of the Year awarded by the residents and cited by the Ministry of Health for his contributions in Vietnam. He is active in mentoring and education and many of his former mentees now hold leadership positions in Vietnam. Dr. Lee earned his Philosophy (Ethics) degree and medical degrees from George Washington University. He completed his Otolaryngology – Head and Neck Surgery Residency and his Head and Neck Oncology Research Fellowship at the Cleveland Clinic Head and Neck Institute. He remained on staff until he was recruited to Duke in 2008. In 2015, he also earned a Masters in Health Sciences from Duke University.

Richard M. Pfohl, D.S.L., is a strategic leadership consultant, educator, and entrepreneur who serves as President of LEAD360 Solutions and Senior Fellow with multiple leadership institutes, focusing on developing leaders, aligning organizations, and cultivating high-performance cultures. With more than two decades of global C-Suite experience, he has advised Fortune 100 and Global 250 organizations across diverse industries, including healthcare, technology, manufacturing, finance, and government, helping them advance strategy, foresight, and organizational transformation. Dr. Pfohl previously held executive roles such as CFO, COO, and Interim CEO within high-growth startups, leading turnarounds and successful exits before transitioning fully into entrepreneurial leadership and consulting. He earned his Doctorate in Strategic Leadership from Regent University, emphasizing global entrepreneurship and strategic foresight, and has since worked extensively with entrepreneurs, mentoring more than a hundred ventures annually through programs connected to SCORE and regional innovation networks. His work integrates evidence-based leadership frameworks and proprietary models designed to strengthen leadership capability, strategic alignment, and long-term organizational performance.

Sarah Prabhu is the Programs Manager at the National Alliance on Mental Illness (NAMI) Santa Clara County. She brings a unique scientific and analytical perspective to her work in mental health advocacy and program management, drawing upon her professional background and a Master of Science in Biochemistry. Prabhu's leadership in regional healthcare policy includes her service as a member of the Mental Health Parity Work Group for Santa Clara County, where she co-created the "Know Your Rights" campaign—an initiative designed to promote the enforcement of mental health parity laws and ensure equitable access to care. At NAMI-SCC, she manages a portfolio of five programs, including the Community Peer Program, a strategic partnership with local hospitals that facilitates the transition of individuals from clinical settings to community-based support networks. Her research and writing are deeply informed by her lived experience as a family member, which helps her connect authentically with those she serves. This personal perspective fuels her focus on early intervention and addressing systemic gaps within the healthcare landscape.

Ray Qian received his M.D. from the Boston University School of Medicine and completed residency training in Internal Medicine at Boston University Medical Center. He subsequently completed a fellowship in Clinical Informatics at Mayo Clinic in Rochester, Minnesota. Dr. Qian is an Assistant Professor of Medicine at Mayo Clinic, where he practices clinically as a hospitalist. His academic work focuses on clinical informatics, with research interests in the design, implementation, and evaluation of health information technologies to improve care delivery, clinical decision-making, and patient outcomes. In addition, he serves as a director and lecturer at the Mayo Clinic Alix School of Medicine and has been an invited speaker at regional and national academic meetings.

Mahendra Ramachandran is a Technologist in the CTO Systems Group at KLA, where he specializes in the strategic development of complex optical systems for the semiconductor industry. Holding a Ph.D. in Electrical Engineering from the University of Electro-Communications in Japan, Mahendra has defined his career by bridging the gap between theoretical concepts and mass production. An accomplished researcher with over 50 publications and multiple patents, he brings a rigorous, systems-oriented approach to evaluating emerging technologies. In addition to his professional leadership in deep tech, Mahendra is a dedicated advocate for systemic improvements in mental health services in corporate settings in Silicon Valley. As a Support Group Facilitator and volunteer leader with the National Alliance on Mental Illness (NAMI) Santa Clara County, he works directly with families navigating the complexities of the healthcare system. His contribution to this volume draws upon a unique dual perspective—combining a technologist's focus on scalable innovation with an advocate's understanding of human barriers—to identify critical opportunities for reform in modern mental healthcare.

Crystal Shannon is the Dean of the College of Health and Human Services and Director of the School of Nursing at Indiana University Northwest.

Index

A

B

C

D

E

F

G

H

I

L

M

N

O

P

Q

R

S

T

U

V

W

www.ingramcontent.com/pod-product-compliance
Lightning Source LLC
LaVergne TN
LVHW080908300926
849162LV00003B/603